Early Onset Scoliosis

Ron El-Hawary • Craig P. Eberson
Editors

Early Onset Scoliosis

A Clinical Casebook

Springer

Editors
Ron El-Hawary
IWK Health Centre
Halifax, Nova Scotia, Canada

Craig P. Eberson
Brown University
Warren Alpert Medical School
Providence, Rhode Island, USA

ISBN 978-3-319-71579-7   ISBN 978-3-319-71580-3 (eBook)
https://doi.org/10.1007/978-3-319-71580-3

Library of Congress Control Number: 2018935675

Printed on acid-free paper

This Springer imprint is published by the registered company Springer International Publishing AG part of Springer Nature
The registered company address is: Gewerbestrasse 11, 6330 Cham, Switzerland

The editors would like to dedicate this book to the children whom we treat, who inspire us every day.
To my amazing wife, Denise, I am "so lucky."
To my boys, Philip, Jake, and Daniel – thanks for never complaining that Dad was on his computer more than usual over the past year.
You guys make me proud every day. Your love and support means everything.

Craig P. Eberson

I would like to thank my parents, Mo and Ferial, for their inspiration and for the example that they have set as true academics.
Thank you to Tricia for her love and support and, of course, to the kids (Alexa, Grace, Kegan, Duncan, and Liam) who make it all worthwhile!

Ron El-Hawary

Preface

Early-onset scoliosis (EOS) is a challenging, potentially life-threatening condition for which there are often myriad treatment options, but no perfect one. The purpose of this volume is to assemble a variety of EOS cases, spanning the spectrum of presentations, and discuss their treatment in a case-based format, highlighting the principles of treatment so that they may be applied to other patients facing similar challenges.

We are grateful to the highly skilled surgeons who contributed their considerable experience to this project, teaching us how they approach the most difficult cases so that we may benefit from their expertise. We are also thankful to our editorial support at Springer for allowing us to be a part of this worthy endeavor. Finally, we consider with respect and gratitude the EOS patients entrusted to our care, who remain a never-ending source of inspiration to continually strive to solve the many challenges their treatment represents.

Halifax, NS — Ron El-Hawary
Providence, RI — Craig P. Eberson

Contents

1 Normal Spine Growth 1
James O. Sanders

2 Classification of Early-Onset Scoliosis 9
Jeremy Doak

3 EDF Casting for Early-Onset Scoliosis 17
Graham Fedorak and Jacques D'Astous

4 Spine-Based Growing Rods for the Treatment of Idiopathic Early-Onset Scoliosis 35
Laurel C. Blakemore and George H. Thompson

5 The Vertical Expandable Prosthetic Titanium Rib (VEPTR) for Idiopathic Early-Onset Scoliosis 47
Daniel J. Miller, Susan E. Nelson, and John M. Flynn (Jack)

6 Treatment of Idiopathic Early-Onset Scoliosis with a Hybrid Growing Rod Construct 59
Haleh Badkoobehi and Lindsay Andras

7 Shilla Growth Guidance Technique for Early Onset Scoliosis 73
Richard E. McCarthy and David B. Bumpass

8 Early Onset Scoliosis Treated with Magnetically Controlled Growing Rods 87
Ryan E. Fitzgerald, Kathleen D. Rickert, Behrooz A. Akbarnia, and Burt Yaszay

9 Modern Trolley Growth Guidance for Early Onset Scoliosis 103
Jean A. Ouellet and Catherine E. Ferland

10 Anterior Vertebral Body Tethering (AVBT) for Early-Onset Scoliosis 117
Firoz Miyanji and Stefan Parent

11 Anterior Vertebral Body Stapling for the Treatment of Idiopathic Scoliosis 135
James T. Bennett, Amer F. Samdani, Robert J. Ames, and Randal R. Betz

12 Congenital Resection for Early-Onset Scoliosis 149
Michael Glotzbecker and John Emans

13 The Vertical Expandable Prosthetic Titanium Rib (VEPTR) for Congenital Scoliosis 167
Daniel J. Miller, Michael R. Eby, Robert M. Campbell, and Patrick J. Cahill

14 Hemiepiphysiodesis for the Treatment of Congenital Scoliosis 183
Senol Bekmez and Muharrem Yazici

15 Congenital Myopathy with Early-Onset Scoliosis 197
Mark C. Lee and Craig P. Eberson

16 Cerebral Palsy with Early-Onset Scoliosis 211
Varun Puvanesarajah and Paul D. Sponseller

17 The Use of the Vertical Expandable Prosthetic Titanium Rib (VEPTR) in Myelomeningocele 221
Graham Fedorak, John A. Heflin, and John T. Smith

18 Early-Onset Scoliosis in Skeletal Dysplasia. 231
David Tager, Suken Shah, and William G. Mackenzie

19 Complications with Early Onset Scoliosis 245
Brandon A. Ramo and Charles E. Johnston

20 Spine Growth Assessment of Growth-Friendly Surgery. 271
Ron El-Hawary and Félix Brassard

21 The Role of Traction in Early-Onset Scoliosis 289
Benjamin Orlik and Craig P. Eberson

22 The End Game for Early-Onset Scoliosis 307
Benjamin Sheffer and Jeffrey R. Sawyer

Index 321

Contributors

Behrooz A. Akbarnia, MD Department of orthopedic Surgery, Rady Children's Hospital and Health Center, San Diego, CA, USA

Department of orthopedic Surgery, San Diego Center for Spinal Disorders, San Diego, CA, USA

Department of Orthopedic Surgery, University of California San Diego (UCSD), La Jolla, CA, USA

Robert J. Ames, MD Temple University Hospital, Philadelphia, PA, USA

Shriners Hospitals for Children, Philadelphia, PA, USA

Lindsay Andras, MD Department of Orthopedic Surgery, Children's Hospital Los Angeles, Los Angeles, CA, USA

Haleh Badkoobehi, MD, MPH Department of Orthopedic Surgery, Children's Hospital Los Angeles, Los Angeles, CA, USA

Senol Bekmez, MD Department of orthopedics and Traumatology, Cankaya Hospital, Ankara, Turkey

Department of Orthopedics and Traumatology, Hacettepe University School of Medicine, Ankara, Turkey

James T. Bennett, MD Temple University Hospital, Philadelphia, PA, USA

Shriners Hospitals for Children, Philadelphia, PA, USA

Randal R. Betz, MD The Institute for Spine and Scoliosis, Lawrenceville, NJ, USA

Laurel C. Blakemore, MD Department of Orthopedics and Rehabilitation, University of Florida School of Medicine, Gainesville, FL, USA

Félix Brassard, MD, FRCS(C) IWK Health Centre, Halifax, NS, Canada

David B. Bumpass, MD Department of Orthopedics, Arkansas Children's Hospital/University of Arkansas for Medical Sciences, Little Rock, AR, USA

Patrick J. Cahill, MD Division of Orthopedic Surgery, The Children's Hospital of Philadelphia, Philadelphia, PA, USA

Robert M. Campbell, MD Division of Orthopedic Surgery, The Children's Hospital of Philadelphia, Philadelphia, PA, USA

Jacques D'Astous, MD, FRCS(C) Shriners Hospital for Children, Salt Lake City, UT, USA

Department of Orthopedic Surgery, University of Utah, Salt Lake City, UT, USA

Jeremy Doak, MD Department of Orthopedic Surgery, State University of New York at Buffalo, Buffalo, NY, USA

Craig P. Eberson, MD Department of Orthopedic Surgery, Connecticut Children's, Hartford, CT, USA

Department of Orthopedic Surgery, Brown University/ Hasbro Children's Hospital, Providence, RI, USA

Michael R. Eby, MD Division of Orthopedic Surgery, The Children's Hospital of Philadelphia, Philadelphia, PA, USA

Ron El-Hawary, MD, MSc, FRCS(C) IWK Health Centre, Halifax, NS, Canada

John Emans, MD Department of Orthopedic Surgery, Boston Children's Hospital and Harvard Medical School, Boston, MA, USA

Graham Fedorak, MD, FRCS(C) Shriners Hospital for Children, Salt Lake City, UT, USA

Department of Orthopedic Surgery, University of Utah, Salt Lake City, UT, USA

Catherine E. Ferland, PhD Department of Paediatric Surgery, McGill University Health Centre and Shriners Hospital, QC, Canada

Department of Anesthesiology, McGill University Health Centre and Shriners Hospital, QC, Canada

Ryan E. Fitzgerald, MD Department of Orthopedic Surgery, Rady Children's Hospital and Health Center, San Diego, CA, USA

Department of Orthopedic Surgery, San Diego Center for Spinal Disorders, San Diego, CA, USA

Department of Orthopedic Surgery, University of California San Diego (UCSD), La Jolla, CA, USA

John M. Flynn, MD[Jack] Division of Orthopedic Surgery, The Children's Hospital of Philadelphia, Philadelphia, PA, USA

Michael Glotzbecker, MD Department of Orthopedic Surgery, Boston Children's Hospital and Harvard Medical School, Boston, MA, USA

John A. Heflin, MD University of Utah, Salt Lake City, UT, USA

Charles E. Johnston, MD Texas Scottish Rite Hospital for Children, Dallas, TX, USA

Department of Orthoapedic Surgery, University of Texas Southwestern, Dallas, TX, USA

Mark C. Lee, MD Department of Orthopedic Surgery, Connecticut Children's, Hartford, CT, USA

Department of Orthopedic Surgery, Brown University/ Hasbro Children's Hospital, Providence, RI, USA

William G. Mackenzie, MD Department of Orthopedic Surgery, Nemours/Alfred I. duPont Hospital for Children, Wilmington, DE, USA

Richard E. McCarthy, MD Department of Orthopedics, Arkansas Children's Hospital/University of Arkansas for Medical Sciences, Little Rock, AR, USA

Department of Neurosurgery, Arkansas Children's Hospital/ University of Arkansas for Medical Sciences, Little Rock, AR, USA

Daniel J. Miller, MD Division of Orthopedic Surgery, The Children's Hospital of Philadelphia, Philadelphia, PA, USA

Firoz Miyanji, MD British Columbia Children's Hospital, Vancouver, BC, Canada

CHU Sainte Justine, QC, Canada

Susan E. Nelson, MD, MPH Division of Orthopedic Surgery, The Children's Hospital of Philadelphia, Philadelphia, PA, USA

Benjamin Orlik, MD Division of Pediatric Orthopedic Surgery, IWK Heath Centre and Dalhousie University, Halifax, NS, Canada

Division of Pediatric Orthopedic Surgery, Hasbro Children's Hospital and Alpert Medical School of Brown University, Providence, RI, USA

Jean A. Ouellet, MD Department of Paediatric Surgery, McGill University Health Centre and Shriners Hospital, QC, Canada

Department of Anesthesiology, McGill University Health Centre and Shriners Hospital, QC, Canada

Stefan Parent, MD British Columbia Children's Hospital, Vancouver, BC, Canada

CHU Sainte Justine, QC, Canada

Varun Puvanesarajah, MD Department of Orthopedic Surgery, Johns Hopkins Hospital, Baltimore, MD, USA

Brandon A. Ramo, MD Texas Scottish Rite Hospital for Children, Dallas, TX, USA

Department of Orthoapedic Surgery, University of Texas Southwestern, Dallas, TX, USA

Kathleen D. Rickert, MD Department of Orthopedic Surgery, Rady Children's Hospital and Health Center, San Diego, CA, USA

Department of Orthopedic Surgery, San Diego Center for Spinal Disorders, San Diego, CA, USA

Department of Orthopedic Surgery, University of California San Diego (UCSD), La Jolla, CA, USA

Amer F. Samdani, MD Shriners Hospitals for Children, Philadelphia, PA, USA

James O. Sanders, MD School of Medicine and Dentistry, University of Rochester, Rochester, NY, USA

Jeffrey R. Sawyer, MD Department of Orthopedic Surgery and Biomedical Engineering, University of Tennessee-Campbell Clinic, Memphis, TN, USA

Le Bonheur Children's Hospital, Memphis, TN, USA

Suken Shah, MD The Spine and Scoliosis Center, Nemours/Alfred I. duPont Hospital for Children, Wilmington, DE, USA

Benjamin Sheffer, MD Department of Orthopedic Surgery and Biomedical Engineering, University of Tennessee-Campbell Clinic, Memphis, TN, USA

Le Bonheur Children's Hospital, Memphis, TN, USA

John T. Smith, MD University of Utah, Salt Lake City, UT, USA

Paul D. Sponseller, MD Department of Orthopedic Surgery, Johns Hopkins Hospital, Baltimore, MD, USA

David Tager, MD West Virginia University Hospital, Morgantown, WV, USA

George H. Thompson, MD Department of Orthopedics and Rehabilitation, University of Florida School of Medicine, Gainesville, FL, USA

Cleveland Medical Center, Rainbow Babies and Children's Hospital, Case Western Reserve University, Cleveland, OH, USA

Burt Yaszay, MD Department of Orthopedic Surgery, Rady Children's Hospital and Health Center, San Diego, CA, USA

Department of Orthopedic Surgery, San Diego Center for Spinal Disorders, San Diego, CA, USA

Department of Orthopedic Surgery, University of California San Diego (UCSD), La Jolla, CA, USA

Muharrem Yazici, MD Department of Orthopedics and Traumatology, Cankaya Hospital, Ankara, Turkey

Department of Orthopedics and Traumatology, Hacettepe University School of Medicine, Ankara, Turkey

Chapter 1
Normal Spine Growth

James O. Sanders

Case Presentation

An 8 month girl who appears otherwise healthy presents with a spinal deformity. Radiographs demonstrate the curve shown in Figure. 1.1. She is neurologically normal and has a normal MRI. She is later found to have a fibrillin-2 abnormality consistent with Beal's syndrome, though she has no contractures or other abnormalities.

The cases in this text focus on the addressing the challenges facing those treating children with spinal deformities. This chapter's goal is to describe the parameters of normal human spinal growth critical for decisionmaking and discusses this girl as an example.

This young girl has no congenital spinal anomalies which are associated with other organ system abnormalities. The spine develops embryologically in conjunction with other organ systems, and congenital anomalies of the spine may be associated with developmental mis-sequences in other organs, particularly of the VACTERL (Vertebral-vascular, Anal atresia, Cardiac, Tracheoesophageal fistula, Esophageal atresia,

J.O. Sanders, MD
School of Medicine and Dentistry, University of Rochester, 601 Elmwood Avenue, Box 665, Rochester, NY, USA
e-mail: James_Sanders@urmc.rochester.edu

R. El-Hawary, C.P. Eberson (eds.), *Early Onset Scoliosis*,
https://doi.org/10.1007/978-3-319-71580-3_1

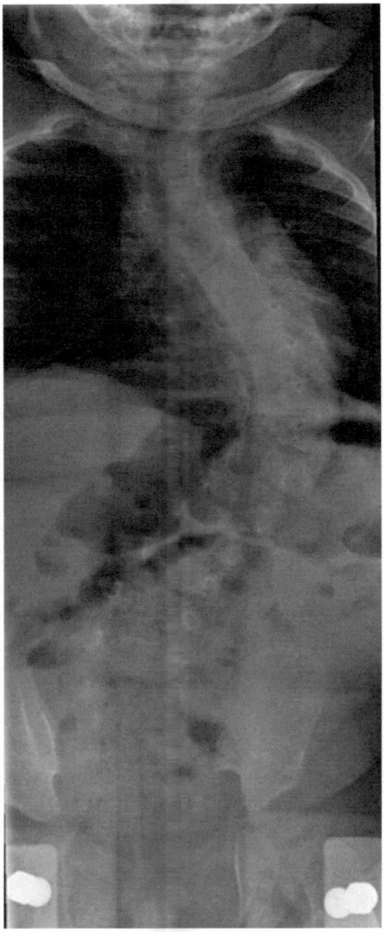

FIGURE 1.1 Supine AP radiographs of an 8 month old girl

Renal-radial, and Limb abnormalities) [1] and spinal cord abnormalities. During gestation, the spinal column grows rapidly compared to the neural elements [2]. Initially, the nerves exit the neuroforamina at their corresponding levels of the cord. By 4 months' gestation, the cord reaches L3 or L4 inferiorly, and by term, the cord is usually at the adult position of L1–L2.

Ultimately, the goals in treating children with early onset scoliosis are normal spine and pulmonary function. For this child, a key goal is her having sufficient pulmonary function at maturity to provide normal adult ventilatory capacity. Her deformity, left untreated, will create abnormal chest walls configuration and mechanics, and an early fusion will result in thoracic insufficiency syndrome [3, 4]. Fusion before age 10 is associated with poor appearance and respiratory function [5]. Karol et al. [6, 7] presented data showing poor pulmonary function when thoracic fusion leaves the thoracic spine length 18 cm or less. However, nearly normal lung function was only achieved with a T1–T12 length of >21 cm. In general, current treatment decision algorithms strive to continue or improve normal spinal growth until a child has achieved 10 years and a T1–T12 length of at least 18 and preferably 22 cm length.

This young girl's deformity is at particular risk of progression during her infant and adolescent growth phases. At birth, the spine is about 19 cm long and grows to about 47 cm at maturity [8] through symmetric superior and inferior end plate endochondral ossification and the cartilaginous caps on the articular processes [9]. Following birth, the trunk grows very rapidly, but the rate of growth diminishes during each succeeding year. The spine gains about 10 cm in length between birth and age 5, a 52% increase, helping account for the rapid progression of congenital and infantile curves often occurring during this time. Growth slows and remains fairly constant from about age 4 until the growth spurt. During the adolescent growth spurt, the maximum rate is often double or triple the earlier childhood rate and occurs earlier but to a lesser degree in girls than in boys but with similar patterns for both.

Figure 1.2, derived cross sectionally from Emans [10] and Bagnall [11], shows the relative length of the thoracic to the lumbar spine by chronological age. The data is nearly identical for boys and girls. At 8 months of age, her thoracic spine has a greater percentage length (72%) than the lumbar spine (28%), but will grow proportionally slower as she reaches childhood when the percentage stabilizes at 63% thoracic

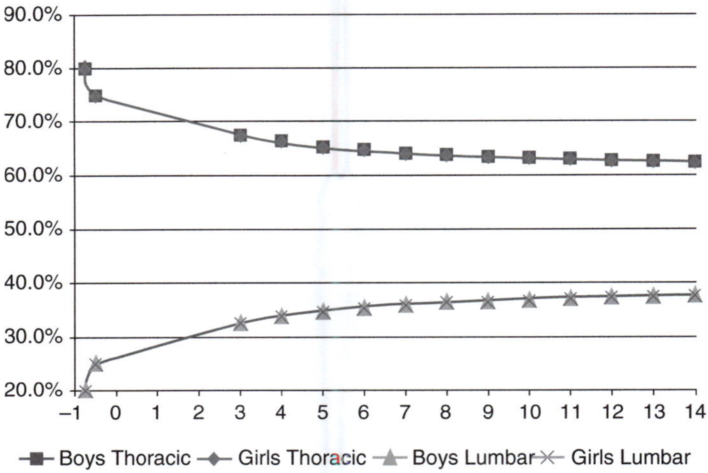

FIGURE 1.2 Percentage length of thoracic to and lumbar spine of T1-S1. Used with permission. Sanders JO. Seminars in spine surgery. Elsevier; 2015

and 27% lumbar. Figure 1.3 shows the lengths of the thoracic spine, lumbar spine, and total spine again combining the data of Emans et al. and Bagnall et al. along with the 5th and 95th percentiles. If the length of the thoracic spine required for adequate adult lung function is 22 cm as described by Karol et al. [7], assuming this patient follows the median, she will reach this at age 10, though it could occur as young as 5 or as old as 12 years. Based on this, a treatment plan should include methods of increasing the length of her thorax by nearly 11 cm before a final fusion.

Assuming some form of growing instrumentation will be needed, how does spinal growth affect the choice of implant? Does she have risk of developing spinal stenosis from pedicle screws crossing the neurocentral synchondrosis? A number of studies have evaluated the anatomic appearance of the neurocentral synchondrosis cross sectionally over various ages [12–17]. But physeal growth may not be directly related

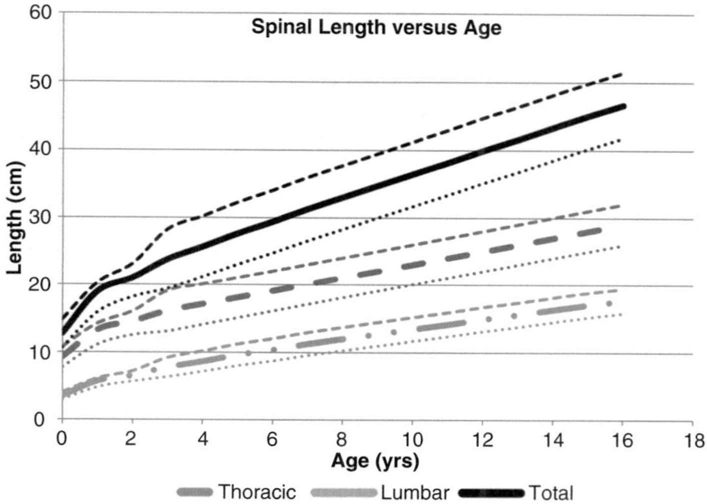

FIGURE 1.3 Percentage length of thoracic to and lumbar spine of T1-S1. Used with permission. Sanders JO. Seminars in spine surgery. Elsevier; 2015

to its appearance on imaging, but clearly once the synchondrosis closes, the canal cannot as easily widen and usually only does so with prolonged pressure such as from a tumor. The canal usually reaches adult size by age 6–8 with closure of the synchondrosis, though the synchondrosis may persist in the thoracic spine until age 10 [17]. The earliest closure is in the lumbar spine followed by the upper thoracic spine and the mid and lower thoracic last. Fortunately, there is little evidence that crossing the neurocentral synchondrosis, even at an early age, is likely to result in symptomatic spinal stenosis.

In summary, by understanding normal growth of the thoracic and lumbar spine, as well as the relationship between spinal growth and pulmonary function, the treatment of children with EOS can be individualized to optimize their functional outcome.

References

1. Solomon BD. VACTERL/VATER Association. Orphanet J Rare Dis. 2011;6:56. Epub 2011/08/19.
2. Vettivel S. Vertebral level of the termination of the spinal cord in human fetuses. J Anat. 1991;179:149–61. Epub 1991/12/01.
3. Campbell RM Jr, Smith MD, Mayes TC, Mangos JA, Willey-Courand DB, Kose N, et al. The effect of opening wedge thoracostomy on thoracic insufficiency syndrome associated with fused ribs and congenital scoliosis. J Bone Joint Surg Am. 2004;86-A(8):1659–74.
4. Campbell RM Jr, Smith MD. Thoracic insufficiency syndrome and exotic scoliosis. J Bone Joint Surg Am. 2007;89(Suppl 1):108–22.
5. Goldberg CJ, Gillic I, Connaughton O, Moore DP, Fogarty EE, Canny GJ, et al. Respiratory function and cosmesis at maturity in infantile-onset scoliosis. Spine. 2003;28(20):2397–406.
6. Karol LA. Early definitive spinal fusion in young children: what we have learned. Clin Orthop Relat Res. 2011;469(5):1323–9. Epub 2010/10/20
7. Karol LA, Johnston C, Mladenov K, Schochet P, Walters P, Browne RH. Pulmonary function following early thoracic fusion in non-neuromuscular scoliosis. J Bone Joint Surg Am. 2008;90(6):1272–81. Epub 2008/06/04.
8. Dimeglio A, Bonnel F. Le rachis en croissance. Paris: Springer; 1990.
9. DiMeglio A, Canavese F, Charles YP. Growth and adolescent idiopathic scoliosis: when and how much? J Pediatr Orthop. 2011;31(1 Suppl):S28–36. Epub 2011/01/05.
10. Emans JB, Ciarlo M, Callahan M, Zurakowski D. Prediction of thoracic dimensions and spine length based on individual pelvic dimensions in children and adolescents: an age-independent, individualized standard for evaluation of outcome in early onset spinal deformity. Spine. 2005;30(24):2824–9.
11. Bagnall KM, Harris PF, Jones PR. A radiographic study of the human fetal spine. 3. Longitudinal growth. J Anat. 1979;128(Pt 4):777–87. Epub 1979/06/01
12. Leemans J, Deboeck M, Claes H, Boven F, Potvliege R. Computed tomography of ununited neurocentral synchondrosis in the cervical spine. J Comput Assist Tomogr. 1984;8(3):540–3.

13. Rajwani T, Bagnall KM, Lambert R, Huang EM, Secretan C, Moreau M, et al. Evaluating MRI as a technique for visualizing the neurocentral junction. Spine (Phila Pa 1976). 2005;30(7):807–12. Epub 2005/04/02.
14. Rajwani T, Bhargava R, Lambert R, Moreau M, Mahood J, Raso VJ, et al. Development of the neurocentral junction as seen on magnetic resonance images. Stud Health Technol Inform. 2002;91:229–34.
15. Schlosser TP, Vincken KL, Attrach H, Kuijf HJ, Viergever MA, Janssen MM, et al. Quantitative analysis of the closure pattern of the neurocentral junction as related to preexistent rotation in the normal immature spine. Spine J. 2013;13(7):756–63. Epub 2013/07/09.
16. Yamazaki A, Mason DE, Caro PA. Age of closure of the neurocentral cartilage in the thoracic spine. J Pediatr Orthop. 1998;18(2):168–72.
17. Zhang H, Sucato DJ, Nurenberg P, McClung A. Morphometric analysis of neurocentral synchondrosis using magnetic resonance imaging in the normal skeletally immature spine. Spine (Phila Pa 1976). 2010;35(1):76–82. Epub 2010/01/01.

Chapter 2
Classification of Early-Onset Scoliosis

Jeremy Doak

Classification of Early-Onset Scoliosis

Hippocrates first introduced the terms kyphosis and scoliosis around 400–500 BC [1, 2]. Beginning with that ancient recognition of spinal deformity, our understanding of the complexities of spinal anatomy and disease has markedly progressed over the last two millennia, allowing us to treat and alter the natural history of these disorders. However; despite our rapidly advancing technology and understanding, consensus regarding the treatment of scoliosis has remained elusive. This in part is likely due to the enormity of the term "scoliosis." Strictly defined, scoliosis is the abnormal lateral curvature of the spine. Certainly this broad terminology offers little to describe the etiology of the spinal asymmetry, the natural history of the disorder, or the effect on the patient.

Early attempts at classification focused on the age of the patient or the etiology of the curvature (Tables 2.1 and 2.2). Historically, early-onset idiopathic scoliosis has been termed infantile if the scoliotic deformity developed between the

J. Doak, MD
Department of Orthopedic Surgery, State University of New York at Buffalo, Buffalo, NY, USA
e-mail: jpdoak@gmail.com

R. El-Hawary, C.P. Eberson (eds.), *Early Onset Scoliosis*,
https://doi.org/10.1007/978-3-319-71580-3_2

Table 2.1 Age-based classification of idiopathic scoliosis

Classification	Age (years)
Infantile	0–3
Juvenile	4–10
Adolescent	11–17
Adult	>18

Table 2.2 Example of etiologic classification of scoliosis

Etiologic classification
Idiopathic
Neuromuscular
Syndrome related
Congenital

ages of 0 and 3 years and juvenile should the curvature of the spine develop between the ages of 4 and 10 years. Adolescent idiopathic scoliosis would be reserved for patients 11 years or older. Scoliosis of neuromuscular, syndromic, or congenital etiologies were classified simply by the etiology without significant attention paid to the age and stage of development of the patient. These classification systems offered no guidance to treatment or correlation with outcomes. A 2-year-old boy with a segmentation anomaly of the vertebrae would be classified as having congenital scoliosis. But no classification system inclusive of multiple components of the disease process or effect on the patient was available.

In 2014, the Scoliosis Research Society offered a definition of the term early-onset scoliosis. In conjunction with the Pediatric Orthopaedic Society of North America, the Growing Spine Study Group, and the Children's Spine Study Group, they defined early-onset scoliosis as "scoliosis with onset less than the age of 10 years, regardless of etiology" [3, 4].

To be clinically useful, a classification system should provide a common language between clinicians that can help guide treatment and standardize reporting of results both of the natural history of the disease process, as well as the results of treatment [3, 5, 6]. The above simplistic age or etiology-based classifications systems did little to accomplish these goals. It also resulted in patients being classified into two competing systems which did not work in concert with one another. To that end, Williams et al. developed the C-EOS (classification of early-onset scoliosis), which was the first published classification scheme specifically for early-onset scoliosis. A panel of 15 surgeons from 13 institutions with significant experience in treating patients with EOS was chosen. The model proposed by Audige et al. for the creation of a fracture classification system was utilized to develop C-EOS [5]. This classification system is composed of multiple variables meant to fully characterize the curvature. This includes the characteristics of EOS that impact treatment directly: Continuous variable of age, etiology, magnitude of the major curve, degree of kyphosis, and the rate of progression [3] (Fig. 2.1).

$$\text{APR} = \{(\text{Major curve} @ t_2) - (\text{Major curve} @ t_1)\} \times \{12\,\text{months}/(t_2 - t_1)\}$$

The value of this system is manifold. To properly manage children with EOS, variables other than Cobb angle are clearly important. In addition to magnitude of the main

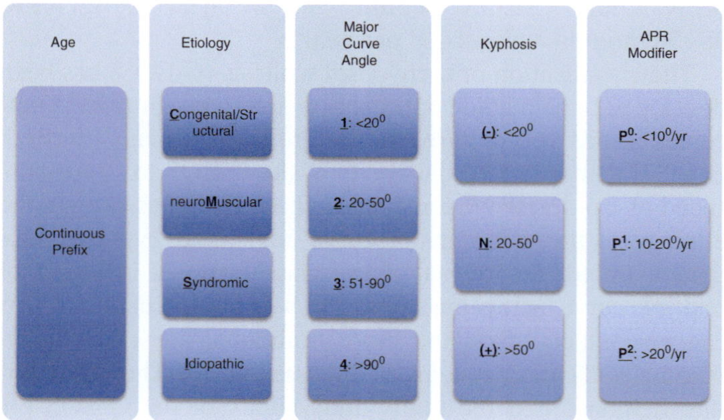

FIGURE. 2.1 The classification of early-onset scoliosis (C-EOS). APR = annual progression ratio. (see Fig. 2.2) [10]

APR = {(Major Curve @ t_2) – (Major Curve @ t_1)} x {12 months/(t_2–t_1)}

FIGURE. 2.2 Annual progression ratio modifier. Progression calculations should be made with two evaluations at times t_1 and t_2 that are a minimum of 6 months apart [3]

curve, the sagittal plane must be considered when planning treatment. When determining the feasibility of continued observation of a patient, understanding the rate of progression is crucial; the APR modifier represents this aspect of curve behavior (Fig. 2.2). Cast treatment of scoliosis has been compared to Ponseti casting of clubfoot deformity. C-EOS allows clinicians to discuss patients and meaningfully evaluate the results of treatment in the same fashion as the Dimeglio scale has permitted a comprehensive description of clubfeet in a manner that has allowed accurate evaluation of the effects of various treatments.

The case of a 4-year-old girl with nemaline myopathy is presented to demonstrate correct application of the C-EOS (Fig. 2.3). At presentation, she had a 35° major curve with 42° kyphosis. At 7 years of age (36 months later), her main curve had progressed to 80° with 60° kyphosis. Her initial C-EOS would be 4M2N. At her follow-up visit, now inclusive of the APR, her C-EOS would be 7 M3(+)P^1 (APR: 38°/36 months = about 13° per year).

The classification of early-onset scoliosis (C-EOS) has been developed to help guide optimal care and to prognosticate outcomes in this very heterogeneous group of patients [3]. Park et al. [7] demonstrated the ability of the C-EOS to stratify the speed of rapid VEPTR proximal anchor failure based upon the etiology of the curve, major curve angle, and kyphosis. This demonstrated the impact of the classification's inclusion of multiple curve factors in its power to help guide treatment. This can be juxtaposed on the more traditional age or etiology-based classification systems as discussed above. This study further demonstrated the utility and validity of the C-EOS [7]. Interobserver and intraobserver reliability is an important aspect of any clinically relevant classification system. These aspects of the C-EOS were verified in a later separate study [8].

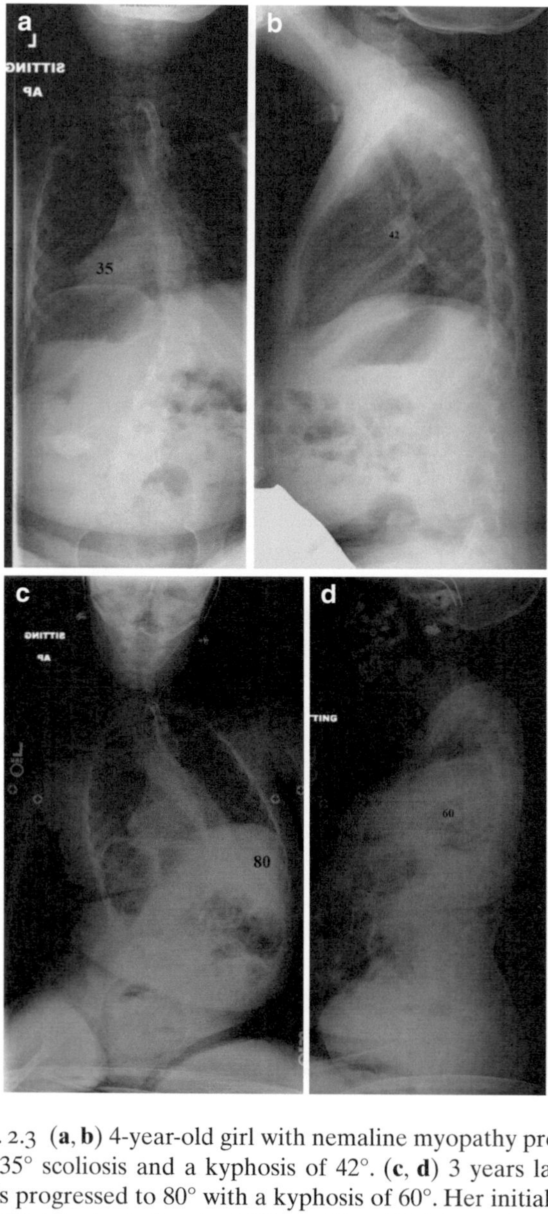

FIGURE. 2.3 (**a**, **b**) 4-year-old girl with nemaline myopathy presented with a 35° scoliosis and a kyphosis of 42°. (**c**, **d**) 3 years later her scoliosis progressed to 80° with a kyphosis of 60°. Her initial CEOS was 4M2N. After including the APR modifier (38°/36 months = approx. 13°/year) and increase in kyphosis classification would be 7M3(+) P[2]

TABLE 2.3 Complications classification system [9]

Grading	Device related	Disease related
I	Does not require unplanned surgery	Outpatient medical management only
II		Inpatient medical management
IIA	Requires 1 unplanned surgery	
IIB	Requires multiple unplanned surgeries	
III	Requires abandoning growth friendly strategy	Requires abandoning growth friendly strategy
IV	Death	Death

Many members of the same group involved in development of the C-EOS have also developed a classification system to grade the severity of complications encountered during growth friendly spine surgery for the treatment of scoliosis (Table 2.3) [9]. Complications were broken down into two groups: those considered device related and those considered disease related. The device-related complications were defined as those directly related to the instrumentation itself or the surgical implantation of the instrumentation. Disease-related complications were defined as those related to repeated surgeries such as pneumonia, persistent pain, and others [9]. This is also a particularly useful instrument to help assess the results, both positive and negative, of our treatment of this difficult cohort of patients. Such a classification can thusly be used, in concert with the C-EOS, to help critically evaluate results of treatment in the hopes of guiding care in the future. Certainly this has utility in both clinical practice and in scientific study and research. This system has yet to be critically validated, and the interobserver and intraobserver reliabilities have yet to be elucidated.

As our understanding of early-onset scoliosis continues to progress, so does the understanding of the complexities and difficulties in treatment that can be expected in this diverse group of patients. As there is significant variability in treatment for patients with EOS, it is crucial that a comprehensive means of classifying patients is used to determine the effectiveness of interventions in preventing the long-term consequence of the disease.

References

1. Kostuik JP. The history of spinal deformity. Spine Deform. 2015;3:417–25.
2. Vasiliadis ES, Grivas TB, Kaspiris A. Historical overview of spinal deformities in ancient greece. Scoliosis. 2009;4:1–13.
3. Wiliams BA, Matsumoto H, McCalla DJ, et al. Development and initial validation of the Classification of Early-Onset Scoliosis (C-EOS). J Bone Joint Surg Am. 2014;96(16):1359–67.
4. Skaggs DL, Guillaume T, El-Hawary R, et al. Early onset scoliosis consensus statement, SRS growing Spine Committee, 2015. Spine Deform. 2015;3:107.
5. Audige L, Bhandari M, Hanson B, Kellam J. A concept for the validation of fracture classifications. J Orthop Trauma. 2005;19(6):401–6.
6. Garbuz DS, Masri BA, Esdaile J, Duncan CP. Classification systems in orthopaedics. J Am Acad Orthop Surg. 2002;10(4):290–7.
7. Park HY, Matsumoto H, Feinberg N, et al. The classification for early-onset scoliosis (C-EOS) correlates with the speed of vertical expandable prosthetic titanium rib (VEPTR) proximal anchor failure. J Pediatr Orthop. 2015;37(6):381–6; epub 1–6.
8. Cyr M, Hilaire TS, Pan Z, et al. Classification of early onset scoliosis has excellent interobserver and intraobserver reliability. J Pediatr Orthop. 2017;37(1):e1–3.
9. Smith JT, Johnston C, Skaggs D, et al. A new classification system to report complications in growing spine surgery: a multicenter consensus study. J Pediatr Orthop. 2015;35(8):798–803.
10. Vitale MG, Trupia E. Classification of early-onset scoliosis. In: Akbarnia BA, Yazici M, Thompson GH, editors. The growing spine. New York: Springer; 2015. p. 113–21.

Chapter 3
EDF Casting for Early-Onset Scoliosis

Graham Fedorak and Jacques D'Astous

Case Presentation

History and Physical Assessment

An 8-month-old female presented with a worsening thoracic scoliosis. She had a past medical history of reflux and developmental dysplasia of the left hip, treated previously with a Pavlik harness. She was otherwise healthy and developmentally appropriate. There was no family history of scoliosis.

- Normal neurologic examination; no signs of spinal dysraphism or other neurocutaneous findings
- C7 plumb line deviated to the right when sitting
- Convex left thoracic curvature noted with left lower thoracic rib prominence.
- Moderately flexible.

G. Fedorak, MD, FRCS(C) • J. D'Astous, MD, FRCS(C) (✉)
Shriners Hospital for Children, Salt Lake City, UT, USA
Department of orthopedic Surgery, University of Utah,
Salt Lake City, UT, USA
e-mail: JDAstous@shrinenet.org

R. El-Hawary, C.P. Eberson (eds.), *Early Onset Scoliosis*,
https://doi.org/10.1007/978-3-319-71580-3_3

Diagnostic Studies

- Sitting AP radiograph demonstrated convex left thoracic scoliosis with a 54° Cobb angle from T6-L1. Apex at T9 (Figure 3.1a—*Initial AP X-ray*)
- Rib vertebral angle difference (RVAD) of 45°, rib phase 2, grade 2 Moe rotation
- Lateral film showed hypokyphosis
- Preoperative supine traction film demonstrated that the curvature decreased to 36° (Figure 3.1b—*supine AP traction)*
- *Presumptive diagnosis of idiopathic early-onset scoliosis (EOS)*
- An MRI was not performed. In children with curves characteristic of idiopathic EOS, who are developing

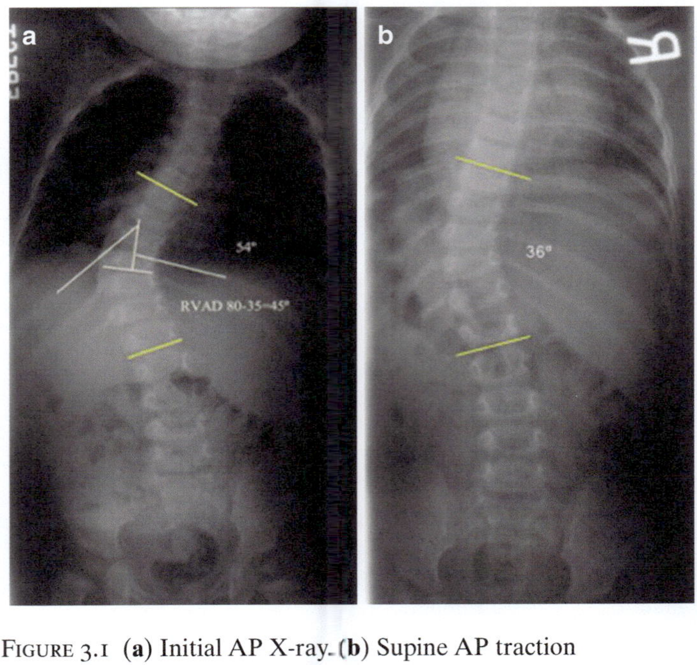

FIGURE 3.1 (**a**) Initial AP X-ray. (**b**) Supine AP traction

normally and have a normal neurologic examination, we typically do not order an MRI prior to beginning cast treatment. The MRI is done at a convenient time. Alternatively, if the curvature is not responsive to cast treatment, if neurologic abnormalities become apparent, or if a change in treatment is being considered (e.g., growing rods), MRI is ordered at that time.

Management Chosen

Based on scoliosis Cobb >20°, RVAD >20°, and phase 2 rib-vertebral overlap, risk of progression is 80% and treatment is deemed necessary to prevent progression of deformity and possibility of eventual thoracic insufficiency syndrome. Options include bracing, EDF (elongation, derotation, flexion) casting as described by Cotrel and Morel [1], adapted and popularized by Mehta [2], or growth-friendly surgery. Bracing may be ineffective at preventing curve progression. We feel that she may be too young for growth-friendly surgery which also has a high rate of complications, particularly in younger EOS patients. Casting can correct spinal deformity in many cases of EOS when instituted before 24 months of age or, at the very least, delay the need for initiation of growth-friendly surgery while allowing for continued growth of the thorax [2–4].

In consultation with the child's parents, a decision was made to proceed with EDF casting. Protocol at our institution is for cast changes under anesthesia every 2 months in children 2 years of age and younger, every 3 months in 3-year-olds, and every 4 months in children who are 4 years of age or older.

Surgical Procedure

Our casting technique has evolved over more than 1200 EDF casts applied; however the core principles described by Mehta have been respected.

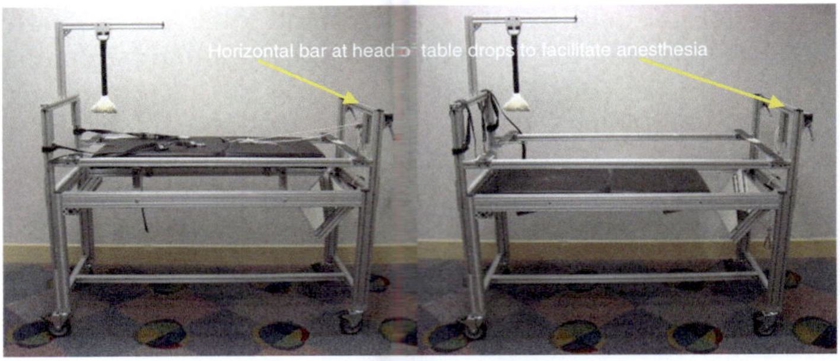

FIGURE 3.2 Table specifically designed for EDF casting

Preoperative Preparation

- A table specifically designed for EDF casting is ideal for optimal results; however, alternatives exist [5] (Figure 3.2).
- In the preanesthetic room, the patient is fitted with a six-way stretch t-shirt, over which two layers of 6 in. stockinette are applied to the torso (cut long enough to shield face) and 2 in. stockinette is applied to both arms to support the arms when the tabletop is dropped (see Appendix A for supplies).

Anesthesia

- Anesthesiologists must be aware of the temporary impairment of ventilation which occurs during cast application. This will resolve upon trimming the cast to open the abdominal window [6].
- General endotracheal anesthesia is preferred, with a bite block to prevent pinching off the ET tube when traction is applied to the head.
- Disposable ear plugs are inserted and tegaderm applied to protect the eyes and ears. Foam padding over the ears prevents pressure from the head halter traction.
- Decompression of the stomach with a nasogastric tube is required. Failure to do so may result in splinting of the diaphragm and further impair ventilation during casting.

Casting Preparation

- Two inch stockinette (~5 ft.) is applied between the layers of body stockinette and cinched over the iliac crests. A simple knot is tied at the level of the greater trochanter and a second overhand knot 6 in. below the simple knot. Pelvic bands are attached to the traction straps at the foot of the casting table. This controls the pelvis (Figure 3.3).
- Body stockinette is brought up over the head with a hole cut for the ET tube. The head halter is applied to grasp the chin and occiput, allowing application of traction to the head. The anterior portion of the halter must just cover the tip of the chin to avoid pressure on the ET tube.
- The patient is moved down the table so that the head rests on a gel cushion on the transverse bar and the sacrum rests on the sacral post.
- The arms are stabilized to the casting table with, for a typical left-sided curve, the right arm being slightly more abducted than the left. Feet are placed in a sling to flex the hips 30°.
- With pelvic traction in place, cervical traction is applied at approximately 40% of the patient's body weight. Pelvic traction is then adjusted to level the pelvis.
- The tabletop is lowered and the rib prominence on the convexity of the scoliosis can be appreciated by looking at the mirror at the head of the table and by palpation.

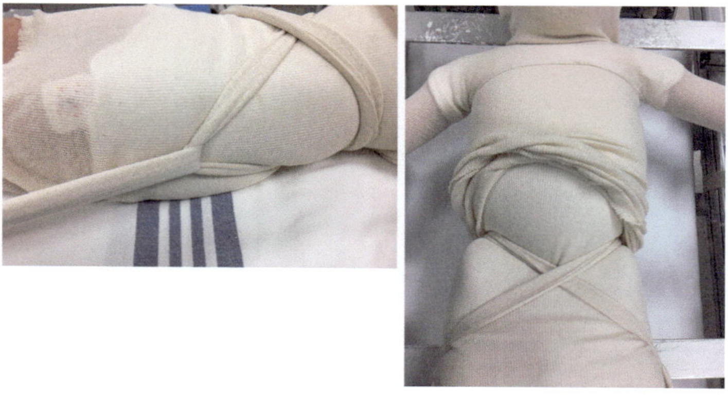

FIGURE 3.3 Straps for pelvic control

- Comma-shaped felt pads are applied over the anterior superior iliac spines (ASIS) and anterior iliac crest. Felt pads are placed in both axillae, asymmetrically, with that on the side of the concavity (typically right side for a left thoracic curve) higher. A felt pad is placed over the rib hump. Pads are held in place with a thin layer of Webril.
- Two-layer thick folded strips of Webril are placed over the sternum anteriorly and over the interscapular region posteriorly. These are held in place with 2 in. Webril straps starting at the lower costal margin anteriorly, going over the shoulder, and ending on the opposite ASIS. The arms are covered with a thin layer of Webril (Figure 3.4).

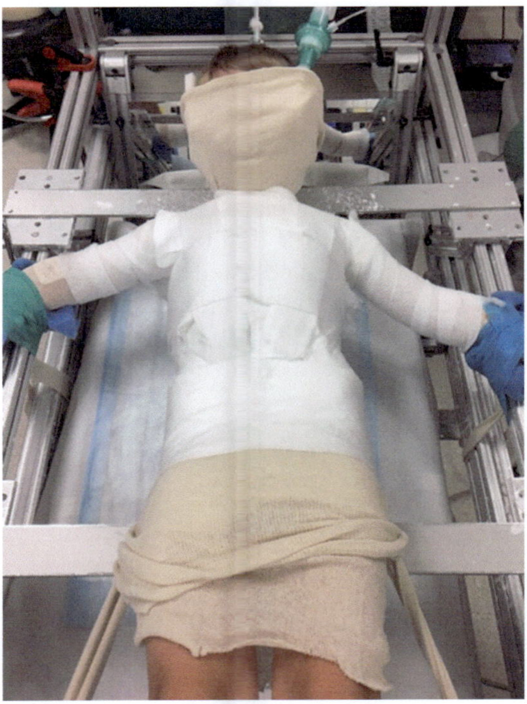

FIGURE 3.4 Layer of Webril

Cast Application

- Required are two sheets of Cellona plaster (anterior and posterior), each four-layer thick, cut into the shape of a camisole, 4 in. rolls of Cellona casting material, fiberglass casting material in 3 and 2 in. widths, and a 4 in. roll of fiberglass casting tape used to fashion shoulder straps. Our preference is to go over the shoulders, but if the apex of the curve is at T8 or below, shoulder straps are optional.
- The sheets comprising the anterior camisole are dipped into tepid water and placed on the anterior torso, followed by application of the posterior sheets. Care is taken to apply tension to the shoulder straps on either side to avoid wrinkles.
- A 4 in. roll of plaster that is applied from distal to proximal is then used to overwrap the plaster sheets. Tension is applied just proximal to the iliac crest to achieve a snug fit to capture the pelvis, which serves as the foundation of the EDF cast.

Correction of Scoliosis (for a Typical Left-Sided Thoracic Curve)

- Right hand—with tips of fingers apply anteriorly directed derotational forces on the left ribs corresponding to the apex of the curvature (pull up on the rib prominence) combined with a medially directed vector. Take care not to laterally compress the ribs with the palm of the right hand (Figure 3.5a).
- Left hand—push down posteriorly and medially on the right ribs cephalad to the apex of the curvature while attempting to elevate the right shoulder to provide lateral flexion
- Two assistants are required: one to stabilize the pelvis and contour the cast over the iliac crests and a second to stabilize the anterior aspect of the left shoulder to prevent it from coming forward with derotation and to

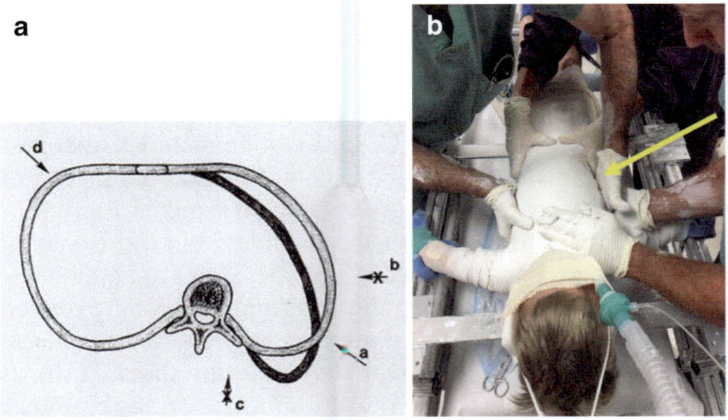

FIGURE 3.5 (**a**) Derotational biomechanics. (**b**) Molding of cast

smooth the posterior interscapular portion of the cast (Figure 3.5b).

- Once the cast is firmly set, it is overwrapped with a thin layer of fiberglass casting tape, after which shoulder straps, fashioned from a 4 in. roll of casting tape, are applied (2–3-layer thick) and the fiberglass layer is completed (Figure 3.6). The fiberglass is then overwrapped with a wet Ace wrap to promote bonding between the fiberglass and the plaster.

Cast Trimming

- The tabletop is raised to support the patient and the two bars are moved away from the patient. Ace wrap is removed, feet lowered, and pelvic straps are cut above the simple knot and removed, thus decreasing pressure on the lower abdomen. We remove all but 2–5 lbs of traction on the head.
- CO_2 levels can rise quickly during casting, particularly with young patients, so the team must proceed quickly and efficiently.

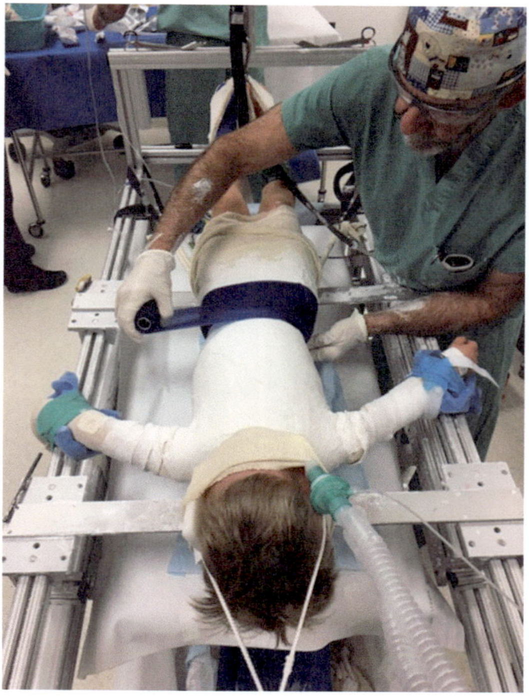

FIGURE 3.6 Application of fiberglass

- Trim lines are drawn, beginning with the neckline at the superior level of the sternal notch. The next line is 1–2 cm above the pubis to allow the hips to flex past 90°. A mushroom-shaped thoracic and abdominal window is drawn with two anterior flanges to capture the lower costal margins. The axillary trim should be higher on the side of the concavity to encourage lateral flexion (Figure 3.7).
- Using a cast saw, we start by cutting out the thoracoabdominal window. Once the chest and abdomen are free, CO_2 levels invariably improve. We then cut out the other trim lines making sure that there is sufficient shoulder

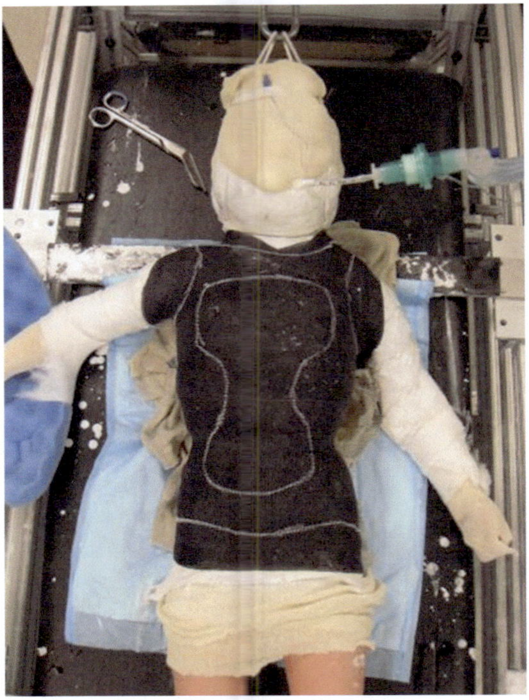

FIGURE 3.7 Anterior trim lines

adduction to get the hands to the mouth and that we have at least 90° of hip flexion.

- The first layer of stockinette is cut in a cross-like fashion followed by the second layer being cut diagonally. Stockinette is then stapled to the cast using a commercially available stapler, and the edges of the felt pads in the axilla are also stapled to the cast. All edges are finished in this fashion (Figure 3.8).
- The patient is turned prone onto two transverse bolsters (aligned with sternal and pubic portions of cast to avoid intra-abdominal pressure), and posterior trimming is performed.

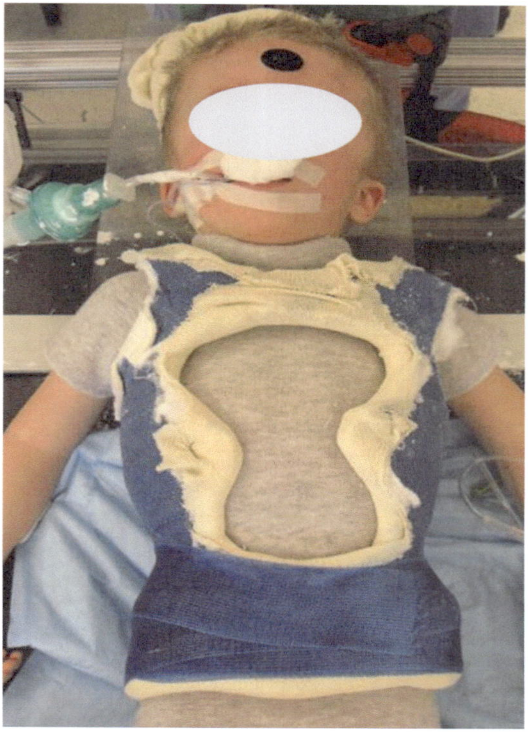

FIGURE 3.8 Thoracoabdominal window with anterior flange

- A posterior window is cut opposite the rib prominence (right side for a left thoracic curve) to allow further derotation (Figure 3.9).
- The duckbill is used to flare the posterior caudal edge of the cast to avoid pressure on the sacrum and to the anterior flanges to avoid too much pressure on the ribs and allow more chest expansion.
- The child is returned to the postanesthetic recovery room, and a standing AP X-ray of the spine is obtained prior to discharge. Supine films in the OR are not done as they tend to overestimate the correction achieved.

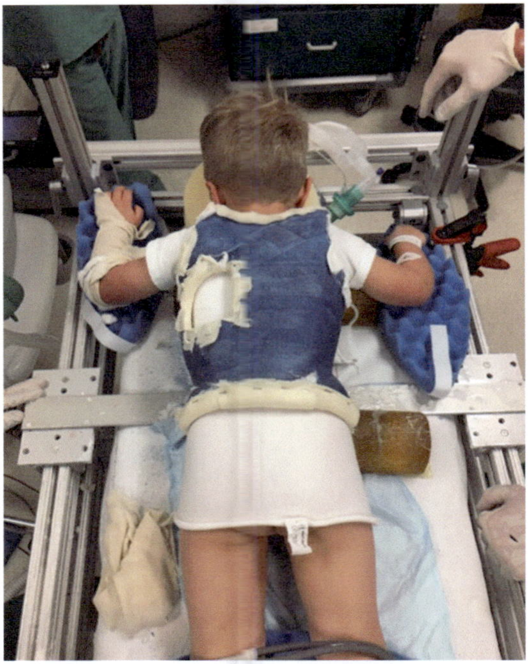

FIGURE 3.9 Posterior thoracic window

- Figure 3.10a illustrates the finished appearance of the casts with Figure 3.10b an example of a cast customized with Gorilla tape.

Clinical Course and Outcome

- The patient tolerated casting well. She underwent six EDF cast applications over a 14-month period.
- At 22 months, with a Cobb angle of 10° (Figure 3.11, out of cast), she was transitioned to a custom TLSO (Figure 3.12 in brace)
- The patient was subsequently followed at an outside hospital. At last follow-up at 10 years and 2 months, she

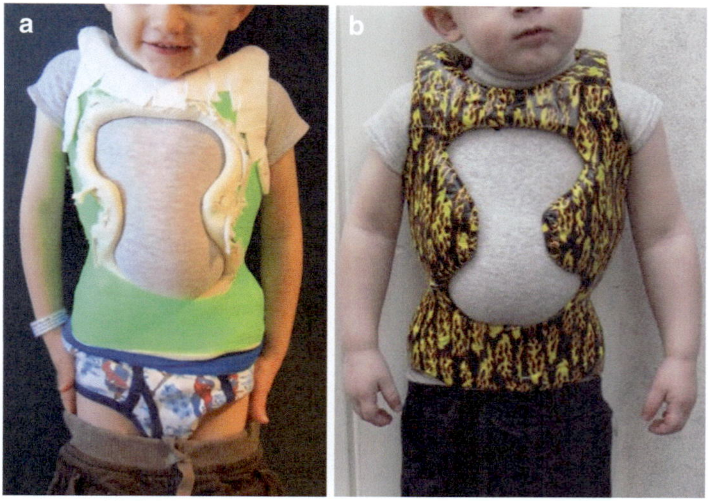

FIGURE 3.10 **a**) illustrates the finished appearance of the casts with **b**) an example of a cast customized with Gorilla tape.

was not wearing a brace and had no residual curvature (Figure 3.13, 9 years after initial cast)

Clinical Pearls and Pitfalls

- When to transition to a brace is debated. We recommend conversion to a TLSO when the curvature is ≤10°, although 15° is used as the threshold by other practitioners. We obtain an in-brace X-ray to ensure that the brace is effective and fitting well. Out-of-brace X-ray is obtained once a year.
- The decision to transition to a brace is typically made at the last cast application. Mold is made under anesthesia just prior to EDF cast application using the same technique. Subsequent EDF braces are custom-made with the child awake in our orthotics department. Children are typically braced full-time with an EDF brace for at least 1 year and then transitioned to a Providence style nighttime brace for at least 6 months afterward.

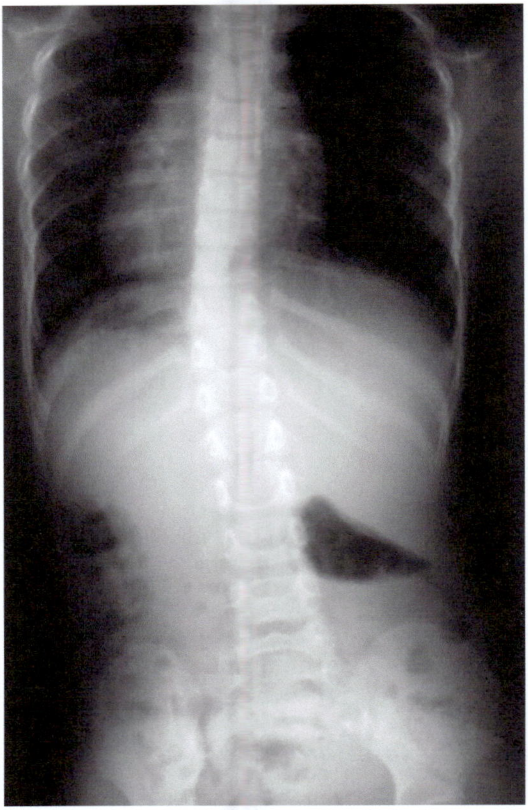

FIGURE 3.11 Out-of-cast film

Literature Review and Discussion

Casting as a potentially curative treatment option for early-onset scoliosis (EOS) was popularized by the work of Mehta, which is based on growth modulation using the technique of elongation-derotation-(lateral) flexion casting (EDF) originally described by Cotrel and Morel [1, 2]. EDF casting places emphasis on correcting the rotational component of the scoliosis and provides a 3D correction of the scoliosis and the chest wall. We adhere to the protocol developed by

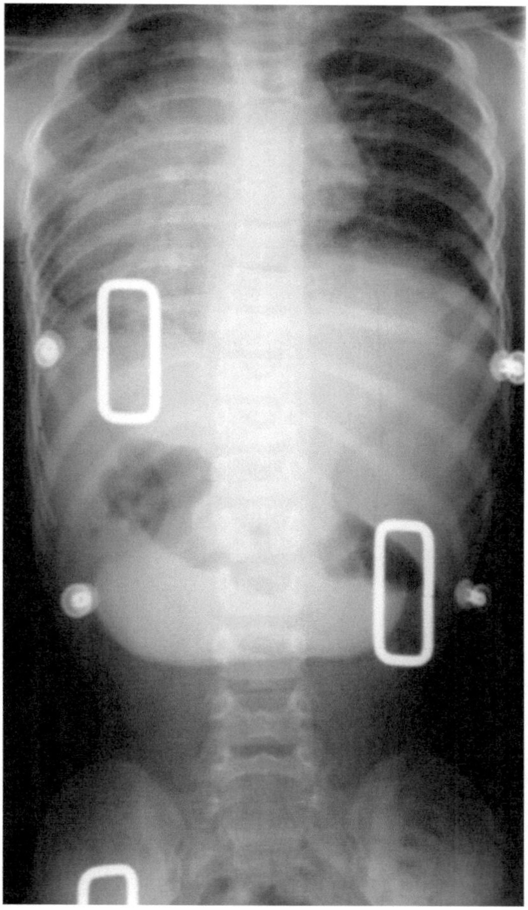

FIGURE 3.12 In-brace film

Mehta, which requires cast changes, every 2–4 months, as outlined above [2].

Risser casts differ from EDF in that they utilize three-point bending forces [7]. In young children with malleable bones, the three-point bend can cause rib deformities and constriction of the chest wall.

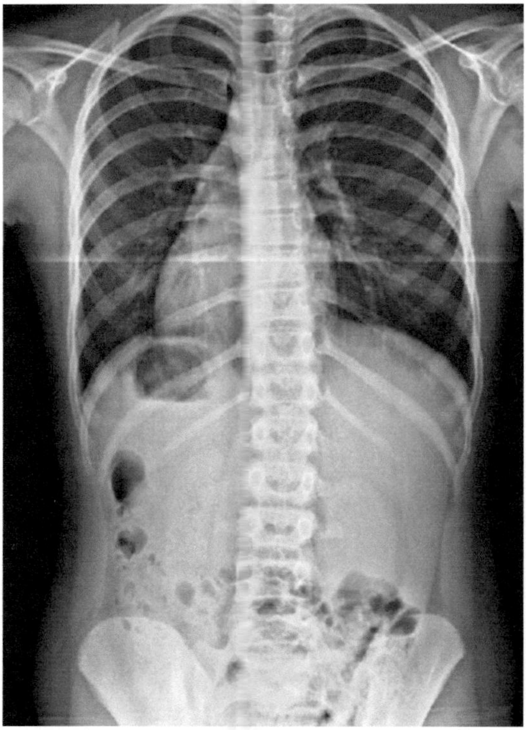

FIGURE 3.13 PA spine 9 years after initial cast

EDF casting has proven effective as a cure for some children with early-onset scoliosis (referred to as "progressive infantile scoliosis" by Mehta and Sanders) [2, 4]. In Mehta's cohort of 136 children treated with EDF casting, the 94 who achieved cure had a mean age of 19 months and a mean Cobb angle of 32°, in contrast to the 42 children in whom casting could reduce but not cure the deformity, who presented at a mean of 30 months with a mean Cobb angle of 52° [2]. The conclusions of Sanders 2009 study, documenting the first North American results, are that EDF casting can result in a cure for patients presenting <2 years of ages with curves <50–60° [4]. In a study on the variability of expert opinion regarding the treatment of EOS, 60°of curvature in infantile idiopathic patients was identified as a point of equipoise between conservative treatment and distraction-based surgery [8].

Closer inspection of the literature demonstrates that EDF casting can be curative in children presenting at older ages and with greater deformity. Mehta's own cohort of "cured" patients included those up to the age of 48 months at the initiation of casting and with curvatures up to 65° [2]. In our experience, we have achieved cure in curves of up to 79° at the initiation of casting and thus feel neither age nor degree of deformity should preclude a trial of several casts. Anecdotally, we have observed that one to two casts may be required to "loosen things up" and that more progress is often made after the second or third cast. In children for whom casting is not curative, casting can still be palliative, effectively buying time, avoiding the early implantation of growing constructs and in many cases controlling the curve long enough to proceed directly to final fusion, or even occasionally avoiding surgery altogether [3, 9]. While most effective in idiopathic EOS, we have achieved cure in some children with syndromic EOS and substantial palliation in both congenital and neuromuscular EOS.

EDF casting is an effective treatment for EOS, providing cure in many cases and delaying the need for "growth-friendly" surgery in the majority of the remainder. We recommend instituting cast treatment once it is clear that the curvature is progressive and have begun casting in children as young as 7 months. While this is a labor-intensive technique, we feel that in an era in which "value" is emphasized in health care, EDF casting is the gold standard for the initial treatment of EOS.

Appendix A

Head halter

- Six way stretch moisture absorbent T-shirt
- Felt pad (3/16″)
- Webril cast padding (4″ and 2″)
- Regular stockinette

Cellona plaster sheets (four layers front and back)
Cellona plaster roll (4″)
Fiberglass casting tape (4″, 3″ and 2″)
Scissors
Duckbill
Stapler (1/4″ staples)

References

1. Cotrel Y, Morel G. The elongation-derotation-flexion technic in the correction of scoliosis. Rev Chir Orthop Reparatrice Appar Mot. 1964;50:59–75.
2. Mehta MH. Growth as a corrective force in the early treatment of progressive infantile scoliosis. J Bone Joint Surg Br. 2005;87-B:1237–47.
3. Fletcher ND, McClung A, Rathjen KE, et al. Serial casting as a delay tactic in the treatment of moderate-to-severe early-onset scoliosis. J Pediatr Orthop. 2012;32:664–71.
4. Sanders JO, D'Astous J, Fitzgerald M, et al. Derotational casting for progressive infantile scoliosis. J Pediatr Orthop. 2009;29:581–7.
5. Halanski MA, Harper BL, Cassidy JA, Crawford HA. Three solutions to a single problem: alternative casting frames for treating infantile idiopathic scoliosis. J Spinal Disord Tech. 2013;26(5):274–80.
6. Dhawale AA, Shah SA, Reichard S, Holmes L Jr, Brislin R, Rogers K, Mackenzie WG. Casting for infantile scoliosis: the pitfall of increased peak inspiratory pressure. J Pediatr Orthop. 2013;33:63–7.
7. Risser JC. The application of body casts for the correction of scoliosis. Instr Course Lect. 1955;12:255–9.
8. Corona J, Miller DJ, Downs J, et al. Evaluating the extent of clinical uncertainty among treatment options for patients with early-onset scoliosis. J Bone Joint Surg Am. 2013;95(10):e67.
9. Demirkiran HG, Bekmez S, Celilov R, Ayvaz M, Dede O, Yazici M. Serial derotational casting in congenital scoliosis as a time-buying strategy. J Pediatr Orthop. 2015;35:43–9.

Chapter 4
Spine-Based Growing Rods for the Treatment of Idiopathic Early-Onset Scoliosis

Laurel C. Blakemore and George H. Thompson

Case Presentation

History and Physical Examination

This 8-year- and 3-month-old female presented for evaluation and treatment of early onset scoliosis (EOS). She was diagnosed with idiopathic scoliosis at approximately 4 years of age and was initially treated with observation for 2 years, followed by TLSO bracing for approximately 18 months. During that time her scoliosis progressed from initial coronal major curve of 68° to 80°.

Past medical history was significant for a mild autism spectrum disorder. Family history was negative for known spinal deformity or significant systemic conditions.

L.C. Blakemore, MD
Department of Orthopedics and Rehabilitation, University of Florida School of Medicine, Gainesville, FL, USA
e-mail: blakelc@ortho.ufl.edu

G.H. Thompson, MD (✉)
Cleveland Medical Center, Rainbow Babies and Children's Hospital, Case Western Reserve University, Cleveland, OH, USA
e-mail: ght@po.cwru.edu

R. El-Hawary, C.P. Eberson (eds.), *Early Onset Scoliosis*,
https://doi.org/10.1007/978-3-319-71580-3_4

Physical examination showed a cooperative child with 30th percentile weight for length for her chronological age. Her right shoulder was elevated approximately 1 cm, and there were no cutaneous changes over the spine. Adam's forward bend revealed a severe right thoracic and moderate left lumbar prominence. Neurologic testing revealed symmetric 5/5 strength throughout the upper and lower extremities, normal lower extremity and abdominal reflexes, and no evidence of clonus.

Diagnostic Studies

Preoperative plain radiographs are shown in Figure 4.1. Coronal major curve measurements showed an 80° right thoracic from T5 to T12 and 56° left lumbar curve from T12 to L4. Bending radiographs showed 44% correction of the thoracic and 61% correction of the lumbar curve. A preoperative magnetic resonance imaging (MRI) of the entire neural axis was obtained which revealed no abnormalities of the central nervous system.

CEOS classification at preoperative evaluation was a I3NP1 (idiopathic curve with a coronal major curve 50–90° and thoracic kyphosis between 20 and 50°, progression at 10–20° per year).

Management Chosen

Surgical options were discussed with the family who elected to proceed with traditional growing rod instrumentation (TGR).

Surgical Procedure

At age 8 years and 4 months, she underwent posterior submuscular dual-rod instrumentation from T2 to L3. Intraoperative neuromonitoring including motor evoked

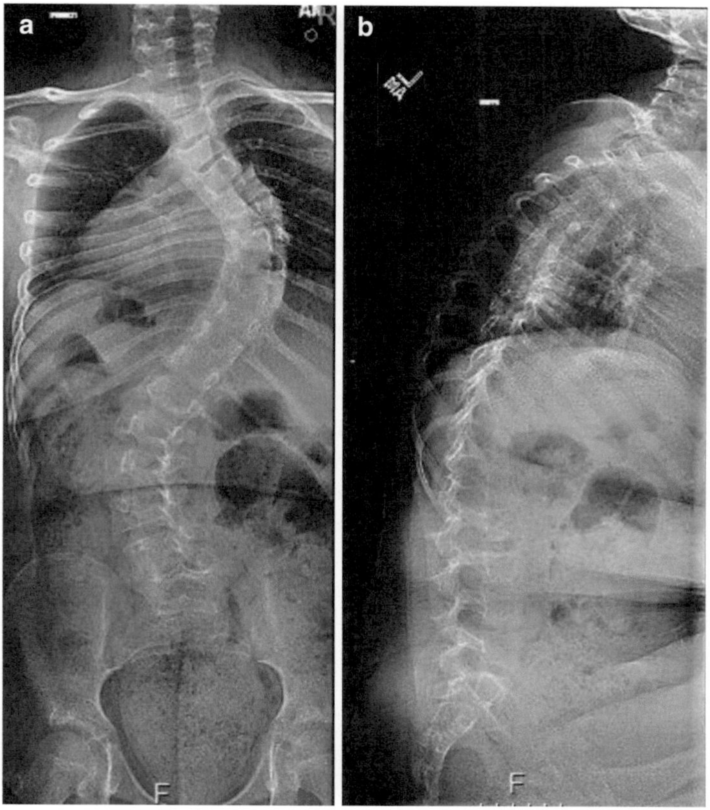

FIGURE 4.1 Preoperative standing plain radiographs of this 8-year-old female with EOS are shown in **a** and **b**. (**a**) Anteroposterior view coronal major curve measurements show an 80° right thoracic from T5 to T12 and 56° left lumbar curve from T12 to L4. Thirteen rib-bearing vertebrae and five lumbar vertebrae are noted. Triradiate cartilages are widely open. **(b)** The lateral view demonstrates 30° of thoracic kyphosis (T1–T12) and 7° of lumbar lordosis (L1–L5)

potentials were initiated, and the patient was positioned prone on a spine operating table. A single midline incision was utilized, exposing subperiosteally from T2 to T3 and L2 to L3 after radiographic confirmation of spinal levels using fluoroscopy. A claw construct was inserted proximally, consisting of bilateral supralaminar hooks at T2 and sublaminar hooks at T3 avoiding subperiosteal exposure these two levels. Distally bilateral facetectomies were performed at L2–L3 followed by placement of bilateral pedicle screws at these levels. Both foundation sites received allograft bone grafting for local fusion. Bilateral 5.5 mm titanium rods were then placed in a submuscular paraspinous plane and distraction applied across the construct. Gentle manual correction of the curve was applied to improve initial correction. The rods were purposefully left long distally to allow for initial the lengthening of the construct. Standard wound closure was performed. She was fit for a postoperative TLSO prior to discharge which she wore when out of bed for 3 months. Postoperative PA and lateral standing radiographs 1 month following postoperative TGR insertion are shown in Figure 4.2. Her right thoracic major curve had been reduced to 33° and the left lumbar curve to 30°. On the lateral radiograph, her thoracic kyphosis measured 37° and lumbar lordosis 27°.

Growing Rod Distraction

Subsequent rod lengthenings were performed on an outpatient basis at mean intervals of 6.1 months. At each lengthening intraoperative neural monitoring was utilized. For the initial two procedures, lengthenings were performed distally at the level of the pedicle screws using the long ends of the rods. At the third lengthening, the rods were divided in the thoracolumbar region and tandem connectors applied. Five additional lengthening procedures were performed through the tandem connectors. She underwent menarche at 12 years 9 months of age. During the 2 years and 6 months between submuscular rod insertion and final fusion, 5.8 cm of coronal height was gained from T1 to T12 and 6.3 cm of overall coronal height from T1 to S1. No complications occurred during this time, and there were no unplanned returns to the operating room.

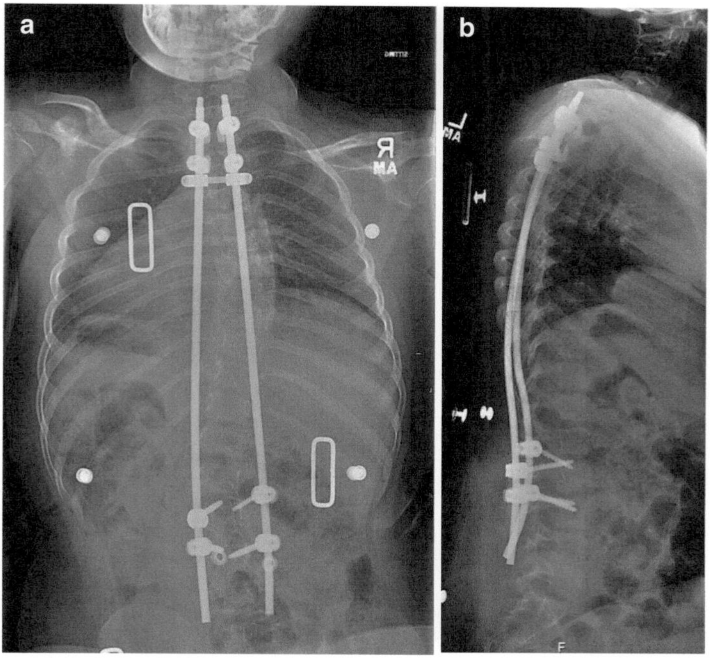

FIGURE 4.2 Postoperative PA and lateral standing radiographs 1 month following TGR insertion are shown in **a** and **b**. (**a**) Her right thoracic (major) curve has been reduced to 33° and the left lumbar curve to 30°. (**b**) The lateral view shows her thoracic kyphosis now measures 37° and her lumbar lordosis measures 27°

Definitive Fusion

At 12 years and 10 months, she was seen prior to definitive final fusion, and radiographs were obtained (Figure 4.3). It was decided to proceed with final fusion because of her excellent correction, advanced secondary sexual characteristics, and recent menarche. Preoperatively her major coronal thoracic curve measured 19° and the lumbar curve 16°. Thoracic kyphosis measured 49° and the lumbar lordosis 46°. Mild increased proximal thoracic kyphosis was also identified and assessed to be 42° from T1 to T3. She underwent definitive instrumentation

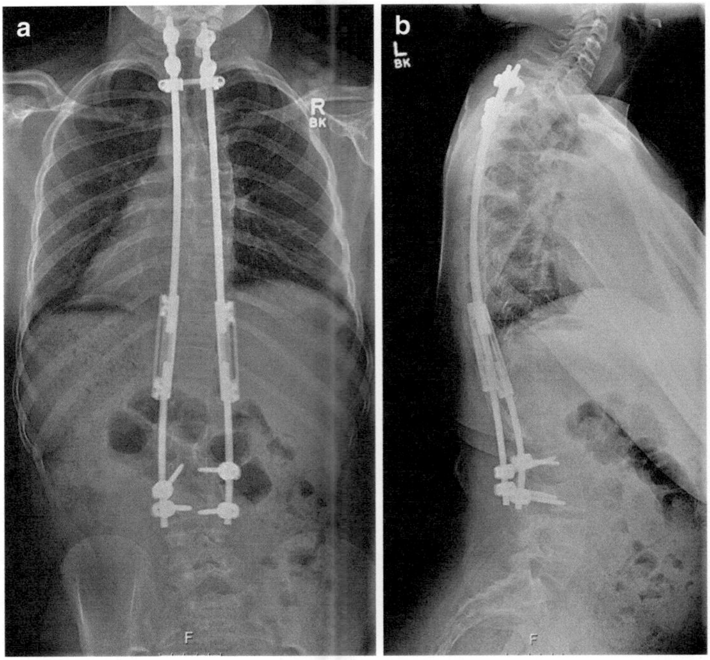

FIGURE 4.3 Preoperative standing radiographs prior to final fusion (**a** and **b**). (**a**) Right thoracic major curve now measured only 19° and the left lumbar curve 16°. (**b**) Lateral radiograph shows her thoracic kyphosis measures 49° and her lumbar lordosis 46°. Observe the moderate PJK

and fusion from T2 to L3 using 5.5 mm titanium segmental spinal instrumentation using pedicle screws. The TGR construct was removed and the lumbar pedicle screws replaced with screws measuring 1 mm larger in diameter. The apical region demonstrated fibrous scarring, but autofusion was not evident other than at the vertebrae of the foundation sites. A small dural tear occurred proximally on the left and was repaired intraoperatively. Autograft obtained during exposure and facetectomies was utilized and supplemented with allograft to complete the fusion. Her postoperative course was uneventful, and she was discharged after 4 days with no apparent sequelae.

Clinical Course and Outcome

Latest follow-up was obtained at 15 years and 7 months of age and 3-year status post final fusion. She denied pain or neurologic symptoms and was active although not participating in organized sports. Radiographs are shown in Figure 4.4

Clinical Pearls and Pitfalls

- TGR fixation options include laminar or transverse process hooks, sublaminar tapes or wires, rib fixation, and pedicle screws.
- Complication rates are relatively high for all growth-friendly instrumentation systems and increase with duration of treatment.
- TGR treatment been associated with high rates of fibrous scarring and autofusion at definitive fusion. This patient gained some progressive correction with lengthenings after initial TGR instrumentation and did not demonstrate autofusion at final surgery.

Literature Review and Discussion

The treatment of idiopathic early onset scoliosis (EOS) continues to evolve. Treatment goals include preservation of spinal growth, maintenance of spinal balance and mobility, and control or correction of spinal deformity. Nonoperative management (casting and bracing) plays an important role in idiopathic EOS; however severe deformities can occur. Delaying TGR or magnetically controlled growing rods (MCGR) with serial or Risser casts in very young children is an excellent method to decrease the total number of procedures and the associated complications of frequent general anesthetics and surgical procedures [1]. If significant growth remains and the curve cannot be controlled with casting or bracing, surgical options must be considered. These include

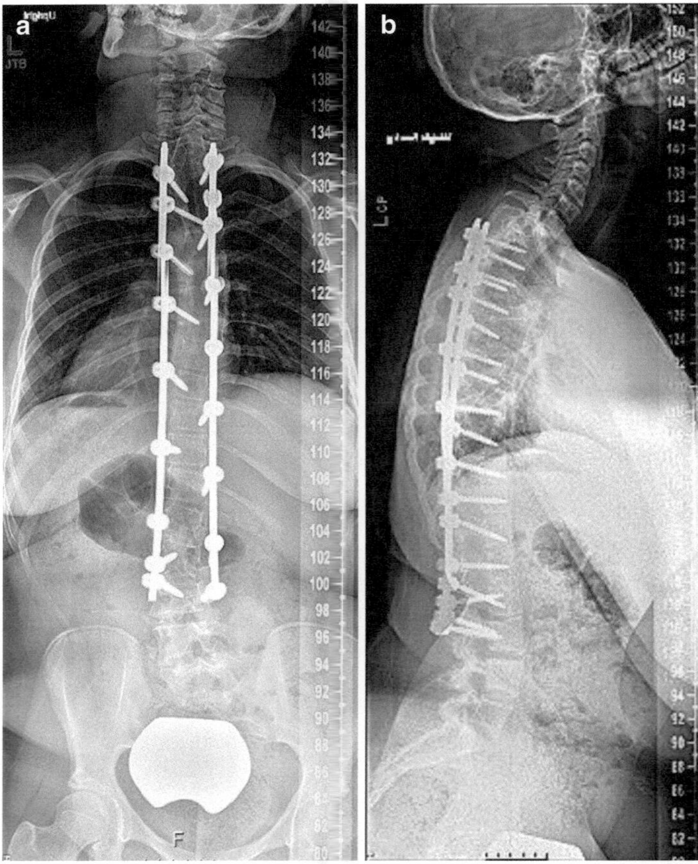

FIGURE 4.4 (**a**) PA standing radiograph at last follow-up at 15 years and 7 months of age and 3-year status post final fusion. Her right thoracic major curve measures 27° and the left lumbar curve 28°. She is Risser stage 4–5. (**b**) Standing lateral radiograph at last follow-up demonstrating 12° of thoracic kyphosis between T1 and T3, 42° of thoracic kyphosis from T3 to T12, and 48° of lumbar lordosis. She still has moderate, but stable, PJK

growth modulating and guided growth treatments, including TGR and more recent MCGR [2]. Although the use of TGR has decreased since the advent of MCGR, there may be some instances in which TGR is a preferred treatment, including very stiff curves, very small children whose spines cannot accommodate the MCGR actuator, and those requiring accurate advanced spinal imaging (e.g., history of spinal neoplasm). Definitive fusion is avoided in children with significant growth remaining, and several authors have demonstrated significant adverse effects after fusion at a young age [3, 4].

First described by Harrington in 1962 and later by others, TGR instrumentation for idiopathic EOS most commonly includes spinal fixation distally and spinal or rib fixation proximally [5, 6]. Rods may be inserted through a single midline incision as in this case, with subsequent exposure through this incision for lengthenings. A two-incision technique can also be employed, tunneling between the proximal and distal incisions to place the rods. This may be of some benefit when self-lengthening or magnetically controlled constructs are utilized, allowing for less soft tissue scarring over the midportions of the instrumentation. Several fixation options including pedicle screws, laminar or transverse process hooks, sublaminar tapes or wires, and rib hooks can be employed. Spinal anchors are typically accompanied by a limited fusion of the instrumented or foundation sites. Concerns for neurologic injury caused by migration of proximal pedicle screw anchors, as well as the preference to avoid proximal thoracic fusion when possible, have led some surgeons to utilize rib fixation with multiple anchor points bilaterally [7, 8]. Tandem or side-by-side connectors are typically utilized to allow progressive lengthening, although one study suggests that failure rates are higher with side-by-side connectors with circular slots [9]. Lengthening can be performed either above or below the trolley by distracting against a rod holder, or through the trolley itself. In this case, lengthening was initially performed at the distal aspect of the construct before inserting tandem connectors, and additional construct revisions were not required. Bilateral rods appear to yield better outcomes than single rod constructs, and the use of at least two proximal anchor points on each rod appears protective against anchor failure [10–12].

The ideal lengthening interval has not been identified, with most surgeons electing to lengthen TGR constructs every 6–9 months. Paloski et al. showed no difference in length gained or major curve correction between patients undergoing growing rod distractions at 9 or more months and patients with shorter times (less than 9 months) between distractions [13]. Higher numbers of distractions are associated with increased complication rates as well as eventually diminished amounts of length achieved, so a larger interval (>9 months) is presently favored.

Our patient demonstrated mild proximal junctional kyphosis (PJK). PJK can occur after distraction-based growth-sparing instrumentation including TGR although it has proven difficult to accurately quantify [14]. El Hawary et al. described a 28% incidence of PJK (defined as proximal junction sagittal angle (PJA) ≥10° and PJA at least 10° greater than preoperative) at 2-year follow-up, with no difference observed between rib-based and spine-based treatment groups [15]. Contouring of the upper end of the rods, minimizing soft tissue disruption and avoiding overcorrection of thoracic hyperkyphosis may decrease the risk of PJK, and children with hyperkyphosis may be at greater risk [16]. Although not performed in this case, in cases of severe PJK, proximal extension of the final fusion may be required.

The ideal definitive management after spine-based growing rod treatment has not been established. Options include observation, implant removal without definitive fusion, fusion in situ, and definitive fusion with re-instrumentation. Autofusion occurs at a high rate [17]. Definitive fusion has been associated with an unexpectedly high complication rate including infection and pseudoarthrosis [18]. Jain et al. compared those undergoing definitive fusion to those who did not at a minimum 2-year follow-up, and recommended fusion could be avoided for selected patients who showed satisfactory final alignment and trunk height, had gained minimal length at last lengthening, and had no implant-related problems [19].

References

1. Fletcher ND, McClung A, Rathjen KE, et al. Serial casting as a delay tactic in the treatment of moderate-to-severe early-onset scoliosis. J Pediatr Orthop. 2012;32(7):664–71.
2. Skaggs DL, Akbarnia BA, Flynn JM, et al. A classification of growth friendly spine implants. J Pediatr Orthop. 2014;34:260–74.
3. Karol LA, Johnston C, Mladenov K, et al. Pulmonary function following early thoracic fusion in non-neuromuscular scoliosis. J Bone Joint Surg Am. 2008;90(6):1272–81.
4. Goldberg CJ, Gillic I, Connaughton O, et al. Respiratory function and cosmesis at maturity in infantile-onset scoliosis. Spine. 2003;28:2397–406.
5. Harrington PR. Treatment of scoliosis. Correction and internal fixation by spine instrumentation. J Bone Joint Surg Am. 1962;44:591–610.
6. Moe JH, Kharrat K, Winter RB, et al. Harrington instrumentation without fusion plus external orthotic support for the treatment of difficult curvature problems in young children. Clin Orthop Relat Res. 1984;35–45.
7. Skaggs KF, Brasher AE, Johnston CE, et al. Upper thoracic pedicle screw loss of fixation causing spinal cord injury: a review of the literature and multicenter case series. J Pediatr Orthop. 2013;33:75–9.
8. Sankar WN, Acevedo DC, Skaggs DL. Comparison of complications among growing spinal implants. Spine. 2010;35:2091–6.
9. Lee C, Myung KS, Skaggs DL. Some connectors in distraction-based growing rods fail more than others. Spine Deform. 2013;1(2):148–56.
10. Yang JS, Sponseller PD, Thompson GH, et al. Growing Spine Study Group. Growing rod fractures: risk factors and opportunities for prevention. Spine. 2011;36(20):1639–44.
11. Thompson GH, Akbarnia BA, Campbell RM Jr. Growing rod techniques in early-onset scoliosis. J Pediatr Orthop. 2007;27:354–61.
12. Akbarnia BA, Marks DS, Boachie-Adjei O, et al. Dual growing rod technique for the treatment of progressive early-onset scoliosis: a multicenter study. Spine. 2005;30:S46–57.
13. Paloski MD, Sponseller PD, Akbarnia BA, et al. Growing Spine Study Group. Is there an optimal time to distract dual growing rods? Spine Deform. 2014;2(6):467–70.

14. Barrett KK, Andras LM, Tolo VT, et al. Measurement variability in the evaluation of the proximal junction in distraction-based growing rods patients. J Pediatr Orthop. 2015;35(6):624–7.
15. El-Hawary R, Sturm P, Cahill P, et al. What is the risk of developing proximal junctional kyphosis during growth friendly treatments for early-onset scoliosis? J Pediatr Orthop. 2017;37(2):86–91.
16. Watanabe K, Uno K, Suzuki T, et al. Risk factors for proximal junctional kyphosis associated with dual-rod growing-rod surgery for early-onset scoliosis. Clin Spine Surg. 2016;29(8):E428–33.
17. Cahill PJ, Marvil S, Cuddihy L, et al. Autofusion in the immature spine treated with growing rods. Spine. 2010;35(22):E1199–203.
18. Poe-Kochert C, Shannon C, Pawelek JB, et al. Final fusion after growing-rod treatment for early onset scoliosis: is it really final? J Bone Joint Surg Am. 2016;98(22):1913–7.
19. Jain A, Sponseller PD, Flynn JM, et al. Avoidance of "Final" surgical fusion after growing-rod treatment for early-onset scoliosis. J Bone Joint Surg Am. 2016;98(13):1073–8.

Chapter 5
The Vertical Expandable Prosthetic Titanium Rib (VEPTR) for Idiopathic Early-Onset Scoliosis

Daniel J. Miller, Susan E. Nelson, and John M. Flynn (Jack)

Case Presentation

History and Physical Examination

The patient presented as a 19-month-old boy who was referred for consultation by his primary care doctor after his parents noted an asymmetric appearance in his back. The parents denied any history of trauma, infection, or back pain. He was born at 38 weeks via normal spontaneous vaginal delivery. He spent 2 days in the NICU for low birth weight (4 lbs 8 oz). He then was discharged after an uneventful hospital course and had been growing and developing as expected at time of presentation (sat at 4 months, crawled at 7 months, and walked at 10 months). His past medical history was unremarkable. There was no family history of spinal deformity.

D.J. Miller, MD • S.E. Nelson, MD, MPH •
J.M. Flynn (Jack), MD (✉)
Division of Orthopedic Surgery, The Children's Hospital of Philadelphia, Philadelphia, PA, USA
e-mail: Millerd9@email.chop.edu; Nelsons2@email.chop.edu; FLYNNJ@email.chop.edu

R. El-Hawary, C.P. Eberson (eds.), *Early Onset Scoliosis*,
https://doi.org/10.1007/978-3-319-71580-3_5

At initial evaluation, the patient was well developed and well nourished. He had normal affect, mood, and age-appropriate judgment. He was normocephalic with no evidence of respiratory distress. There was no tenderness on palpation of the spine. Adam's forward bend demonstrated a right thoracic prominence which was flexible in nature. Iliac crest height was symmetric and the sagittal contour of the spine was normal. There were no hairy patches, sacral dimples, café au lait spots, or other cutaneous abnormalities about the spine with no concerning cutaneous findings on the upper and lower extremities. Muscle bulk, strength, and tone were normal throughout bilateral upper and lower extremities. Gait was reciprocal and non-antalgic, and the patient was able to walk with normal strength and coordination.

Diagnostic Studies

Initial radiographic evaluation demonstrated a right thoracic curve measuring 58° and a left thoracolumbar curve measuring 49° (Figure 5.1a).

Management Chosen

The patient underwent an MRI to rule out neuraxial lesions and was fitted with a thoracolumbosacral orthosis (TLSO) in an attempt to delay progression of spinal deformity and need for surgical intervention. Full-time brace wear was recommended. He was followed every 4 months with full-length spine X-rays. His spinal deformity was maintained for 1 year, after which he demonstrated evidence of curve progression from 58 to 71° (Figure 5.1b). At this point, the decision was made to proceed with a unilateral, right-sided VEPTR (DePuy Synthes Spine, Raynham, MA) rib to spine construct. The VEPTR was subsequently distracted seven times over the next 4 years, with exchange for a new VEPTR device required after 2.5 years after he had reached full excursion of the VEPTR implant.

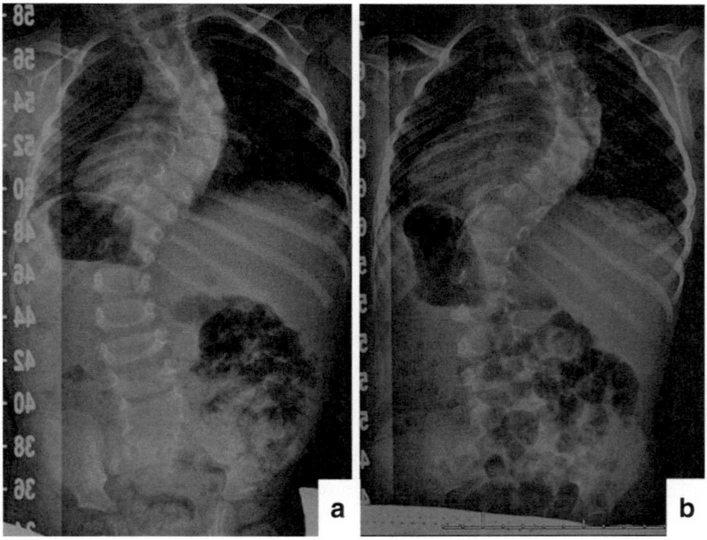

FIGURE 5.1 Initial PA (**a**) radiograph demonstrating a right thoracic curve measuring 58° and a left thoracolumbar curve measuring 49°. After 1 year of bracing with a TLSO, radiograph demonstrates evidence of curve progression to 71° and 57° (**b**)

Surgical Procedure

VEPTR Insertion

The patient was positioned prone on gel rolls on a Jackson frame (Mizuho OSI, Union City, CA) after induction of anesthesia and neuromonitoring. A curvilinear incision was made between the spine and the medial border of the left scapula. The trapezius and rhomboids were split in line with the incision. The paraspinal muscles were elevated lateral to medial to the tips of the transverse processes. Inadvertent exposure of the spine should be avoided to prevent fusion. The cranial surface of the third rib and the caudal of the fourth rib were subperiosteally exposed, and a VEPTR cradle was placed.

An incision was made over the planned distal anchor sites. The subcutaneous tissues carefully elevated the left-sided paraspinal muscles of the L1 and L2 vertebrae. A rongeur was used to create an opening in the ligamentum flavum and the channel for the down-going laminar hooks. These hooks were placed at the L1 and L2 level. A 220 mm radius VEPTR lumbar extension rod and rib support construct was sized, cut, and contoured based on the distance between the proximal anchors and the caudal rib cage (in this case size 7). A uterine packing forceps was used to create a subcutaneous tunnel, and a chest tube was used to shuttle the VEPTR device. The device should be passed in a cranial to caudal direction to minimize the chance of thoracic penetration. The VEPTR was subsequently engaged in the cradle proximally and hooks distally and in provisional distraction was performed distally to tension the laminar hooks. Bone graft was applied at the rib 3–4 level in order to get a spot fusion at this site. After final tightening, the wounds were irrigated copiously and closed in layers. No complications occurred. Postoperative images are provided in Figure 5.2.

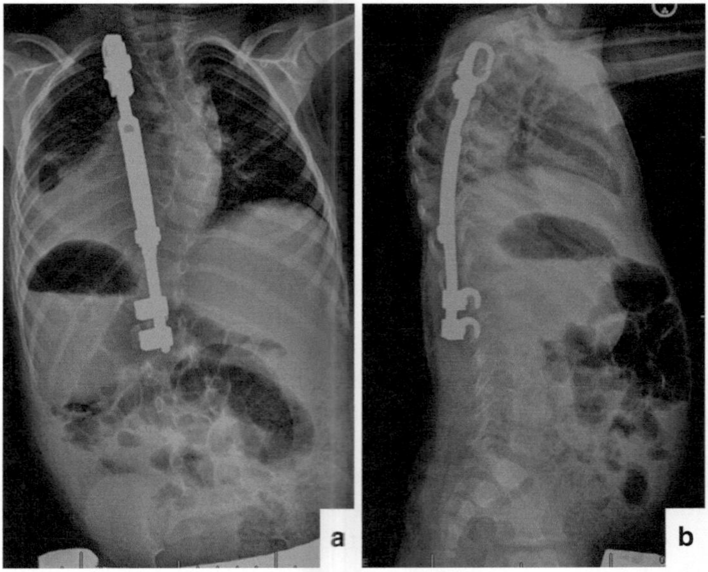

FIGURE 5.2 PA (**a**) and lateral (**b**) radiographs taken 1 week following the initial VEPTR implantation

VEPTR Lengthening

Six months after the index implantation procedure, the VEPTR construct was distracted to allow for thoracic growth and continued control of spinal deformity. Subsequent lengthening procedures occurred at intervals of approximately 6 months and were performed on an outpatient procedure (Figure 5.3). During each lengthening procedure, distraction of 0.5–1.0 cm was accomplished.

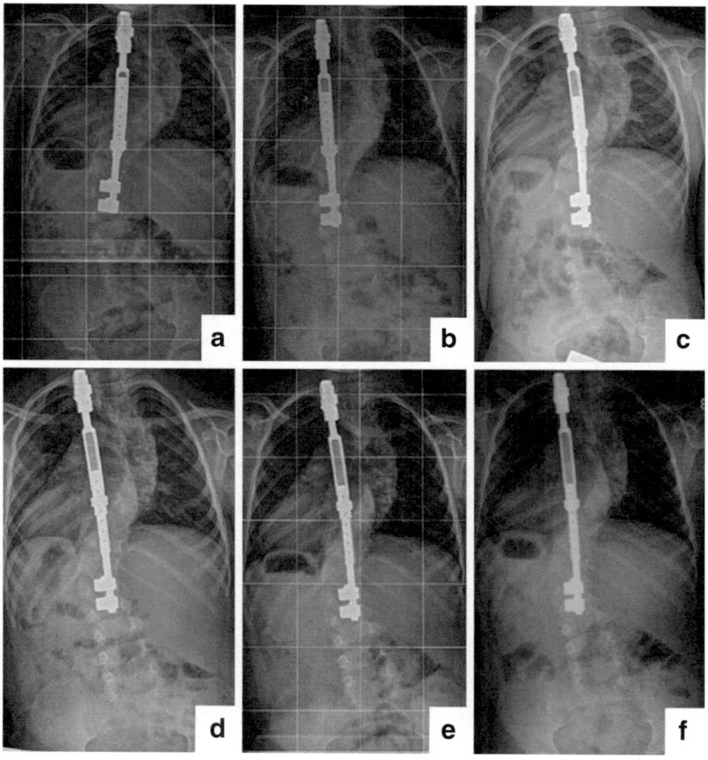

FIGURE 5.3 PA radiographs from before the first distraction (**a**, 5 months following initial surgery), after the first distraction (**b**, radiograph taken 11 months following initial surgery), after the second distraction (**c**, radiograph taken 17 months following initial surgery), after third distraction (**d**, radiograph taken 23 months following initial surgery), after fourth distraction (**e**, radiograph taken 29 months following initial surgery), after fifth distraction (**f**, radiograph taken 36 months following initial surgery)

VEPTR Exchange

After five lengthening procedures, the VEPTR device reached maximal excursion; therefore an exchange procedure was performed (size 7 to size 11). Proximal and distal anchors were stable and were unchanged during the revision. The patient tolerated the exchange without complication and was discharged home on postoperative day 1. Postoperative images are provided in Figure 5.4.

VEPTR Lengthening

Six months after the VEPTR exchange, subsequent lengthening procedures resumed at intervals of approximately 6 months.

Clinical Course and Outcome

Radiographs demonstrate interval correction and maintenance of alignment over 4 years of follow-up (Figure 5.5). During the course of treatment and subsequent follow-up thus far, no complications have been noted. At most recent follow-up, a 35° right-sided curve from T3 to T11 and a 33° left-sided curve from T11 to L4 were present. T1–S1 height gained from pre-initial to final was 7.2 cm, with 6.5 cm gained from post-initial to most recent follow-up. His care plan moving forward will include continued serial lengthening every 6–9 months with a plan for eventual instrumented fusion near skeletal maturity.

Clinical Pearls and Pitfalls

- Control of spinal deformity while preserving growth of the spine and thorax is the chief aim of surgery in patient with early-onset idiopathic scoliosis.
- Complete correction of deformity is not required.

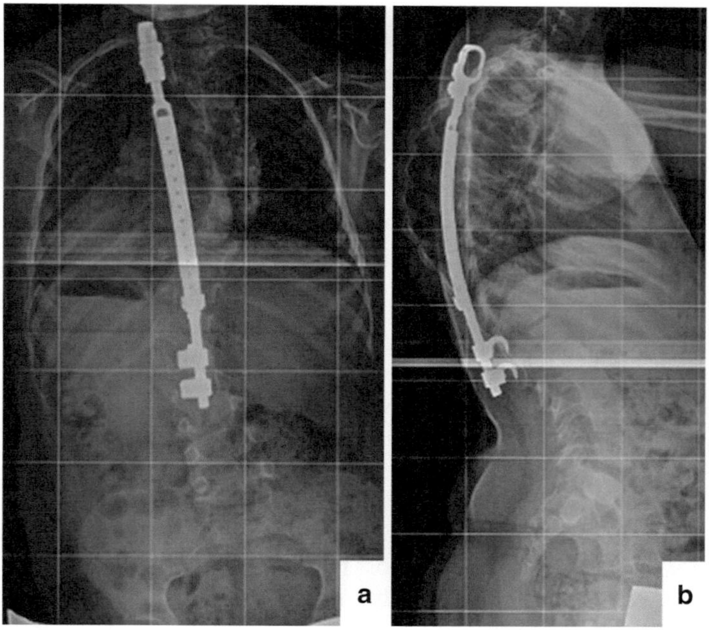

FIGURE 5.4 PA (**a**) and lateral (**b**) radiographs taken following VEPTR device exchange

- The VEPTR represents a valuable tool in the arsenal of treatment for EOS.
- Multiple surgeries, including revisions, are required when initial implantation is done in young children. Families need to understand this when discussing treatment options.

Literature Review and Discussion

Infantile idiopathic scoliosis (IIS) represents a small percentage of all EOS diagnoses. Patients are more likely to be male, and convex left curves predominate compared to adolescent idiopathic scoliosis. Idiopathic etiology specifically has been found to resolve spontaneously in up to 92% of cases [1–4].

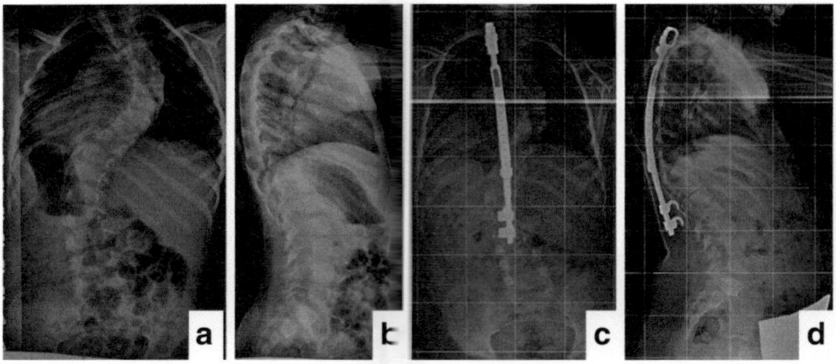

FIGURE 5.5 Preoperative PA (**a**) and lateral radiographs (**b**); PA (**c**) and lateral radiographs (**d**) at most recent follow-up 4 years after initial VEPTR implantation. A total of 7.2 cm in T1–S1 length was gained from pre-initial surgery to most recent follow-up

However, progressive curves during early life negatively impact development of the lungs, spine, and chest wall and are potentially fatal. The most reliable predictors of progression were described by Mehta in 1972 [3] including scoliosis >20°, a rib-vertebra angle difference (RVAD) ≥20°, and a phase 2 rib-vertebra relationship.

Historically options for management of infantile idiopathic scoliosis have varied including casting, bracing, growing instrumentation, and fusion. Typically, formal fusion should be delayed until at least 8–10 years of age due to detrimental effects of pulmonary function when fusion is performed earlier [5]. In younger patients with progressive deformities refractory to nonoperative techniques, or too severe for nonoperative management, growing constructs may be used to control or correct the deformity while allowing thoracic growth. The VEPTR indications have expanded beyond the primary intended scope for thoracic insufficiency and can be included under the umbrella of growing constructs.

VEPTR has been used successfully for controlling scoliosis and increasing thoracic volume in patients with congenital scoliosis and fused ribs [6, 7]. However, there are few reports regarding the use of VEPTR to control deformity in idiopathic infantile scoliosis. VEPTR use in idiopathic cases has been examined in heterogeneous samples of EOS patients without rib abnormalities including neuromuscular, syndromic, and congenital scoliosis [8–10] and independently [11, 12].

Most recently, El-Hawary in a multicenter prospective study reported on the radiographic outcomes of VEPTR in EOS patients without rib abnormalities at 2-year follow-up [8]. Of 63 EOS patients, including 17 with IIS, 54 (86%) had a successful outcome, defined as scoliosis magnitude less than or equal to preoperative magnitude at 2-year follow-up or trunk height/spinal length greater than or equal to immediate postoperative trunk height or spinal length. Although overall mean kyphosis was similar at 2-year follow-up to preoperative measurements (47.9 vs. 48°), the idiopathic group had a 23% increased kyphosis at follow-up. 49% of patients had at least one complication (26% device related, 14% pneumonia, 14% wound complications, 14% pneumonia, 11% infection). The authors conclude that VEPTR allowed spine growth while controlling progression of the scoliosis in this heterogeneous population without rib abnormalities [8].

Schultz reported on the results of VEPTR in IIS from a single institution. Eight IIS patients were identified retrospectively over a 9-year period and followed for an average 32 months [11]. Patients had VEPTR instrumentation either rib to spine or rib to pelvis, unilateral or bilateral depending on curve and patient characteristics. No deep wound infections or other wound complications were reported, and 37% of cases had hardware complications. They found coronal curve radiographic measurement improved from an average of 84–56°; an average curve correction of 35.1%. Although VEPTR is thought to be a kyphosis inducing instrumentation, average kyphosis improved from 55.7 to 32.4° at most recent follow-up. The mean length per extension gained was 6.4 mm over average four lengthenings. They conclude VEPTR is a growth-friendly treatment alternative in IIS patients that presents or progresses beyond what is recommended for nonoperative management and suggest the minimally invasive nature of insertion may diminish autofusion caused by other growing spinal instrumentation [11].

The limited results of VEPTR use in IIS are in part due to the rarity of the condition, in addition to the spontaneous resolution and the success of nonoperative treatment such as Mehta casting. VEPTR may be used as a growing construct in IIS patients with severe curves, with the benefit of limiting dissection and potentially autofusion. However, complications associated with VEPTR implantation and repeated operative lengthening remain a concern as does the kyphosis inducing potential of construct. Careful patient selection and review of all options remain essential for successful treatment of IIS.

References

1. Ceballos T, Ferrer-Torrelles M, Castillo F, Fernandez-Paredes E. Prognosis in infantile idiopathic scoliosis. J Bone Joint Surg Am. 1980;62(6):863–75.
2. Diedrich O, von Strempel A, Schloz M, Schmitt O, Kraft CN. Long-term observation and management of resolving infantile idiopathic scoliosis a 25-year follow-up. J Bone Joint Surg Br. 2002;84(7):1030–5.
3. Mehta MH. The rib-vertebra angle in the early diagnosis between resolving and progressive infantile scoliosis. J Bone Joint Surg Br. 1972;54(2):230–43.
4. Gillingham BL, Fan RA, Akbarnia BA. Early onset idiopathic scoliosis. J Am Acad Orthop Surg. 2006;14(2):101–12.
5. Karol LA, Johnston C, Mladenov K, Schochet P, Walters P, Browne RH. Pulmonary function following early thoracic fusion in non-neuromuscular scoliosis. J Bone Joint Surg Am. 2008;90(6):1272–81.
6. Campbell RM Jr, Hell-Vocke AK. Growth of the thoracic spine in congenital scoliosis after expansion thoracoplasty. J Bone Joint Surg Am. 2003;85-A(3):409–20.
7. Emans JB, Caubet JF, Ordonez CL, Lee EY, Ciarlo M. The treatment of spine and chest wall deformities with fused ribs by expansion thoracostomy and insertion of vertical expandable prosthetic titanium rib: growth of thoracic spine and

improvement of lung volumes. Spine (Phila Pa 1976). 2005;30(17 Suppl):S58–68.
8. El-Hawary R, Kadhim M, Vitale M, Smith J, Samdani A, Flynn JM, et al. VEPTR implantation to treat children with early-onset scoliosis without rib abnormalities: early results from a prospective multicenter study. J Pediatr Orthop. 2017.
9. Hasler CC, Mehrkens A, Hefti F. Efficacy and safety of VEPTR instrumentation for progressive spine deformities in young children without rib fusions. Eur Spine J. 2010;19(3):400–8.
10. Samdani AF, Ranade A, Dolch HJ, Williams R, St Hilaire T, Cahill P, et al. Bilateral use of the vertical expandable prosthetic titanium rib attached to the pelvis: a novel treatment for scoliosis in the growing spine. J Neurosurg Spine. 2009;10(4):287–92.
11. Schulz JF, Smith J, Cahill PJ, Fine A, Samdani AF. The role of the vertical expandable titanium rib in the treatment of infantile idiopathic scoliosis: early results from a single institution. J Pediatr Orthop. 2010;30(7):659–63.
12. Smith JR, Samdani AF, Pahys J, Ranade A, Asghar J, Cahill P, et al. The role of bracing, casting, and vertical expandable prosthetic titanium rib for the treatment of infantile idiopathic scoliosis: a single-institution experience with 31 consecutive patients. Clinical article. J Neurosurg Spine. 2009;11(1):3–8.

Chapter 6
Treatment of Idiopathic Early-Onset Scoliosis with a Hybrid Growing Rod Construct

Haleh Badkoobehi and Lindsay Andras

Case Presentation

History and Physical Examination

The patient was diagnosed with idiopathic infantile scoliosis at 7 months of age with a curve magnitude of 44° (Fig. 6.1). He was treated with a thoracolumbar sacral orthosis (TLSO) that was poorly tolerated and did not control the curve. At age 2, the patient presented to us with progressive scoliosis that measured 102° and kyphosis that measured 73° (Fig. 6.2). Review of systems, family, and social history were noncontributory.

At 2 years of age, the patient was noted to be of average height and BMI. He could sit independently on the examination table and was ambulatory. The C7 plumb line was to the left, and his pelvis was level. He actively moved all four extremities symmetrically, without any apparent neurologic

H. Badkoobehi, MD, MPH • L. Andras, MD (✉)
Department of Orthopedic Surgery, Children's Hospital Los Angeles, Los Angeles, CA, USA
e-mail: halehbad@gmail.com; lindsayandras@gmail.com

R. El-Hawary, C.P. Eberson (eds.), *Early Onset Scoliosis*,
https://doi.org/10.1007/978-3-319-71580-3_6

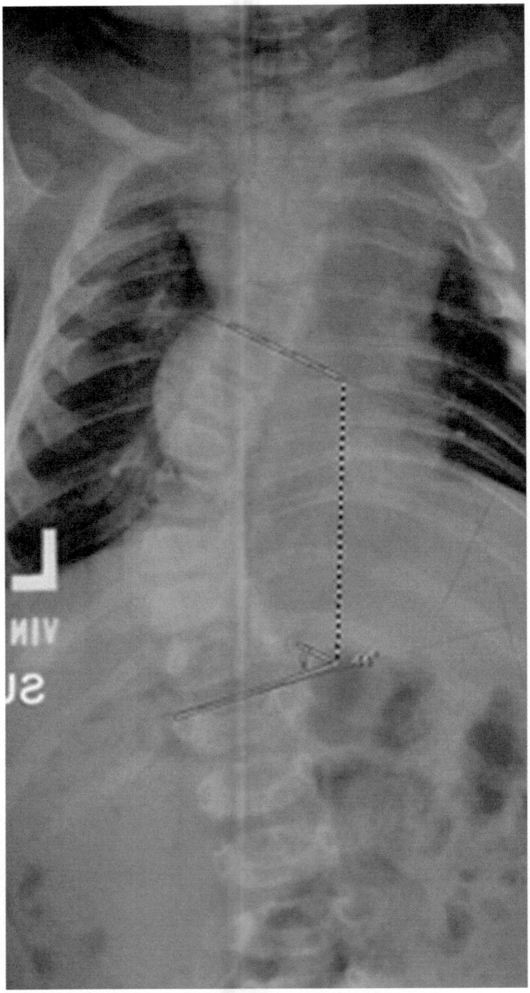

FIGURE 6.1 Initial PA radiograph demonstrating a left thoracic curve, measuring 44°

issues. His elbows, wrists, hips, and knees were flexed and extended fully, and his feet dorsiflexed past neutral bilaterally. There were no deformities noted in his extremities. Tone and reflexes were within normal limits.

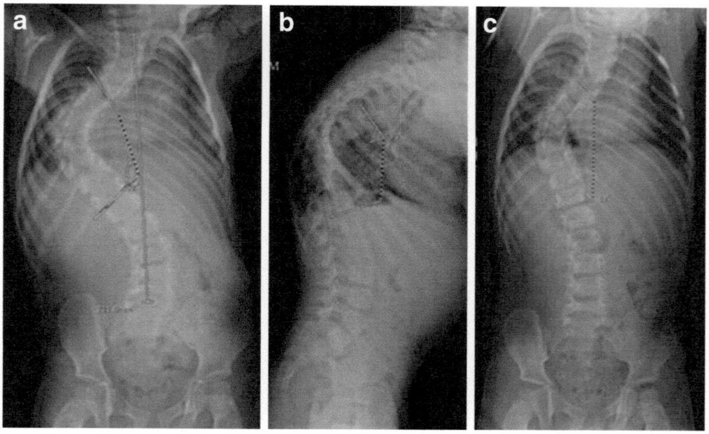

FIGURE 6.2 PA (**a**) and lateral (**b**) spine radiographs at 2 years of age demonstrating 102° scoliosis and 73° kyphosis. T1–S1 height measured 22.2 cm. Traction PA (**c**) of the spine shows correction to 61° scoliosis prior to initiation of EDF casting

Diagnostic Studies

At 7 months, upright PA and lateral spine radiographs demonstrated a left thoracic curve, which measured 44° (Fig. 6.1). At age 2, standing PA and lateral spine radiographs showed that the curve had progressed to 102° of scoliosis and 73° of kyphosis, with a T1–S1 height of 22.2 cm. A traction PA of the spine showed correction of the scoliosis to 61° (Fig. 6.2). MRI of the cervical, thoracic, and lumbar spine was obtained which was negative for intraspinal pathology or congenital anomalies.

Management Chosen

EDF casting was initiated in an attempt to control the progression of scoliosis and kyphosis and to delay the need for open surgical intervention (Fig. 6.3). In total, 12 serial casts were applied over 3 years. Although there was improvement in the coronal plane from 102 to 55° of scoliosis, there was

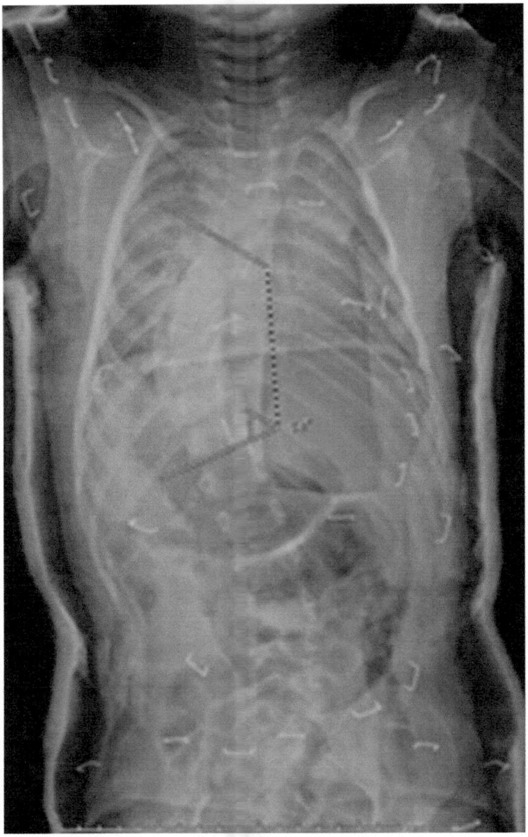

FIGURE 6.3 PA spine radiograph demonstrating a 53° scoliosis after first EDF cast placement

significant progression in the sagittal plane, with kyphosis worsening from 73 to 102°. There was also increased spinal rotation and a worsening rib deformity. At this point, the decision was made to abandon EDF casting and intervene surgically with a hybrid construct, magnetically controlled growing rods (MCGR) from T2 to L3, with proximal rib-based hook anchors and distal pedicle screw spinal anchors (Fig. 6.4).

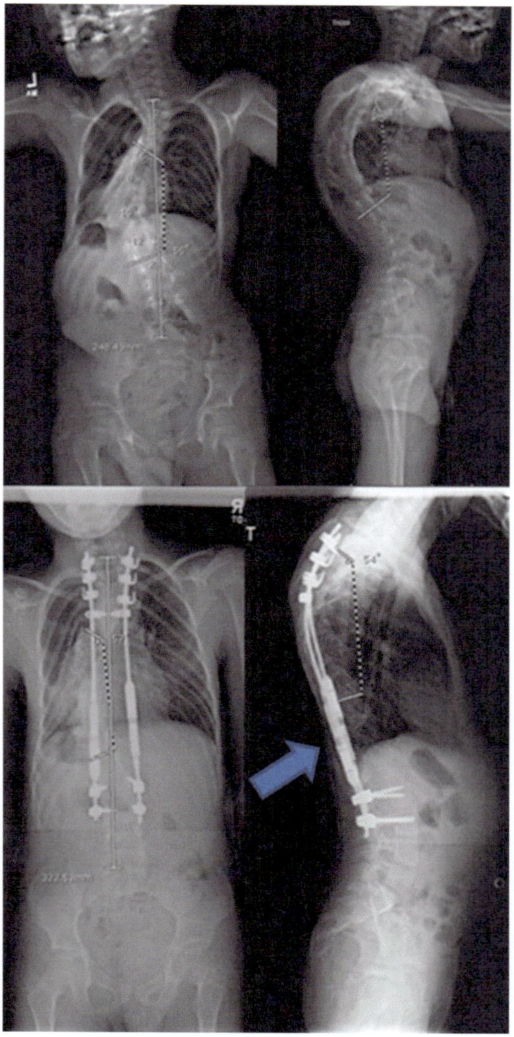

FIGURE 6.4 Preoperative PA and lateral spine radiographs and most recent PA and lateral spine radiographs after hybrid growing MCGR placement after three lengthening procedures, with T2–T4 rib anchors and L2–L3 pedicle screws. T1–S1 height was 24.8 cm preoperatively and 32.3 cm at most recent follow-up. The *blue arrow* demonstrates where the (straight) magnet was placed on the relatively straight thoracolumbar spinal segment, close to the distal anchor

Surgical Procedure

A Mayfield head holder was applied and torqued to the 40-pound line. The patient was then positioned prone on a Jackson Table. A 10-pound weight was applied to the Mayfield, and a 5-pound weight was applied to each lower extremity via tape (Fig. 6.5). Of note, the patient weighed approximately 40 pounds. We generally aim to have the total weight in traction be 50% of the patient's body weight and divide this equally between the weight on the head (25% of the patient's body weight) and the weight on the lower extremities. If there is fixed pelvic obliquity, we place all of the weight on the side of the elevated hemipelvis (25% of the patient's body weight). In cases such as this one where the pelvis is level on the traction film, we place an equal amount of weight on each thigh (12.5% of the patient's body weight). We have moved toward using tape rather than distal femur traction pins due to many of the patients complaining of knee discomfort postoperatively. Additionally this eliminates problems with skeletal traction pins cutting through poor quality bone and potential for physeal injury. Neuromonitoring showed

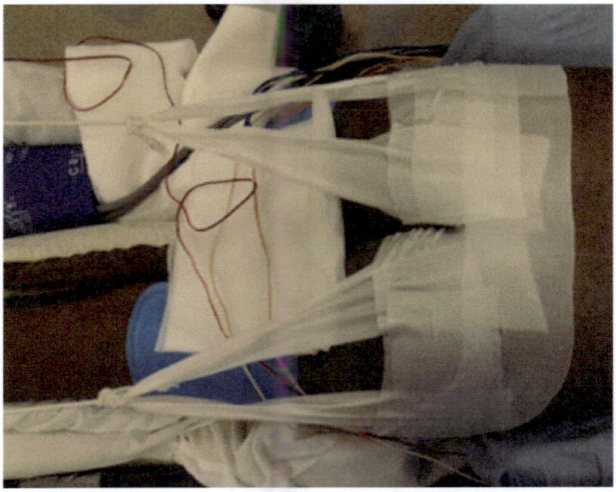

FIGURE 6.5 Intraoperative photograph demonstrating taping used for halofemoral traction

present SSEPs and TcMEPs in all extremities. This did not change after positioning or with the addition of the weight.

Technical note: In cases in which there is a change in the neuromonitoring signals with addition of the weight for traction, consideration is given to staging the procedure and using preoperative halogravity traction for a more gradual correction. We have also used preoperative halogravity traction in cases where the preoperative traction film demonstrated a large amount of deformity (especially kyphosis) that would not be able to accommodate placement of the straight magnetic segment. In these cases, preoperative halogravity traction may not only improve the correction achieved with growing rod insertion but also may allow a child to have MCGR placed who would not otherwise have been a candidate.

With fluoroscopy, T2 to T4 and L2 to L3 were marked. We began with placement of the distal anchors. An incision was made to allow for exposure of the L2 and L3 pedicle screw starting points. Facetectomies were performed at L1/L2 and L2/L3. Care was taken to preserve the intraspinal ligament distal to L3 to guard against junctional kyphosis and autofusion. Positioning of the screws was confirmed with fluoroscopic images, and the screws were stimulated.

Attention was then turned proximally. The skin was incised above T2 to T4 bilaterally, and then the fascia was incised just lateral to the transverse processes. The overlying muscle was bluntly dissected. Fluoroscopy was used to confirm position of ribs 2–4. Hooks were placed bilaterally at those levels (Fig. 6.6).

The magnetic rods were then cut and contoured, using one standard and one offset actuator. Prior to implantation, the magnetic rod distraction function was confirmed. A tonsillar forceps was used to tunnel below the fascia and the muscle layers while staying just above the ribs to the level of the lumbar screws. A chest tube was then passed through this tract with a tonsillar forceps. Care was taken to ensure that this tract did not violate the chest wall. The right magnetic rod was then passed in this tract using the chest tube. The rod was secured first proximally to the rib hooks and then distally to the lumbar screws, and distraction was performed. The left rod was then placed in the same manner. Of note, care was taken to place the straight segment of the magnet at the distal aspect of the construct to allow room for kyphotic contouring proximally.

After placing both magnetic rods, a T-square was used to evaluate coronal balance. Additional distraction was performed to level the shoulders. The area at L2–L3 was decorticated to provide a limited fusion at the base. A Valsalva maneuver was performed to evaluate for evidence of pneumothorax. Corticocancellous allograft was combined with autograft and vancomycin powder and was packed around L2–L3 for fusion. Also, vancomycin powder was coated along the implants proximally and on the fascia. Postoperatively, the patient was fitted with a TLSO brace. We have generally used a postoperative brace for 3 months when out of bed to prevent excessive bending and twisting in rambunctious youngsters in order to allow for healing of the limited fusion at the distal anchor site.

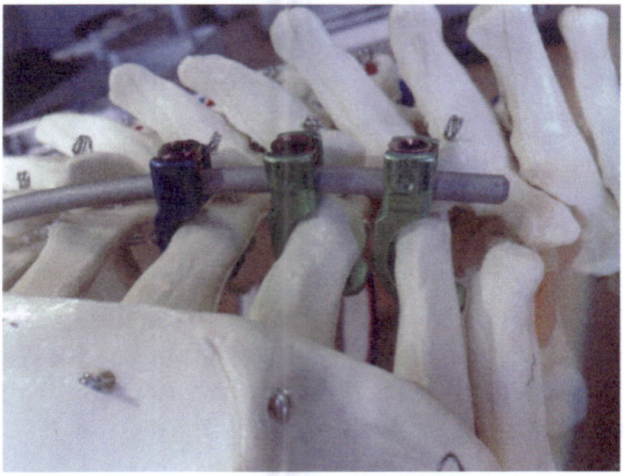

FIGURE 6.6 Photograph showing position of rib anchors

Clinical Course and Outcome

The patient is currently 6 years old. Since implantation, the construct has been distracted 3 times at 3-month intervals. At his last follow-up, PA and lateral spine radiographs measured 57° scoliosis and 54° kyphosis. T1–S1 height has increased from 24.8 cm preoperatively to 32.3 cm at most recent follow-up (Fig. 6.4). There have been no complications or return trips to the operating room since the index surgical procedure. Definitive instrumented spinal fusion is anticipated around age 10 years, but may not be necessary if his spine is autofused and well-balanced at that point.

Clinical Pearls and Pitfalls

- EDF casting can delay initiation of growing rod surgery, but patients should be monitored for continued curve progression or development of iatrogenic chest wall deformity.
- Proximal rib hook anchors may allow for more mobility than proximal pedicle screw anchors. Proximal rib hooks theoretically decrease the stiffness of the construct and may be protective against rod breakage.
- Intraoperative positioning including use of halo traction can facilitate deformity correction while minimizing stress placed on anchors during correction.
- Respect sagittal profile with kyphosis bent into upper aspect of rods and straight connector (or MCGR) at the thoracolumbar junction (see arrow in Fig. 6.4).
- Magnetically lengthening rods are FDA approved for 1.5 T MRI but limit the ability to image adjacent areas due to metal artifact and thus are contraindicated in children with intraspinal pathology such as a syrinx or tethered cord, which require MRI monitoring.

Literature Review and Discussion

Idiopathic EOS is defined as curvature of the spine in the coronal plane ≥10° with age of onset before 10 years, without any other associated condition [1]. Idiopathic EOS is rare, accounting for <1% of all scoliosis diagnoses [2].

There are a variety of treatment options for idiopathic EOS, including bracing, casting, distraction-based guided growth including traditional or hybrid constructs, single or dual spine growing rod constructs, MCGR, Shilla guided growth constructs, tethering, and definitive spinal fusion.

While definitive fusion may effectively control spinal deformity, arresting spinal growth and tethering the thorax will adversely affect pulmonary development and function in patients with remaining growth potential [3, 4]. An attractive alternative to early definitive fusion is a distraction-based growth-friendly construct, both to control the spinal deformity and to optimize growth of the thorax. Distraction-based spinal growth constructs have been shown to prevent progressive decline of pulmonary function [5–7].

This case illustrates the use of a hybrid construct consisting of rib-based proximal anchors, which are low-profile upgoing hooks placed on the ribs. Distally, pedicle screws serve as spinal anchors. Only the distal anchor segments are fused, and care is taken not to disrupt the periosteum at any other level to prevent unintentional fusion. Either a traditional connector or a magnetically controlled rod is placed between the anchors.

Rib-based proximal anchors have multiple benefits over pedicle screws. They are technically less challenging to place when compared to thoracic pedicle screws and have less fluoroscopic demand [8], without compromise in strength. Rib hooks have shown equivalent ultimate strength to failure when compared to pedicle screws [9], and the use of ≥5 proximal rib anchors prevents loss of fixation and migration of anchors [10]. Importantly, the use of rib hooks eliminates the need for limited proximal fusion and allows for mobility through this segment. Decreased rigidity in the proximal segment of the hybrid construct lowers stress concentration and theoretically decreases implant failures. A lower incidence of rod fracture with the use of hybrid constructs with proximal rib anchors has been demonstrated when compared to proximal spine anchors [11].

MCGR represent a significant advance in distraction-based growing rod constructs due to cost neutrality and the reduced number of complications such as infection and trips to the operating room for serial lengthenings. Traditional growing rod constructs consist of proximal and distal spinal anchors with a connector and limited fusion at anchor levels. This technique requires repeated surgical procedures for lengthening through the connector at 6-month intervals. In contrast, MCGR eliminate the need for surgical lengthening procedures, as serial lengthenings are performed in the clinic setting with the use of a magnet. Initially, MCGR were thought to be a more expensive alternative to traditional growing rods, but multiple economic analyses have shown that after 3–6 years, the total cost of treatment with magnetic rods becomes equal to treatment with traditional growing rods [12, 13]. Implant complications such as proximal hook pullout and rod breakage still occur with magnetic rods [14]. Parental counseling of the possibility of multiple complications requiring return trips to the operating room should occur prior to placement of any growth construct.

Traditional growing rod constructs with spine anchors have demonstrated diminishing returns in spinal length increases over time due to suspected autofusion [15, 16]. Autofusion has been seen in up to 89% of patients treated with growing rods [17]. The Growing Spine Study Group (GSSG) reported on 58 patients who went on to instrumented spinal fusion after treatment of scoliosis with growing rods. At the time of surgery they noted that 20% of spines were mobile, 40% had segments of autofusion, and 40% were completely autofused. Osteotomies were needed in 15% of these patients [18]. In our case, final instrumented fusion is planned at around age 10. If at that time there is a well-balanced spine, the need for definitive fusion may be obviated.

In summary, a hybrid growth construct with proximal rib-based anchors and distal pedicle screws with MCGR is an effective treatment option in severe progressive cases of idiopathic EOS. The mobility provided by the proximal rib-based anchors when compared to proximal pedicle screws aids in minimizing implant issues such as rod fracture. MCGR represents a significant advancement, allowing for lengthening in the clinic setting and decreased surgical complications such as infection. Though management of EOS continues to present challenges, as these growth-friendly constructs evolve, we continue to move toward the goal of controlling spinal deformity without sacrificing spinal growth and thoracic development and improving the quality of life for our patients.

References

1. El-Hawary R, Akbarnia BA. Early onset scoliosis—time for consensus. Spine Deform. 2015;3(2):105–6.
2. Riseborough EJ, Wynne-Davies R. A genetic survey of idiopathic scoliosis in Boston, Massachusetts. J Bone Joint Surg Am. 1973;55(5):974–82.
3. Karol LA, et al. Pulmonary function following early thoracic fusion in non-neuromuscular scoliosis. J Bone Joint Surg Am. 2008;90(6):1272–81.
4. Goldberg CJ, et al. Respiratory function and cosmesis at maturity in infantile-onset scoliosis. Spine (Phila Pa 1976). 2003;28(20):2397–406.
5. Motoyama EK, et al. Effects on lung function of multiple expansion thoracoplasty in children with thoracic insufficiency syndrome: a longitudinal study. Spine (Phila Pa 1976). 2006;31(3):284–90.
6. Mayer OH, Redding G. Early changes in pulmonary function after vertical expandable prosthetic titanium rib insertion in children with thoracic insufficiency syndrome. J Pediatr Orthop. 2009;29(1):35–8.
7. Dede O, et al. Pulmonary and radiographic outcomes of VEPTR (vertical expandable prosthetic titanium rib) treatment in early-onset scoliosis. J Bone Joint Surg Am. 2014;96(15):1295–302.
8. Miller DJ, Vitale MG. Rib-based anchors for growing rods in the treatment of early-onset scoliosis. Oper Tech Orthop. 2016;26(4):241–6.

9. Akbarnia BA, et al. Biomechanical evaluation of 4 different foundation constructs commonly used in growing spine surgery: are rib anchors comparable to spine anchors? Spine Deform. 2014;2(6):437–43.
10. Myung KS, David L, Yazici M, Diab M, Noordeen Hilali H, Vitale MG, Johnston CE. Hybrid growth rods using spinal implants on ribs. Abstract presented at the 45th Annual Scoliosis Research Society Meeting. 2010. p. 105–6.
11. Yamaguchi KT Jr, et al. Are rib versus spine anchors protective against breakage of growing rods? Spine Deform. 2014;2(6):489–92.
12. Su AW, Milbrandt TA, Larson AN. Magnetic expansion control system achieves cost savings compared to traditional growth rods: an economic analysis model. Spine (Phila Pa 1976). 2015;40(23):1851–6.
13. Polly DW Jr, et al. Cost analysis of magnetically controlled growing rods compared with traditional growing rods for early-onset scoliosis in the US: an integrated health care delivery system perspective. Clinicoecon Outcomes Res. 2016;8:457–65.
14. Choi E, et al. Implant complications after magnetically controlled growing rods for early onset scoliosis: A multicenter retrospective review. J Pediatr Orthop. 2017 Dec;37(8):e588–e592.
15. Sankar WN, et al. Lengthening of dual growing rods and the law of diminishing returns. Spine (Phila Pa 1976). 2011;36(10):806–9.
16. El-Hawary R, et al. Rib-based distraction surgery maintains total spine growth. J Pediatr Orthop. 2016;36(8):841–6.
17. Cahill PJ, et al. Autofusion in the immature spine treated with growing rods. Spine (Phila Pa 1976). 2010;35(22):E1199–203.
18. Akbarnia BA, et al. Fusionless procedures for the management of early-onset spine deformities in 2011: what do we know? J Child Orthop. 2011;5(3):159–72.

Chapter 7
Shilla Growth Guidance Technique for Early Onset Scoliosis

Richard E. McCarthy and David B. Bumpass

Case Presentation

History and Physical Examination

A 3-year 1-month-old boy presented after his mother noted a slight deviation in his stance and brought this to the attention of his primary care physician who referred him to a pediatric spine specialist. Birth history was normal, although he was 3 weeks premature. Developmental milestones were met on time. Family history includes scoliosis in several cousins, and he lives with both parents who do not have scoliosis and do not smoke.

R.E. McCarthy, MD (✉)
Department of orthopedics, Arkansas Children's Hospital/
University of Arkansas for Medical Sciences, Little Rock, AR, USA

Department of Neurosurgery, Arkansas Children's Hospital/
University of Arkansas for Medical Sciences, Little Rock, AR, USA
e-mail: rmccarthy@uams.edu

D.B. Bumpass, MD
Department of orthopedics, Arkansas Children's Hospital/
University of Arkansas for Medical Sciences, Little Rock, AR, USA

R. El-Hawary, C.P. Eberson (eds.), *Early Onset Scoliosis*,
https://doi.org/10.1007/978-3-319-71580-3_7

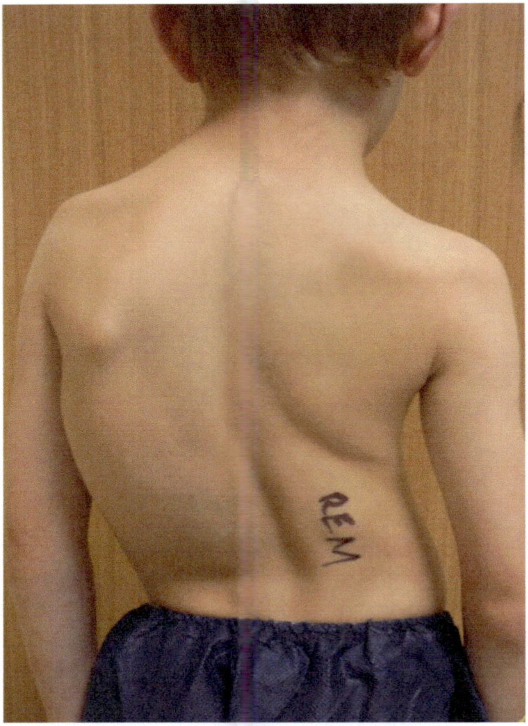

FIGURE 7.1 Preoperative clinical photograph

The standing view from behind demonstrated a left truncal shift with a rib prominence (Fig. 7.1) which measured 15° with a scoliometer on forward bend test. Neurologic examination was normal, with symmetric abdominal reflexes and no clonus. The arch of the palate was somewhat high, but no cutaneous lesions were noted on his body. His examination was otherwise normal.

Diagnostic Studies

The initial standing PA film revealed a curve of 54° (Fig. 7.2). A full spinal MRI was normal without spinal cord or brainstem abnormalities.

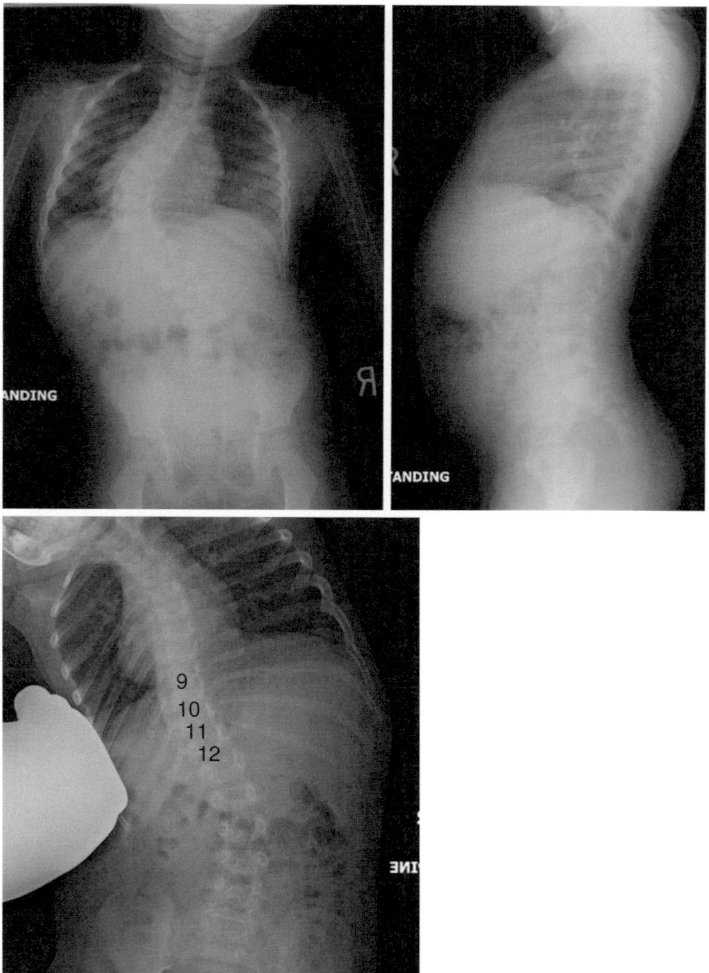

FIGURE 7.2 Preoperative standing PA and lateral radiographs of the entire spine with supine flexibility film. Curve measures 72°.

Management Chosen

Options for treatment were discussed with the family and included casting, distraction-based surgery, and growth guidance. The family preferred to postpone a decision until the full spine MRI was performed; however, because of his age, a general anesthetic was necessary for this study. These arrangements took time, further delaying his treatment and resulting in a worsening of the curve.

Upon return to the clinic 4 months after initial presentation, the curve as measured from T2 to L2 had increased to 72°. Flexibility films showed correction by approximately 50%. After further discussion, the family decided to proceed with surgical treatment using a growth guidance method of instrumentation.

Surgical Procedure

Overview

The premise of the Shilla technique is that once the apical segments are corrected to a neutral position in the coronal, sagittal, and axillary planes, the remaining vertebral levels involved in the curve will follow into a neutral position and add height to the spine through vertebral growth. The apical segments are fused together and fixed to the midsection of the two vertical rods. Growth occurs cephalad and caudad to the apex, guided by "growing screws" placed into the pedicles in a minimally invasive trans-muscular fashion to not disrupt the vertebral periosteum or facet capsules. The growing screws slide along the parallel rods, enabling movement and growth [1, 2].

Selecting the Apical Fusion Levels

Flexibility films denote the three or four apical segments that least correct with bending. These vertebrae will be treated in a manner sufficient to derotate and align the curve to a straight alignment. This requires posterior column osteotomies or anterior disc releases, typically the former. Curve stiffness and the surgeon's skill set will determine where and how to achieve the necessary apical flexibility. Severely rigid or congenital curves may even necessitate a pedicle subtraction osteotomy or vertebral column resection to maximally realign the apex. The patient in this case report had a supine, assisted bend film which determined the apex to be T9–T12. These levels were approached subperiosteally and loosened with Ponte osteotomies at T9–T10, T10–T11, and T11–T12. Bilateral fixed-head pedicle screws 5.5 mm in diameter were placed into these vertebrae at maximal length.

Placing Growing Screws

With fluoroscopic or navigational imagery, large polyaxial (6.5 mm) screws are placed through the muscle layer after the fascial release 1 cm off the midline. Jamshidi needles placed into the center of the pedicle will permit a flexible guidewire over which a cannulated tap and screw can be driven deep into the vertebral body. Lumbar screws are usually placed bilaterally at the same levels, while thoracic levels are staggered.

Corrective Maneuvers

Deformity correction begins with a provisional rod across the convex apical screws, as well as one growing screw above and below the apical fusion segment. The rod is pre-contoured to the correct sagittal profile, laid into the convex screws loosely to match the coronal deformity, and derotated. Two of the apical screws are tightened. Coronal benders are then used to push the apex toward the concavity; only then are the permanent rod lengths measured. The rods are roughly the same length, and at least 2 cm of additional length are added at each end to accommodate spinal growth. If the patient is large enough, 5.5 mm rods are used, but, if the patient is particularly small, 4.5 mm rods can be used (as in our case example). Based on high breakage rates in the senior author's experience, 3.5 mm rods are not suggested for Shilla use. Sagittal contours are applied with extra upper proximal thoracic kyphosis and relatively minimal lordosis at the lower end, to reduce screw pullout and junctional kyphosis. The permanent concave rod is then applied to the screw heads and rolled into proper sagittal position; the provisional rod can then be removed and the permanent convex rod placed.

The final corrective maneuver is apical derotation, with a counter-rotational force applied above and/or below the apex. Regardless of the derotation instrument/technique chosen, the two rods must be firmly held and prevented from rotating until a cross-link is applied distal to the apex to join the rods securely together, preventing spring back. Minor changes in rod alignment can be made with rod benders (Fig. 7.3).

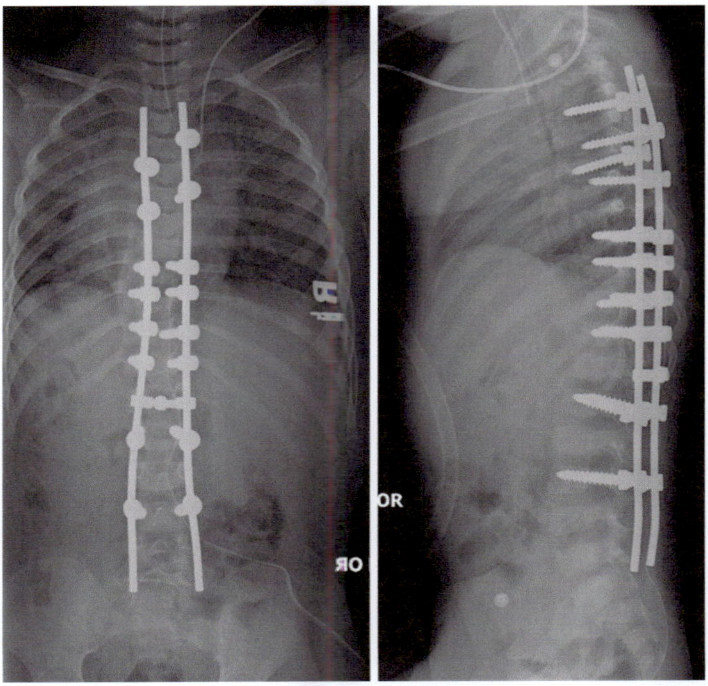

FIGURE 7.3 Supine AP and lateral radiographs immediately after index surgery

Clinical Course and Outcome

In our case, growth was evidenced at 1 year by the shortened distance between the end of the rod and the proximal screw. There was a slight tendency toward rotation of the apex (Fig. 7.4). At 2 years, more growth was evident. The rotation has stabilized. His improved clinical appearance has been maintained (Fig. 7.5). At 4-year postop, he was starting to grow off the rod at the top with slight implant prominence (Fig. 7.6).

At 5-year 2-month postop, coupled with a sizable weight gain, the 4.5 mm diameter rod on the left broke (Fig. 7.7). Both rods were replaced with 5.5 mm diameter rods, necessitating screw exchange to accommodate the larger rod. Any screws found with a loose bone-screw interface were replaced with larger diameter screws.

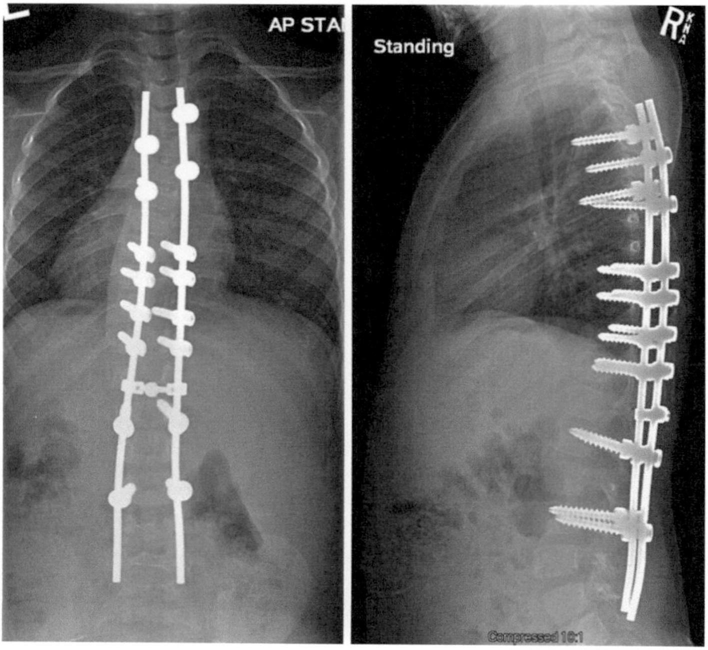

FIGURE 7.4 One year after surgery

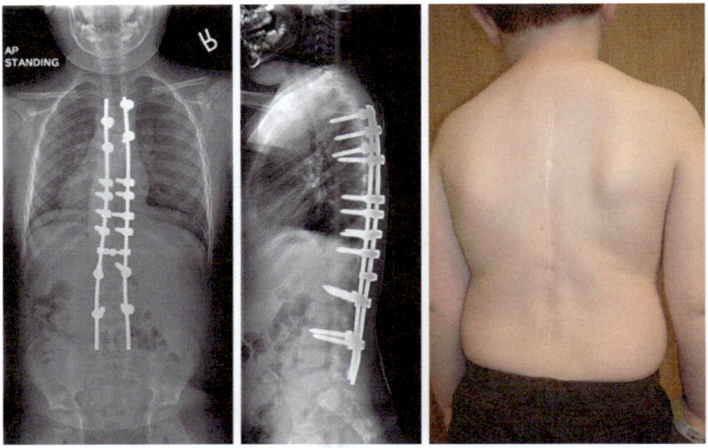

FIGURE 7.5 Two years after surgery

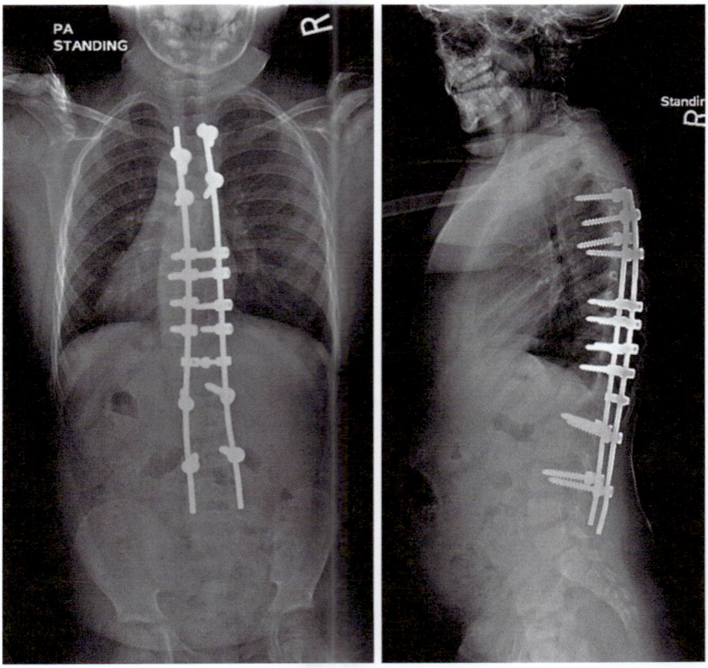

FIGURE 7.6 Four years after surgery

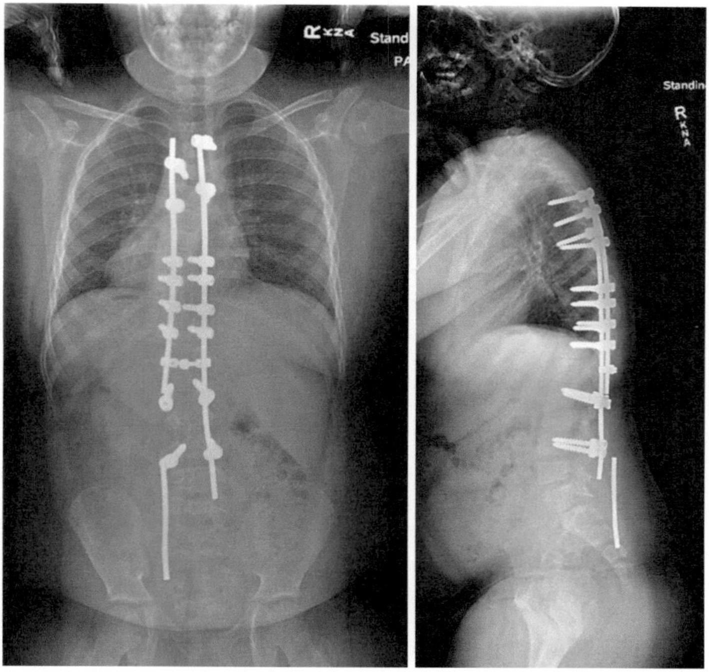

FIGURE 7.7 Five years after surgery with broken 4.5 mm rod

At 1 year post revision and 10½ years of age, he has excellent pulmonary function tests with a FVC of 96% and FEV1 of 97% (Fig. 7.8). He has remained actively involved in noncontact sports. He attends school and is developing a good sense of his potential as an adult having avoided repeated trips to the hospital. We expect to follow him through adolescence and remove his implants at maturity without further treatment.

Clinical Pearls and Pitfalls

- Careful selection of apical levels is crucial, based on upright and flexibility radiographs; apical screws should be placed bilaterally into three (moderate curve) or four (severe curve) apical vertebra.
- Use screw sizes that maximize length and diameter, for both apical and growing screws.

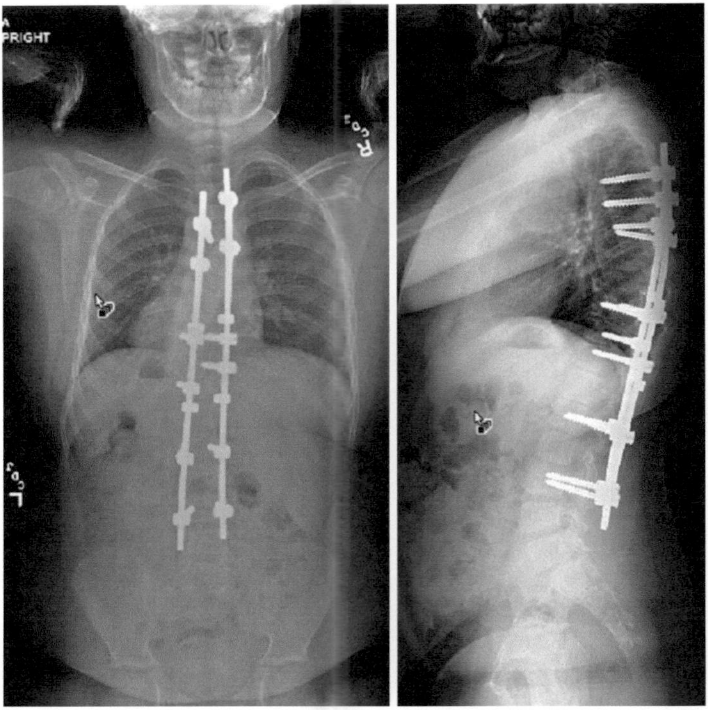

FIGURE 7.8 One year post revision for broken implant. Patient is now 10½ years of age

- Use fixed-head or monoaxial (unidirectional) screws at all apical levels.
- If navigation is used, then the registry antenna can be placed directly on a convex apical pedicle screw placed at the outset in freehand fashion (as these are typically the largest-diameter pedicles encountered in a Shilla case).
- Use of a convex provisional rod for initial coronal apical correction is very useful to bring the deformity under initial control and more accurately measure/contour the final rods.
- Add at least 2 cm of length onto each end of the rods to allow for growth.
- Use 4.5 mm rods in small children and 5.5 mm rods in larger children (>30 kg). Do not use 3.5 mm rods, as they will break early.

- Bend in significant kyphosis to the proximal portion of the rod, so that the rod is not exerting a posteriorly directed vector on the proximal screws that might dislodge them.
- Additional protection against proximal screw pullout can be achieved by passing a fiber wire tether in a sub-laminar fashion and tying this tether over the proximal rod/screw interface.
- Derotation of the apex should be performed with both Shilla rods in place, and then a cross-link secured distal to the apex prior to releasing the derotational force.
- A turtle-shell thoracolumbosacral brace should be used postoperatively for 3 months to minimize stress on implants during initial healing and fusion incorporation, particularly in ambulatory children.
- In the case of a rod breakage, replace both rods; if the patient is >30 kg, then convert rods from 4.5 to 5.5 mm at time of revision.

Literature Review and Discussion

Initial 2-year multicenter outcomes (38 patients) for the Shilla technique demonstrated that deformity was decreased from a mean of 71° preoperatively to 27° postoperatively, and that correction was well-maintained. Spinal height (C7–S1) increased at a mean of 12%, and space available for the lungs increased at a mean of 13% [3].

Single-center 5-year follow-up (40 patients) demonstrated continued curve control, with a mean curve magnitude of 38°. Spinal height increased at a mean of 80 mm over the 5-year study period, and mean space available for the lungs increased approximately at 30%. Six patients (15%) experienced wound infections, and three patients (8%) developed proximal junctional kyphosis. Eighteen patients had reached skeletal maturity, with 15 who were converted to definitive fusion and 3 who had implant removal with a well-maintained correction without definitive fusion [4].

A comparison of 19 Shilla and 6 distraction-based growing rod (GR) patients found equivalent outcomes for percent curve correction over a 4-year timeframe. T1–S1 growth and growth per month were similarly equivalent. The 19 Shilla patients underwent a total of 29 operations, in 63% of the patients. Conversely, the 6 GR patients underwent 40 reoperations, with 100% of these patients returning to surgery during the course of their treatment. Thus, there were, on average, 1.5 reoperations per Shilla patient and 6.7 reoperations per GR patient ($p = 0.0003$) [5].

In a matched multicenter analysis of 36 Shilla and 36 distraction-based GR patients, Andras et al. found that the GR patients had a greater mean deformity correction (36° vs. 23°, $p = 0.012$), and T1–S1 spinal height increased by 8.8 cm in the GR patients as compared to 6.4 cm in the Shilla patients ($p = 0.017$) [6]. However, the Shilla patients did have a notably fewer number of operative procedures, with a mean of 2.8 surgeries vs. 7.4 surgeries for the GR patients ($p < 0.001$). There was no difference in the overall complication rate between Shilla and GR patients. However, Luhmann et al. published a similar matched multicenter cohort study of 18 Shilla and 18 GR patients that did not demonstrate differences between treatment groups in curve correction and T1–T12 growth [7]. Shilla patients had threefold fewer operations than the GR patients. The difference between the Andras et al. study and the Luhmann et al. study was that the patients in the latter were followed until their definitive treatment, with 2 years of additional mean follow-up.

By every criterion established by the Scoliosis Research Society Growing Spine Committee for a successful treatment, this patient has realized those criteria [8]:

- Minimize spinal deformity.
- Maximize thoracic volume and function.
- Minimize fusion.
- Minimize complications, procedures, hospitalization, and burden to family.
- Consider overall development of the child.

By minimizing his trips to the hospital, clinic, and especially the operating room, he has been allowed the freedom from the burden of disease imposed on so many families with spinal deformity patients. He has been able to develop a sense of self and confidence separate from what could have been a life-shortening chronic disease.

References

1. McCarthy RE. The Shilla growth guidance technique. Oper Tech Orthop. 2016;26:268–72.
2. Morell SM, McCarthy RE. New developments in the treatment of early-onset spinal deformity: role of the Shilla growth guidance system. Med Devices. 2016;9:241–6.
3. McCarthy RE, Luhmann S, Lenke L, McCullough FL. The Shilla growth guidance technique for early-onset spinal deformities at 2-year follow-up: a preliminary report. J Pediatr Orthop. 2014;34(1):1–7.
4. McCarthy RE, McCullough FL. Shilla growth guidance for early-onset scoliosis: results after a minimum of five years of follow-up. J Bone Joint Surg Am. 2015;97:1578–84.
5. Luhmann SJ, McCarthy RE. A comparison of Shilla growth guidance system and growing rods in the treatment of spinal deformity in children less than 10 years of age. J Pediatr Orthop. 2016; 2017;37(8):e567–e574 [epub ahead of print].
6. Andras LM, Joiner ERA, McCarthy RE, McCullough FL, Luhmann SJ, Sponseller PD, et al. Growing rods versus Shilla growth guidance: better Cobb angle correction and T1-S1 length increase but more surgeries. Spine Deform. 2015;3:246–52.
7. Luhmann SJ, Smith JC, McClung A, McCullough FL, McCarthy RE, Thompson GH, et al. Radiographic outcomes of Shilla growth guidance system and traditional growing rods through definitive treatment. Spine Deform. 2017;5:277–82.
8. Scoliosis Research Society Growing Spine Committee. Early onset scoliosis Consens Statement June 2014. http://www.srs.org/about-srs/quality-and-safety/position-statements/early-onset-scoliosis-consensus-statement. Accessed 21 Aug 2017.

Chapter 8
Early Onset Scoliosis Treated with Magnetically Controlled Growing Rods

Ryan E. Fitzgerald, Kathleen D. Rickert, Behrooz A. Akbarnia, and Burt Yaszay

Case Presentation

History and Physical Examination

The patient was a 6-month-old male with a known diagnosis of Prader-Willi syndrome. He presented with a thoracolumbar curvature of 31°. On serial examination, the curvature was noted to be increasing in magnitude. Despite custom TLSO bracing, it continued to progress over a 2-year time interval to 78°. At 2 years and 7 months, he was treated with

R.E. Fitzgerald, MD • K.D. Rickert, MD • B.A. Akbarnia, MD (✉)
B. Yaszay, MD
Department of Orthopedic Surgery, Rady Children's Hospital and Health Center, San Diego, CA, USA

Department of Orthopedic Surgery, San Diego Center for Spinal Disorders, San Diego, CA, USA

Department of Orthopedic Surgery, University of California San Diego (UCSD), La Jolla, CA, USA
e-mail: rfitzgerald@rchsd.org; akbarnia@ucsd.edu; byaszay@rchsd.org

R. El-Hawary, C.P. Eberson (eds.), *Early Onset Scoliosis*,
https://doi.org/10.1007/978-3-319-71580-3_8

Risser casts which corrected his curvature to 41° in cast. After 6 months, he could not tolerate casting any longer. He then returned to bracing and had continued progression of his kyphoscoliosis until the age of 4.

At the time of preoperative evaluation, the patient was 4 years and 6 months of age, 102 cm, and 20.3 kg and had a BMI of 19.1 kg/m^2. On examination, he was hypotonic, developmentally delayed, nonverbal, and unable to ambulate. He had pronounced, fairly flexible thoracolumbar kyphosis, an asymmetric waist with a deep crease on the right, and a high left shoulder. Outside of his hypotonia and inability to cooperate with examination, he is otherwise neurovascularly intact.

Diagnostic Studies

Initial preoperative radiographic analysis prior to growing rod insertion demonstrated a left thoracolumbar curvature of 109° and kyphosis of 67° (Fig. 8.1). An MRI was completed with no evidence of spinal dysraphism. We typically do not encourage the use of MRI once the MCGR is implanted. Although studies of a 0.3 T MRI indicate that it may be possible, it is against manufacturer's recommendations due to concerns of a higher-strength MRI's effect on the rare earth magnets found within the MCGR [1].

Management Chosen

Surgical management for this patient was initiated prior to the availability of magnetically controlled growing rods in the United States. Secondary to his progression, lack of ability to tolerate more non-operative management, it was decided that his scoliosis would best be treated with "growth-friendly" spinal instrumentation. At the age of 4 years and 6 months, he had traditional spine-based growing rods inserted from T3–

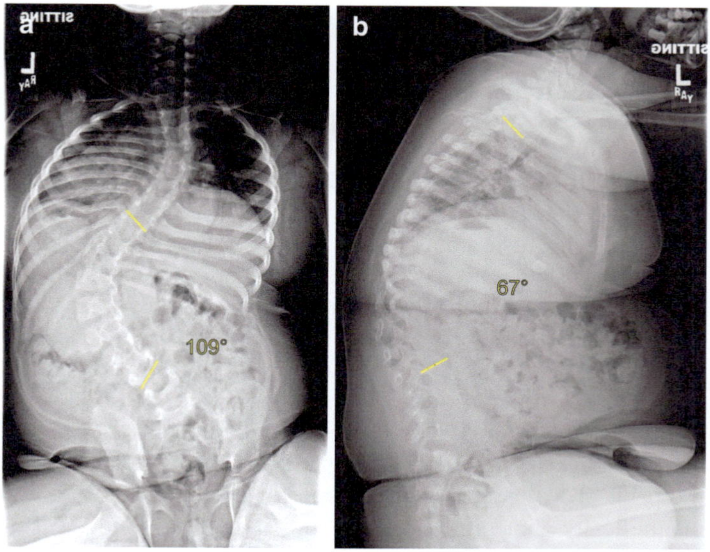

FIGURE 8.1 Preoperative posteroanterior (**a**) lateral (**b**) radiographs at 4 years and 6 months of age demonstrating progressive coronal left 109° thoracolumbar curve and 67° of kyphosis

T4 to L5–L6 (with six lumbar vertebrae). He subsequently underwent open distraction five times over 2.5 years with no subsequent complications.

Three years after placement of the original growth-friendly construct, the patient underwent conversion to magnetically controlled growing rods. This was 4 months after the implant's introduction to the United States. At the time of his conversion, the curvature was a 52° left thoracolumbar curve with 60° of kyphosis. The lead authors of this chapter believe that conversions are indicated in patients that still have potential for growth, in order to save subsequent surgeries and anesthetic events prior to final fusion. If the patient has reached or is close to maximum potential chest size and lung maturity, then we would recommend continuation of management with TGR until final fusion is recommended.

Surgical Procedure

The patient was placed prone on the Jackson table in the standard fashion. No traction was applied during the procedure. Using prior incisions, localized to the upper thoracic levels (T3–T4) and the lumbar levels (L5–L6 with six lumbar vertebrae), we exposed and removed the prior traditional growing rods. The prior fusion masses and instrumentation at the upper and lower instrumented segments were explored and found to be stable. The magnetically controlled growing rods were measured, cut, and contoured appropriately. We tested each rod's actuator individually prior to insertion to confirm their function. Of note, the contouring of the rods should be done prior to testing the actuator to be sure that the mechanism has not been damaged during contouring. The subfascial tunnels from the prior growing rods were utilized for placement of the new magnetically controlled growing rods into the previous fused proximal and distal level's pedicle instrumentation. New set screws were placed. Gentle distraction was placed distally across the base after the proximal set screws were tightened. We then tightened the distal set screws and completed final tightening. A proximal cross connector was applied between the rods. Final irrigation, topical vancomycin powder, and a standard closure were then completed. No complications occurred. Pre- and postoperative images are provided in (Fig. 8.2).

Some technical points about the abovementioned procedure should be noted. The MCGR should not be used in patients less than 2 years of age or less than 25 lbs. (11.4 kg). Rod selection should be based off of the patient's weight. Please consult the company's insert for this detailed information. With contouring each rod, it is crucial that no contour be placed through the actuator or within 10 mm of the actuator on either side. This translates to maintaining a 90 mm flat segment of MCGR for the 70 mm actuator or 110 mm for the 90 mm actuator. By doing so it may damage the mechanism by which the MCGR distracts. It is important to note that when using a dual rod construct, the actuators should be placed at the same height. We recommend that at least one cross connector be used between the rods either proximally or distally if there is poor bone quality or question of

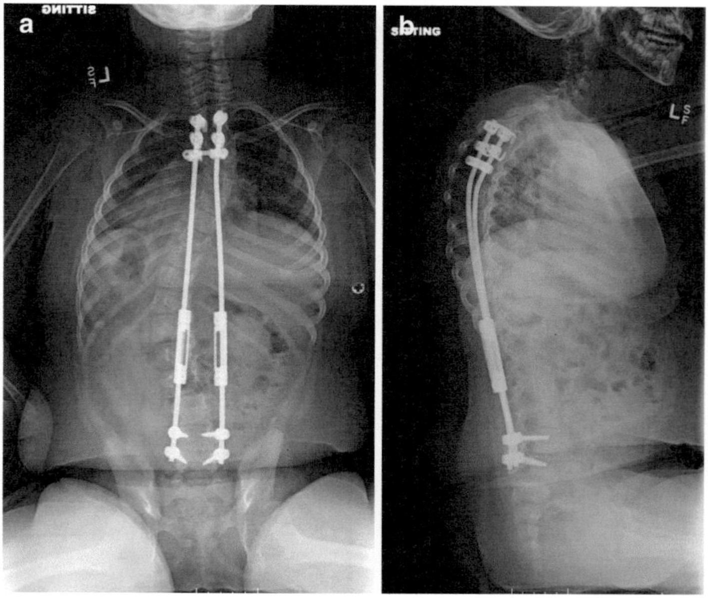

FIGURE 8.2 Preoperative and postoperative imaging of TGR to MCGR conversion shown respectively (**a–d**) with thoracolumbar curve of 52° with 60° of kyphosis prior to conversion and improved postoperative curvature of 40° with 50° of kyphosis

foundation strength. Cross connectors are added to these constructs to help add rigidity to an inherently less stable construct than traditional pedicle-based posterior spinal instrumented fusion. We recommend doing this at the upper foundation. It is important to not use cross connectors proximally and distally, as this will lock the device and not allow distraction.

Subsequent Steps

Over 3 years following the MCGR insertion, 12 lengthenings were completed. During each office-based distraction, we gained 1–2.5 mm of length with each rod. It should be noted that earlier lengthenings yielded greater results.

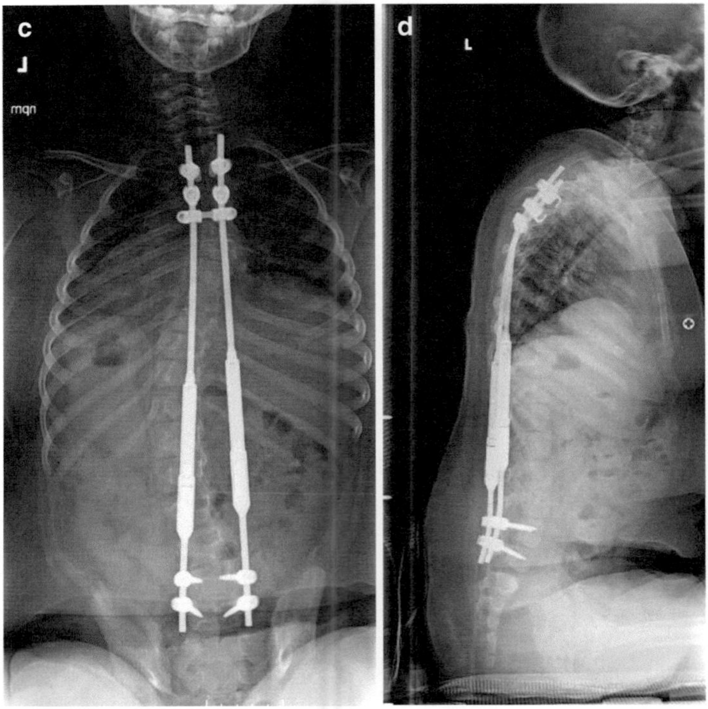

FIGURE 8.2 (continued)

During the lengthening visits, the magnetic portion of the MCGR is found by the use of ultrasound or a magnet locator. An electrically powered, motor driver called an external remote control (ERC) is held over the back with the patient prone on the exam table (Fig. 8.3). This position allows for maximum lengthening as it decreases the force required to lengthen the rod by removing the effect of gravity and weight of the upper thoracic cavity. If difficulties arise during lengthening, the first course of action is to reposition the patient. There are multiple positions that may allow for further lengthenings of the rod when other positions have failed. Some options to try include placing a pillow under the abdomen, traction, lateral decubitus position, or even sitting.

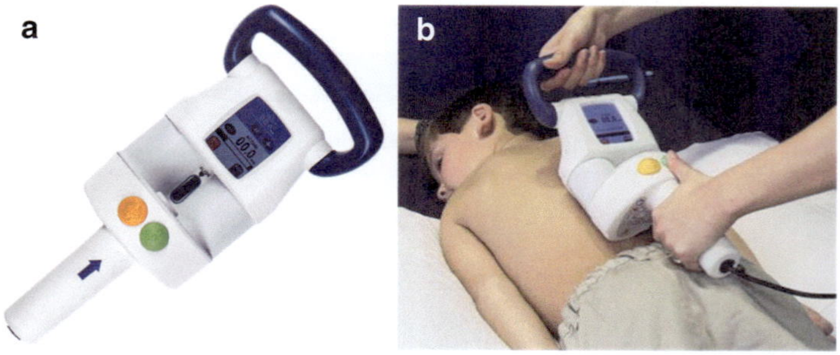

FIGURE 8.3 External remote control used to distract the MCGR (**a**) and an example of an external remote control being used on a patient (**b**)

If none of these techniques work, the surgeon may need to wait a few months to attempt lengthening again as there may not have been adequate spinal growth in the interim to allow for distraction of the MCGR. The ERC activates the magnet within the rods causing them to rotate and lengthen the rod. If the magnet and the ERC are not at the same level, the ERC will not be able to engage the actuator, and no lengthening will occur. Lengthenings can be scheduled as often as desired by the treating surgeon. We personally recommend lengthenings every 2–3 months. To determine the amount of lengthening per distraction, calculations based on Dimeglio's work should be performed. On average, T1–S1 increases 1 cm per year from the ages of 5–10 [2]. Then divide this by spinal segments included and the length of time between distractions. On average, this calculation ends up being 3 mm per lengthening if attempting lengthening in 3-month intervals. The preferred method for checking the magnet's length pre- and post-lengthening is with the use of ultrasound (Fig. 8.4) [3]. If ultrasound is not available or radiographic imaging is needed, we prefer the use of microdose EOS to reduce overall radiation to the patient. If EOS were to be used, we would recommend taking one image per clinic visit prior to lengthening. We then compare the images from the subsequent visit to measure the length gained from the prior visit. This also helps to minimize radiation exposure to the patient.

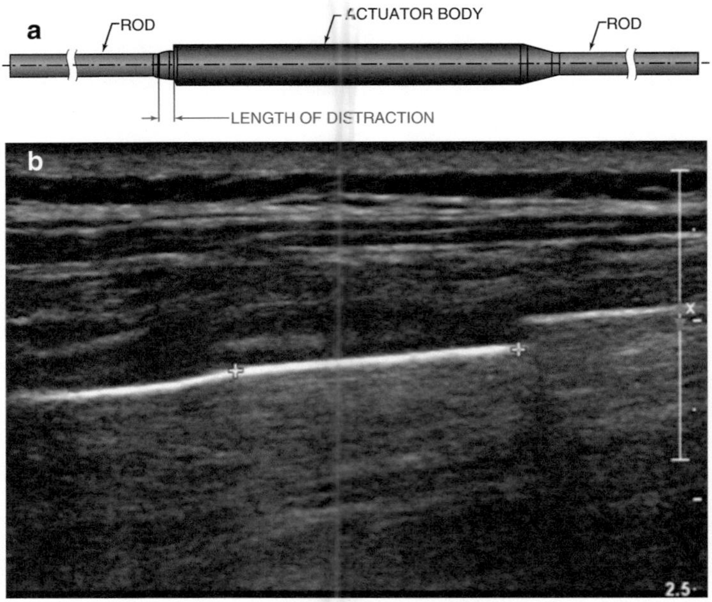

FIGURE 8.4 Representation of MCGR and the distractible segment (**a**) and an ultrasound image demonstrating measurement of the MCGR distractible segment after an office-based lengthening (**b**)

Clinical Course and Outcome

Our patient has had no complications and no further operative interventions since the conversion to magnetically controlled growing rods. The obvious benefits to this method include more frequent, smaller lengthenings without the risk, morbidity, and cost of surgery. At last follow-up, the patient had a 30° curve from T10 to L2 and 46° of kyphosis from T2 to T7. Of note, the majority of the kyphosis is in the proximal portion of the construct. The T1–T12 and T1–S1 height gained from initial growing rod insertion to final magnetically controlled growing rod length was 5.6 and 11.9 cm, respectively. Please reference Table 8.1 for measurements completed at significant treatment intervals. During the last

TABLE 8.1 Cobb and spinal length measurements during treatment.

Event	Initial	Pre-TGR[a]	Pre-MCGR[b]	Post-MCGR[b]	Most recent
Age	6 m	4y + 6 m	7y + 2 m	7y + 3 m	9y + 1 m
Cobb angle	31°	109°	52°	40°	30°
Kyphosis (max)	[c]	67°[d]	60°[d]	50°[d]	46°[e]
T1–T12	112.5 mm	147.8 mm	172.4 mm	192.8 mm	204.3 mm
T1–S1	192.2 mm	252.9 mm	309.2 mm	335.6 mm	372.4 mm

[a]*TGR* traditional growing rods
[b]*MCGR* magnetically controlled growing rods
[c]Supine film
[d]Seated film
[e]Standing film

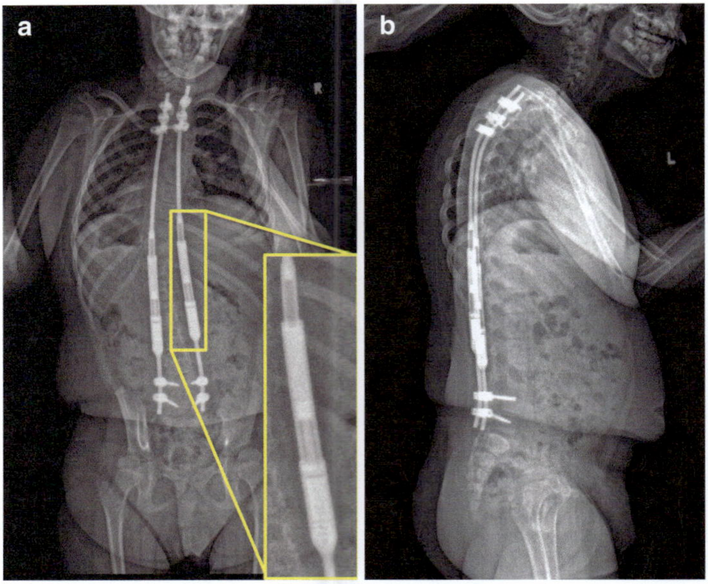

FIGURE 8.5 Latest follow-up, posteroanterior (**a**) lateral (**b**) radiographs with the magnified image showing the actuator demonstrating correction of the left thoracolumbar curve to 30° with 46° of kyphosis

3 years, there has been an increase in the axial rotation around the magnetically controlled growing rods as can be seen in Fig. 8.5. We are nearing the age of final fusion, which is typically after the age of 10 at our institution.

Clinical Pearls and Pitfalls

- This technique should be used in young patients with increasing deformity, who have significant chest and lung development remaining.
- Magnetically controlled growing rods are able to maintain deformity correction and be growth friendly through a noninvasive method.
- Noninvasive lengthening procedures have decreased complication rates, avoidance of anesthetic events, and decreased overall cost, despite the up-front cost of implants.

- Office-based lengthening helps the patient and family to avoid social stigma to decrease the pressures of missed school and work days and overall helps the patient from a psychological standpoint.
- It is unclear if magnetically controlled growing rods will be subject to diminishing returns as seen with traditional spine-based growing rods.
- There is a risk of high radiation exposure through serial imaging with this treatment as treatment intervals are typically shorter than traditional growing rods.
- By using ultrasound technology to measure the magnet pre- and post-lengthening, the surgeon can monitor the distraction while minimizing the radiation risk.

Literature Review and Discussion

Early onset scoliosis is a challenge for both the patient and treating surgeon. The greatest issue is managing the magnitude of curvature, while attempting to allow the thoracic cavity and therefore pulmonary system to develop and grow [4]. This technique is one that should be considered in EOS patients younger than 10 years of age, with significant growth remaining and curve progression despite conservative measures. Extensive exposure, instrumentation, and fusion of the spine at this young age would result in a short trunk, decreased thoracic growth, and pulmonary insufficiency [5, 6]. Significantly reduced pulmonary function has been shown in comparison to a normal age-matched cohort, for patients that undergo posterior spinal fusion prior to the age of 9. Patients with fusion prior to this age had an average FVC of <60% of their age-matched cohort. The reason for this dramatic difference is that the alveolar number per terminal lung unit increases from approximately 1370 at 22 months of age to 2630 alveoli by age 10 [7]. It has been shown that a thoracic height, which can be correlated to lung maturity, of 18 cm is required to avoid severe respiratory insufficiency [8]. For this reason, it is recommended to strive for a thoracic height (T1–T12) of 22 cm. When this thoracic height is achieved, it is reasonable to proceed to final spinal fusion.

Multiple treatment strategies have been developed for this disease process. Harrington described attempting to preserve growth with internal fixation without fusion through subperiosteal dissection with rod placement against the bony posterior spinal elements. Moe described the first subcutaneous Harrington rod placement technique to control severe curves in young patients [9–11]. Since that time these techniques have been refined. TGR, Shilla, VEPTR, and now MCGR have been created as an attempt to improve growth preservation, curve control, and lung development and decrease complications [12].

The MCGR was created and initially marketed in Europe in October of 2009. By 2014, when the FDA approved the use of MCGR, it had been used in more than 500 patients in 20 countries worldwide [13]. In most published reports, it has shown favorable results with much less morbidity than traditional growing rod techniques. In 2014, Akbarnia et al. compared 12 matched patients who were treated with TGR (follow-up of 4.1 years) to 12 patients treated with the MCGR technique (follow-up of 2.5 years). There were 57 fewer operative procedures in the MCGR group, which is an average of 4.75 fewer procedures per patient [14]. Due to the replacement of surgical lengthenings with office-based lengthenings, it appears that surgical complications such as infection (3.7% vs. 11.1%), anesthetic complications, blood loss, and wound complications are all decreased with MCGR [15]. Despite this, the MGCR patient population is still at risk of infection, rod breakage, implant pullout, prominent implants, or junctional kyphosis inherent in patients with growth-friendly treatment [16–18]. One article found that all patients with single rod constructs required revision procedures and therefore concluded that these constructs should not be used [16]. Inaparthy et al. looked at a cohort of 21 patients with MCGR and showed the incidence of PJK (>10° increase of kyphosis) to be 28.6% at final follow-up of 33 months [17].

Aside from the diminished surgical complications and number of subsequent procedures, there are many other benefits that must be considered when discussing MCGR vs. TGR constructs. The most significant from a patient perspective is most likely psychosocial in nature [19]. With less surgery looming in the near future, there are significantly less psychosocial stressors, including decreased time out of school for the patient and time out of work for the parents. It can be psychologically difficult to be away from social networks and support as well as financially detrimental for the entire family unit. When taking all of these variables into consideration, it is apparent that having frequent surgery decreases quality of life.

Finally, treating surgeons need to evaluate and keep in mind the cost to the healthcare system. In a study by The National Institute for Health and Care Excellence in the United Kingdom, a cost analysis was completed. This research showed that after 6 years of treatment with MCGR vs. TGR, that overall cost savings per patient is around £12,000 (~$15,000) for patients treated with MCGR [20]. Since the United Kingdom is a socialized healthcare system, there may be doubts as to its applicability to a U.S. market. Polly et al. looked further into this issue in 2016 by constructing an economic model of cumulative costs of MCGR vs. TGR. They concluded that cost offsets accrue over time and that in order to achieve cost neutrality, the patient needs to be treated for 6 years [21]. In either model, it appears that the up-front cost of MCGR should not be a hindrance to its use, as it is at least economically neutral in the long term.

Early onset scoliosis is a difficult problem that has many potential treatment modalities. Magnetically controlled growing rods are a recent technological advancement and appear to have a promising future in the care for these complex patients. Deformity control, while permitting continued growth of the spine, is the goal of treating this disease process. With current short-term follow-up, MCGR has demonstrated that it can accomplish these goals without requiring serial operative procedures [10, 22–26].

References

1. Eroglu M, Demikiran G, Kocyigit IA, et al. Magnetic resonance imaging safety of magnetically controlled growing rods in an in vivo animal model. Spine. 2017;42(9):e504–8.
2. Canavese F, Dimeglio A. Normal and abnormal spine and thoracic cage development. World J Orthop. 2013;4(4):167–74.

3. Yoon WW, Chang AC, Tyler P, et al. The use of ultrasound in comparison to radiography in magnetically controlled growth rod lengthening measurement: a prospective study. Eur Spine J. 2015;24(7):1422–6.
4. Dimeglio A. Growth of the spine before age 5 years. J Pediatr Orthop. 1993;1(B):102–7.
5. Kesling KL, Lonstein JE, Dennis F, et al. The crankshaft phenomenon after posterior spinal arthrodesis for congenital scoliosis: a review of 54 patients. Spine. 2003;28:267–71.
6. Winter RB, Moe JH. The results of spinal arthrodesis for congenital spinal deformity in patients younger than five years old. J Bone Joint Surg Am. 1982;64:419–32.
7. Emery JL, Mithal A. The number of alveoli in the terminal respiratory unit of man during late intrauterine life and childhood. Arch Dis Child. 1960;35(184):544–7.
8. Karol LA, Johnston C, Mladenov K, et al. Pulmonary function following early thoracic fusion in non-neuromuscular scoliosis. J Bone Joint Surg Am. 2008;90:1272–81.
9. Akbarnia BA, Cheung K, Noordeen H, et al. Next generation of growth-sparing techniques. Spine. 2013;38(8):665–70.
10. Moe JH, Kharrat K, Winter RB, et al. Harrington instrumentation without fusion plus external orthotic support for the treatment of difficult curvature problems in young children. Clin Orthop Relat Res. 1984;185:35–45.
11. La Rosa G, Oggiano L, Ruzzini L. Magnetically controlled growing rods for the management of early-onset scoliosis: A preliminary report. J Pediatr Orthop. 2017;37(2):79–85.
12. Akbarnia BA, Marks DS, Boachie-Adjei O, et al. Dual growing rod technique for the treatment of progressive early-onset scoliosis: a multicenter study. Spine. 2005;30:S46–57.
13. Akbarnia B. Magnetically controlled growing rods (MCGR) for the treatment of progressive early-onset scoliosis (EOS). Spineuniverse Case Study Library. 2013. http://www.spineuniverse.com/professional/case-studies Accessed 21 Feb 2017.
14. Akbarnia BA, Pawelek JB, Cheung K, et al. Traditional growing rods versus magnetically controlled growing rods for the surgical treatment of early-onset scoliosis: a case-matched 2-year study. Spine Deform. 2014;2(6):493–7.
15. Choi E, Yaszay B, Mundis G et al. Implant complications after magnetically controlled growing rods for early onset scoliosis: a multicenter retrospective review. J Pediatr Orthop. (epub). 2016.

16. Teoh KH, Winson D, James S, et al. Magnetic controlled growing rods for early onset scoliosis: a 4-year follow up. Spine J. 2016;16(4):S34–9.
17. Inaparthy P, Queruz JC, Bhagawati D, et al. Incidence of proximal junctional kyphosis with magnetic expansion control rods in early onset scoliosis. Eur Spine J. 2016;25(10):3308–15.
18. Bess S, Akbarnia BA, Thompson GH, et al. Complications of growing-rod treatment for early-onset scoliosis: analysis of one hundred and forty patients. J Bone Joint Surg Am. 2010;92:2533–43.
19. Thompson W, Thakar C, Rolton DJ. The use of magnetically-controlled growing rods to treat children with early-onset scoliosis: early radiological results in 19 children. Bone Joint J. 2016;98-B(9):1240–7.
20. Jenks M, Craig J, Higgins J, et al. The MAGEC system for spinal lengthening in children with scoliosis: a NICE Medical Technology Guidance. Appl Health Econ Health Policy. 2014;12(6):587–99.
21. Polly DW, Ackerman SJ, Schneider K, et al. Cost analysis of magnetically controlled growing rods compared with traditional growing rods for early-onset scoliosis in the US: an integrated health care delivery system perspective. Clinicoecon Outcomes Res. 2016;8:457–65.
22. Hickey BA, Towriss C, Baxter G, et al. Early experience of MAGEC magnetic growing rods in the treatment of early onset scoliosis. Eur Spine J. 2014;23(S1):61–5.
23. Rolton D, Thakar C, Wilson-Macdonald J, Nnadi C. Radiological and clinical assessment of the distraction achieved with remotely expandable growing rods in early onset scoliosis. Eur Spine J. 2015;25(10):3371–6.
24. Cheung J, Cahill P, Yaszay B, et al. Special article: update on the magnetically controlled growing rod: tips and pitfalls. J Orthop Surg. 2015;23(3):383–90.
25. Cheung K, Man-Chee K, Pui-Yin Cheung J, et al. Magnetically controlled growing rods for severe spinal curvature in young children: a prospective case series. Lancet. 2012;379(9830):1967–74.
26. Lebon J, Batailler C, Wargny M, et al. Magnetically controlled growing rod in early onset scoliosis: a 30-case multicenter study. Eur Spine J. 2016. https://doi.org/10.1007/s00586-016-4929-y.

Chapter 9
Modern Trolley Growth Guidance for Early Onset Scoliosis

Jean A. Ouellet and Catherine E. Ferland

Case Presentation

History and Physical Examination

A 5-year-old boy presented with his parents to the outpatient scoliosis clinic for evaluation of his spinal deformity. The parents had noted that over the last 2 years, they were having more and more difficulties keeping him upright in his stroller and his wheelchair. Patient was known to have a severe axonal neuropathy that had led to his progressive neuromuscular scoliosis. His past medical history was unremarkable during the prenatal period, uncomplicated birth history, though it was noted to be quite hypotonic at birth. Patient has had recurrent pneumonia since birth thought to be secondary to poor cough. A series of investigations, including muscle and nerve biopsy, were inconclusive with an ill-defined diagnosis

J.A. Ouellet, MD (✉) • C.E. Ferland, PhD
Department of Paediatric Surgery, McGill University Health Centre and Shriners Hospital, Montreal, QC, Canada

Department of Anesthesiology, McGill University Health Centre and Shriners Hospital, Montreal, QC, Canada
e-mail: jaouellet@hotmail.com

R. El-Hawary, C.P. Eberson (eds.), *Early Onset Scoliosis*,
https://doi.org/10.1007/978-3-319-71580-3_9

of diffuse axonal neuropathy that appeared to be nonprogressive. At baseline, the patient had a mild developmental delay and was able to crawl in the house, although he required a wheelchair to mobilize outside for any long distance. Patient had no prior orthopedic issues and has never had any prior surgeries.

Physical exam did not reveal any dysmorphic features. The patient was sitting with an obvious pelvic obliquity and a global kyphoscoliosis and fairly good head control. Reflexes were diminished both in the upper and lower extremities. Neither clonus nor any Babinski could be elicited. Patient was small for stated age with a low body mass.

Lower extremity exam did not reveal any contractures and had voluntary motor function of both upper and lower extremities with diminished tone and strength throughout. Sensation appeared to be intact.

Diagnostic Studies

Serial radiographs revealed a progressive collapsing kyphoscoliosis (Figure 9.1). Preoperative imaging including the supine bending films revealed a flexible left thoracolumbar curve measuring 75° able to be reduced to 35° on bending films with leveling of the pelvis (Figure 9.2).

Management Chosen

In light of his poor respiratory status, the patient's family wished to avoid repetitive general anesthetics required for repetitive surgical interventions. After discussing different options with the family, it was decided to proceed with a growth guidance spine-based construct in keeping with modern Luque trolley concepts. The concept of self-growing rods by using VEPTR rods (DePuy Synthes, Raynham, MA) is an off-label technique. One intentionally does not place the locking clips, which allows for expansion of the telescopic rods as the spine grows. The added benefits of using this

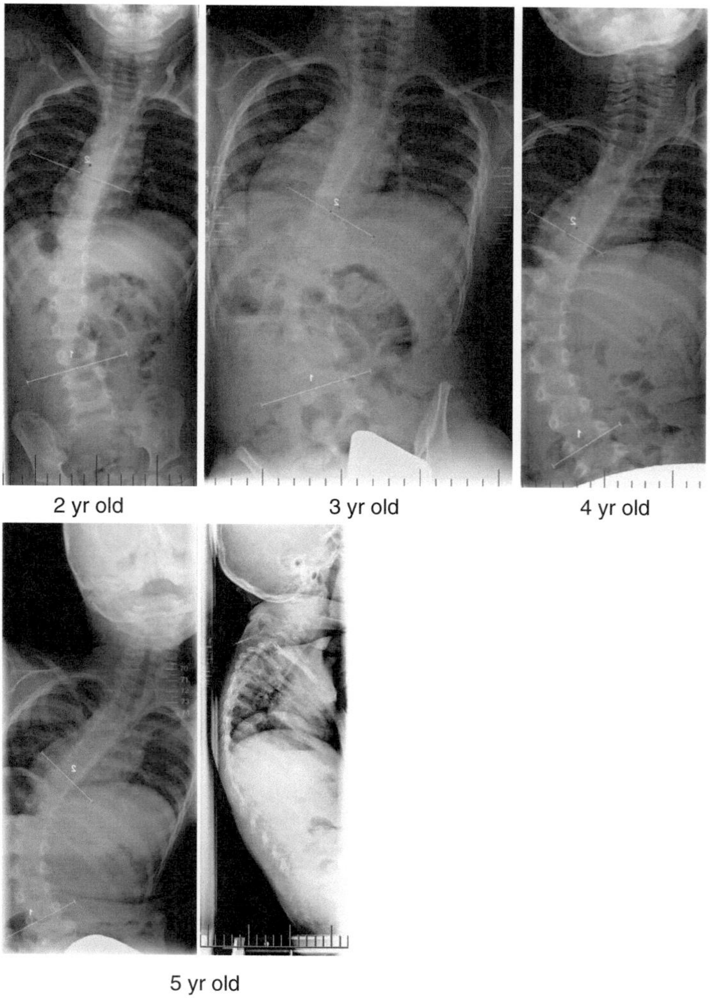

FIGURE 9.1 Serial X-rays from the age of 2–5 years of age illustrating that despite bracing, this child developed a progressive collapsing kyphoscoliotic deformity

implant are that it is extremely robust and also confers some anti-rotational stability because the I-beam design of the VEPTR minimizes rotation.

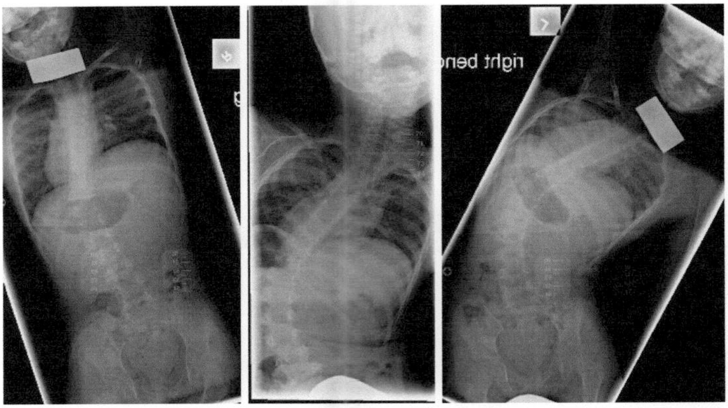

FIGURE 9.2 Preoperative radiographs illustrate a flexible left thoracolumbar curve

Surgical Procedure

The patient, under a general anesthetic on a radiolucent table with appropriate bolsters, was prepared and draped in a sterile fashion exposing the entire spine. Using intraoperative fluoroscopy, the location of the fixed proximal and distal anchor points were marked on the skin (Figure 9.3a, b). The pedicles of the apical vertebra, as well as all planned location of gliding anchors, should be identified by fluoroscopy to minimize surgical exposure. Using a midline incision, a classic subperiosteal dissection was performed to insert bilateral pedicle screws into T3 and T4 proximally and into L4 and L5 distally (Figure 9.3c, d). These segments were decorticated, and a formal interlaminar and intra-articular fusion was undertaken. Great care was taken to ensure that each fixed angle screw was perfectly placed both in the sagittal and coronal plan to facilitate rod coupling. In addition, pedicle screw diameter is carefully chosen to fill the lumen of the pedicle to optimize immediate fixation (Figure 9.3d).

Once the proximal and distal fixed anchors were placed, we turned our attention to capturing the apical vertebra. For the gliding anchors, preoperative planning and execution are crucial. Incisions must be planned to ensure that no incision lies directly over any spinal implant. Location and density of

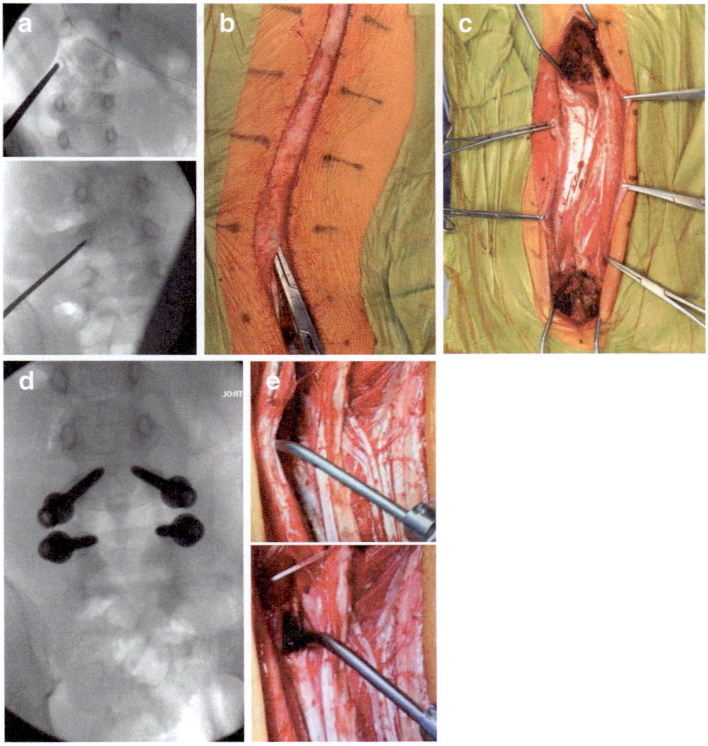

FIGURE 9.3 Using fluoroscopy, (**a**) Location of the fixed distal and proximal anchor points are marked on the skin. (**b**) A midline skin incision is made along the entire planned instrumented spine. (**c**) Subperiosteal dissection is performed at the proximal and distal fixation. (**d**) Proximal and distal fixed anchors must be perfectly placed. If pedicle screws are used, they should fill the lumen of the pedicle and should have some convergence of the screw to add purchase. (**e**) A Wiltse type approach is performed to ensure a thick layer of muscle and fascia over the gliding anchors without exposing the bone

gliding anchors are dictated by the type and the severity of the deformity. Considering this deformity was very flexible, we choose to only capture the apical vertebra at T12. The overall number of vertebra to be captured by gliding anchors is related to the rigidity of the curve. Flexible curve requires little gliding anchors, while slightly more stiff curves should have greater gliding anchors. Care must be taken not to insert too many gliding anchors as the risk of spontaneous fusion increases. The incision was made directly over the spinous process of T12, thus avoiding the risk that an implant be located below the incision. Once the skin was incised, the fascia was open along the midline and an oblique transmuscular dissection was taken down toward the transverse process on the convexity of the curve. This left a good cuff of muscle and fascia above the planned implant, still ensuring that there is still a layer of the paravertebral muscles and periosteum covering the lamina to avoid spontaneous fusions (Figure 9.3e).

Specific to this case, we used a "post" technique that allowed us to cantilever the apical vertebra across midline which maximizes correction. This was possible by placing a pedicle screw on the convexity of the apical vertebra. This post is a standard non-articulated pedicle screw that is *not* connected to the rod but acts as a fulcrum for the rod to reduce the deformity. The convex VEPTR rod is attached to the proximal anchor points, tunnelled in a transmuscular fashion, and is then translated to align with the distal anchor points. The "post", acting as a fulcrum, translates the apex and corrects the deformity. One must take advantage of the kyphotic sagittal shape of the rod to facilitate capturing the apex. By rotating the rod in the appropriate sagittal orientation, the coronal deformity is corrected as the distal end of the rod is cantilevered and connected to the distal anchors.

After the convex rod was inserted, the concave rod was inserted and an apical sublaminar wire was tensioned in order to achieve additional correction. Of note, in an effort to avoid spontaneous fusion, this sublaminar wire was inserted by performing two small laminotomies in T11 and L1 while avoiding taking down the interlaminar ligament.

Wounds were thoroughly irrigated, and meticulous facial closure above the implants was done taking care not to injure the soft-tissue envelope covering the implants.

Clinical Course and Outcome

This patient has had only one surgical procedure at 5 years of age and has been followed every sixth month for the last

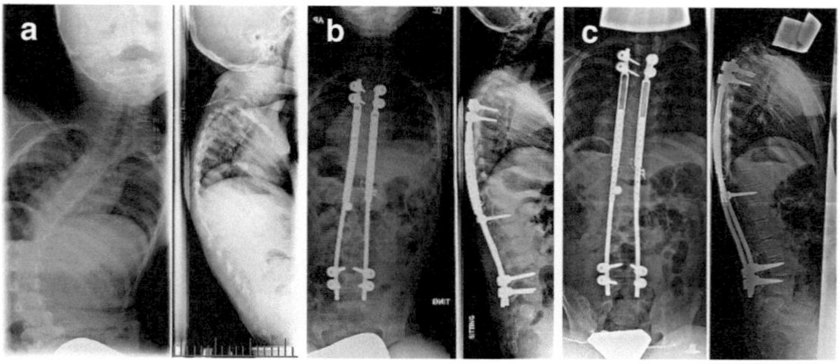

FIGURE 9.4 (**a**) Preoperative AP/Lat X-ray at the age of 5 years. (**b**) Immediate postoperative X-ray illustrates the power of the "post" cantilever reduction technique. (**c**) Postoperative X-ray at the age of 11 years without the need for any lengthening or any revision surgery. Curve remains controlled, and the spine has grown 5 cm across the instrumented spine as illustrated by the space now seen in the female VEPTR chamber

6 years. Immediate postoperative X-rays confirm almost complete resolution of his scoliotic deformity with maximal apical translation. The subsequent imaging illustrates that without any distraction or revision surgeries, the VEPTR has expanded while maintaining the scoliotic deformity to a minimum (Figure 9.4). This patient has achieved 95% of his expected growth with no revision surgeries, no complications, and complete control of his spinal deformity. At last follow-up, a 10° left -sided curve from T1 to L5 remains with no residual pelvic obliquity. T1–S1 height gained from pre-initial surgery to final follow-up was 8 cm, with 5 cm gained across the instrumented spine from initial postop to final follow-up.

Clinical Pearls and Pitfalls

- Patient selection is crucial to have a predictable outcome with modern Luque trolley constructs.
- Patients with hypotonic collapsing spinal deformities are ideal candidates for modern Luque trolley technique.
- Flexible curves and apical translation are crucial to have good outcome. Capturing and controlling the apex is essential.

- Meticulous preoperative planning and execution is key to avoid complications in this patient population.
- If the apex is not repositioned to midline, curve progression will occur and expected spinal growth will be less.
- By avoiding repetitive lengthening procedures, the overall complication rates are lower.

Literature Review and Discussion

Eduardo Luque described the first self-growing rod construct in 1977 [1] followed by Moe in 1984 [2]. They used segmental sublaminar wires and U- or L-shaped rods to treat young patients (<11 years) that had severe scoliosis that did not respond to bracing. The Luque trolley was described as a rigid internal brace that would allow the spine to grow along the rods as the spine was instrumented but not fused. Luque published his early results showing that the technique had good corrective power decreasing average scoliosis from 72° to 22° while still allowing on average 2.5 cm growth over 2 years [1]. Subsequent long-term results showed poor maintenance of spinal growth (range, 32–49% of expected growth) [3, 4], high spontaneous fusion (range, 4–100%) [3], and a high implant failure rate of 32% [5]. In 1999, Pratt et al. published a 5-year follow-up retrospective study looking at 26 patients with a diagnosis of EOS treated with Luque trolleys where 18 had anterior apical epiphysiodesis in addition to the posterior segmental growth guidance technique. They concluded that the Luque trolley prevented curve progression (from 48° to 25° to a final scoliosis of 43°). They also showed that the Luque trolley allowed for 50% of expected growth if the epiphysiodesis was not done. The addition of the anterior epiphysiodesis improved curve control by decreasing the average preop scoliosis from 65° to 26° to a final scoliosis of 32°; however, the apical hemiepiphysiodes had worse growth potential with an average of 32% of expected growth [5]. Complications remained high mainly secondary to implant failures. The authors concluded that there was a need for improved instrumentation and for new surgical measures to allow better spinal growth and curve control. Patients who did poorly with the classic Luque trolley were those with large rigid curves preoperatively and/or patients who had large residual postoperative curves.

In 2011, Ouellet and et al. published a small series of five patients with EOS treated with a modern version of the Luque trolley that had been followed for 4.5 years. They described a new surgical technique that instrumented the apex of the deformity via minimal invasive muscle sparing exposure coupled with solid proximal and distal anchors [6]. In contrast to the original Luque trolley, where every level was captured with a sublaminar wire and bound to the rod (Figure 9.6a), the new approach used modern spinal implants (pedicle screws) for solid proximal and distal fixed spinal anchors. They used off label modern spinal implants to allow for gliding anchors. For example, using pedicle screws designed for a 6 mm rod were used with a 5 mm rod allowing for motion. At the apex, these mismatched oversized pedicle screws or sublaminar wires allow the rods to glide across the apex (Figure 9.6b). Off-label use of the VEPTR, as illustrated in Figure 9.4, was also used (Figure 9.6c). With a mean follow-up of 4.5 years, the scoliotic deformity on average was decreased from 61° (range, 38–94°) to a mean of 21° (range, 10–33°) with gradual increase back to 35° at the last follow-up. During the same interval, the spine grew on average 67% (range, 26–91%) of expected growth [6]. This small case series demonstrated that self-lengthening growth guidance systems could indeed be successful in reducing the overall number of surgical procedures and to prevent progression of spinal deformity, while maintaining spinal growth. We recently reviewed an additional ten patients with self-growing constructs and found similar results with an average scoliosis reduction of 50% at an average 4-year follow-up. Patients' spines grew on average 63% of the calculated growth and were found to be inversely proportional to the residual post-operative Cobb angle (Pearson's R score of −0.546; $p = 0.035$). Residual Cobb angle less than 25° had close to normal expected spinal growth and had the least amount of correction loss (Table 9.1).

Self-growing rod constructs can vary significantly depending on the type and rigidity of curve. In general, we recommend that a greater number of gliding anchors are used above and below the apex for large deformities. However; if there are too many anchors used, there is a greater risk of spontaneous fusion. For such large and rigid deformities, then classic dual growing rods requiring active distraction may be more appropriate [7, 8]. One can use off-label modern spinal implants to achieve gliding construct as the case we illustrated (Figure 9.4) or use specific implants that have been developed to allow for gliding anchors. Medtronic (Medtronic, Memphis, TN) has obtained FDA approval for its Shilla screws, while DePuy Synthes (Raynham, MA) has an EU mark for the trolley gliding vehicle (TGV) (Figure 9.5). Via the Health Canada's Special Access Program, trolley gliding vehicles are available in Canada. The advantage of using such pedicle-based gliding anchor is its low-profile rod capturing mechanism. To avoid spontaneous spinal fusion, it is critical to keep the rods away from the lamina; hence the gliding screws must be left proud. However, the screw heads must not be prominent as patients with EOS often have little muscle mass and subcutaneous tissue. In addition, the system has been developed with the intent to have the least

FIGURE 9.5 (**a**) Five-year-old girl with Prader-Willi that failed conservative treatment for her progressing 50° neuromuscular scoliosis. (**b**) New gliding implant: trolley gliding vehicle. It is a pedicle screw with a PEEK cable tie and a ultrahigh-molecular-weight polyethylene liner that captures the rods. (**c**) Transmuscular insertion of the trolley gliding anchors. (**d**) Intraoperative photograph of the final construct with the proximal and distal fixed anchors at T3/4 and L3/4 and gliding anchors at T7,10, and 12. (**e**) Intraoperative X-ray showing the three gliding anchors capturing the apex of the deformity. (**f**) Postoperative X-rays 2 years after surgery, no revision nor lengthening surgery. The spine has grown 1.5 cm across the 10 instrumented vertebra representing 100% of expected growth based on Dimeglio calculation (2 year × 10 vertebral × 0.7 mm = 14 mm)

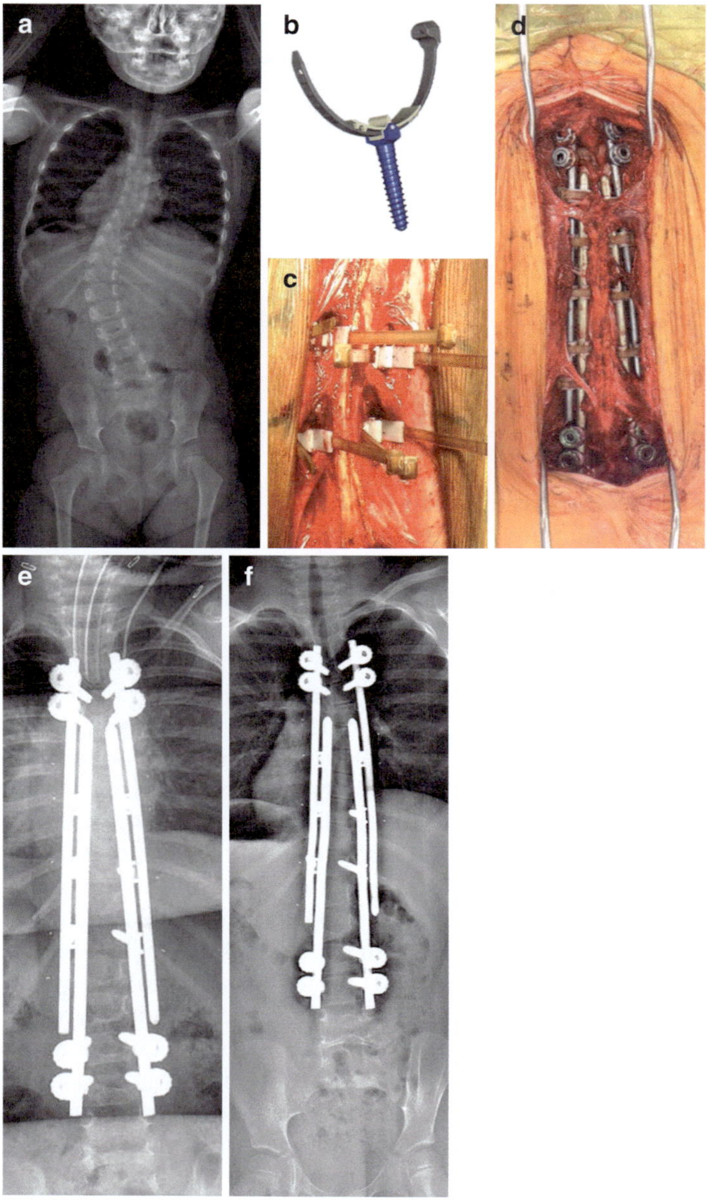
a
b
c
d
e
f

TABLE 9.1 Instrumented spinal height gain in cm per year of follow-up

Group	PO Cobb range	Mean (cm)	*N*	Std. deviation	Minimum (cm)	Maximum (cm)
1	≤15	2.41	2	2.34	0.76	4.06
2	15.1–25.0	1.44	4	0.61	0.62	2.08
3	25.1–35.0	0.51	6	0.29	0.03	0.91
4	35.1–45	0.47	1	NA	0.47	0.47
5	>45	0.27	2	0.38	0.00	0.53
	Total	0.98	15	1.02	0.00	4.06

resistance across the gliding parts. The rods have been highly polished and are captured by a lined polyetheretherketone (Peek) cable tie with ultrahigh molecular weight polyethylene (UhmwPE). Both systems have been tested in animals showing the systems grow with little to no local inflammatory response [9, 10].

Granted that both the Shilla and the modern Luque trolley are guided growth techniques, they are technically as well as conceptually different. The Shilla-guided growth system is based on a two-rod construct with apical fusions while having the end vertebrae grow away from the apex. In contrast, classic modern Luque trolley relies on solid proximal and distal anchors (similar to those used with traditional spine-based growing rods) with intercalated apical gliding anchors translating the apex back to midline with a four-rod construct (Fig 9.6d). Long-term clinical follow-up remains sparse on either constructs; however guided growth surgery remains an attractive option for specific patients with early onset scoliosis. Skeletally immature patients (younger than 10 years old with open triradiate cartilage) with collapsing progressive flexible scoliosis who are unable to tolerate repetitive anesthesia are ideal candidate for the modern Luque trolley.

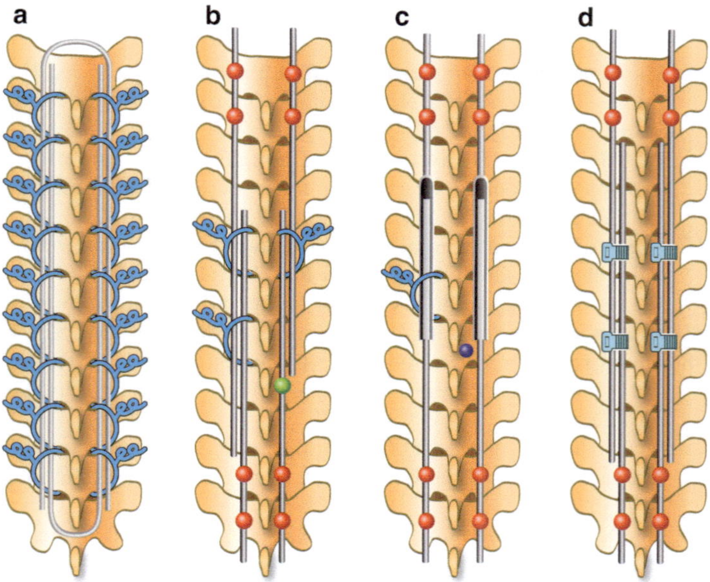

FIGURE 9.6 (**a**) Original Luque trolley. No segment of the spine is fused, but every level is captured with a sublaminar wire and is bound to the rod. (**b**) Modern Luque trolley with off-label use of mismatched oversized pedicle screws and sublaminar wires allowing the rods to glide across the apex. (**c**) Modern Luque trolley with off-label use of an unlocked VEPTR and a post allowing apical translation. (**d**) Modern Luque trolley with new apical gliding spinal implant—trolley gliding vehicle

References

1. Luqué ER, Cardoso A. Treatment of scoliosis without arthrodesis or external support: preliminary report. J Orthop Transl. 1977;1:37–8.
2. Moe JH, Kharrat K, Winter RB, et al. Harrington instrumentation without fusion plus external orthotic support for the treatment of difficult curvature problems in young children. Clin Orthop Relat Res. 1984:35–45.
3. Yang JS, McElroy MJ, Akbarnia BA, Salari P, Oliveira D, Thompson GH, Emans JB, Yazici M, Skaggs DL, Shah SA, Kostial PN, Sponseller PD. Growing rods for spinal deformity:

characterizing consensus and variation in current use. J Pediatr Orthop. 2010;30(3):264–70.
4. Mardjetko SM, Hammerberg KW, Lubicky JP, Fister JS. The Luque trolley revisited. Review of nine cases requiring revision. Spine. 1992;17(5):582–9.
5. Pratt RK, Webb JK, Burwell RG, Cummings SL. Luque trolley and convex epiphysiodesis in the management of infantile and juvenile idiopathic scoliosis. Spine. 1999;24(15):1538–47.
6. Ouellet J. Surgical technique: modern Luque trolley, a self-growing rod technique. Clin Orthop Relat Res. 2011;469(5):1356–67.
7. Skaggs DL, Akbarnia BA, Flynn JM, et al. A classification of growth friendly spine implants. J Pediatr Orthop. 2014;34:260–74.
8. Thompson GH, Akbarnia BA, Campbell RM Jr. Growing rod techniques in early-onset scoliosis. J Pediatr Orthop. 2007;27:354–61.
9. McCarthy RE, Sucato D, Turner JL, et al. Shilla growing rods in a caprine animal model: a pilot study. Clin Orthop Relat Res. 2010;468(3):705–10.
10. Ouellet JA, Ferland CE, Klein K, Racloz G, Klein K, Richter H, Steffen T, von Rechenberg B. Evaluation of the modern Luque trolley construct for treatment of early onset scoliosis using a gliding implant in an immature animal model. Clin Spine Surg. 2017;30(4):E460–5.

Chapter 10
Anterior Vertebral Body Tethering (AVBT) for Early-Onset Scoliosis

Firoz Miyanji and Stefan Parent

Case Presentation

History and Physical Examination

An otherwise healthy 8 + 6-year-old female, with strong family history of scoliosis, presented with her mother for evaluation. She had no complaints with respect to her back, denied any neurological symptoms to her upper and lower extremities, and there were no concerns regarding her bladder and bowel habits. Her developmental history was otherwise unremarkable, and she reached all of her milestones appropriately. Family history was positive in that her older brother presented at the age of 7 years with a 70° right main thoracic idiopathic curve that has been since managed with growing rods. He was now 9 years of age at the time his younger sister presented.

F. Miyanji, MD (✉) • S. Parent, MD
British Columbia Children's Hospital, Vancouver, BC, Canada

CHU Sainte Justine, Montreal, QC, Canada
e-mail: fmiyanji@cw.bc.ca; stefan.parent@umontreal.ca

R. El-Hawary, C.P. Eberson (eds.), *Early Onset Scoliosis*,
https://doi.org/10.1007/978-3-319-71580-3_10

- The patient's gait was normal and was able to heel, toe, and tandem gait walk without difficulty.
- Examination of her back revealed a right-sided curvature of her thoracic spine with subtle elevation of her right shoulder.
- There was no significant trunk shift and C7 plumb line was well-compensated.
- Forward bend revealed an obvious right-sided rib prominence that measured 9° with a scoliometer; there were no significant upper thoracic or lumbar prominences noted.
- Neurologically, the patient had no deficits to sensory and motor testing of her upper and lower extremities; abdominal reflexes were symmetric bilaterally, as were upper and lower extremity reflexes.
- Her integument was unremarkable and there was no evidence of spinal dysraphism.

Diagnostic Studies

- PA and lateral full-length scoliosis series X-rays showed a right main thoracic curve which measured 29° with no measurable upper thoracic and lumbar curves. Her lateral profile showed a T2–T12 kyphosis of 42° (Figure 10.1).
- Her MRI was normal with no intraspinal pathology demonstrated (Figure 10.2).

Management Chosen

This young girl presents with juvenile onset idiopathic scoliosis with an older sibling that presented with a fairly malignant curve at a young age and has been managed with growing rods. Her risk of progression is high and treatment options were discussed with the patient and family. At this point, bracing therapy was recommended but the patient declined. She was then carefully monitored at 6-month intervals with serial X-ray and physical exam.

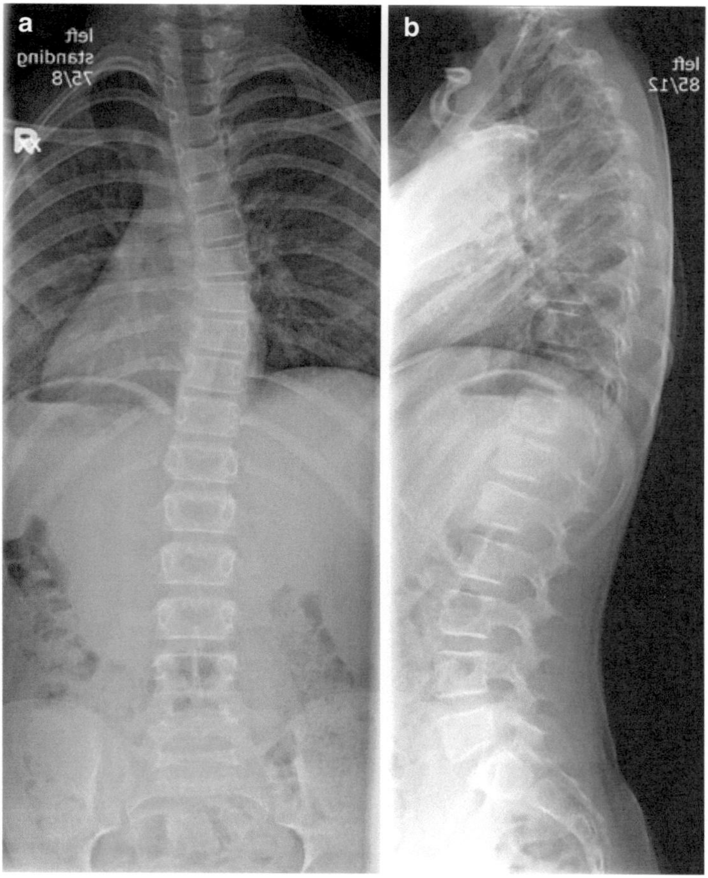

FIGURE 10.1 PA (**a**) and lateral (**b**) radiographs confirming moderate scoliosis on the first presentation

Her scoliosis continued to progress as documented by clinical exam and X-rays. She was now 10 years of age, remained premenarchal, and continued to voice no concerns with her back. Her clinical exam showed a larger curvature to the right of her thoracic spine with elevation of her right shoulder now 1 cm higher than the left. Her trunk was shifted to the right by 1.5 cm, and her right rib prominence measured

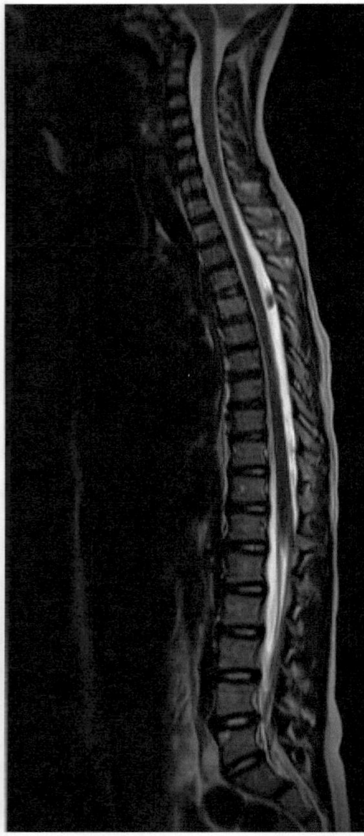

FIGURE 10.2 Midsagittal MRI shows no intraspinal pathology

14° with the scoliometer. She did not have any significant upper thoracic or lower lumbar curvatures or prominences on forward bend.

Her most recent upright PA and lateral radiographs showed progression of her right main thoracic curve to 44° with a proximal thoracic curve measuring 24° and a subtle lumbar curve of 21°. Her lateral T2–T12 kyphosis was 44°. She was a Risser 0 with closing triradiates.

Treatment options were discussed with the family and patient; given her age, skeletal immaturity, size, and location of the curve, an anterior vertebral body tethering (AVBT) procedure was discussed. Options around bracing were again dismissed by the patient, and the likelihood of requiring a fusion was high. The family and patient agreed to move ahead with AVBT.

Surgical Procedure

The procedure described here is for a typical right thoracic curve. Although a left curve could theoretically also be treated with this approach, most of our patients have right thoracic curves. The procedure is performed under general anesthesia with the patient intubated with a double-lumen tube when possible to allow for single-lung ventilation and right-lung deflation intraoperatively. If the patient's size is not amenable to double-lumen intubation, a bronchial blocker can also be used. The disadvantage of a bronchial blocker is that this is more difficult to position and that it can get dislodged during the procedure (especially after positioning) which makes it more difficult to control the right lung during the procedure. Once the patient is intubated, the patient is positioned in the lateral decubitus position with the convex side (usually the right side) facing upwards and a soft gel roll under the axilla to protect the brachial plexus. The patient is usually secured to the table using tape or with the use of a pelvic pad. The right arm should be positioned on an armrest taking care not to cause trauma to the ulnar nerve. Care should be taken not to elevate/extend the arm too high superiorly.

Once the patient is properly positioned, identification of the entry points should be done to insure proper visualization and instrumentation of each vertebral body to be instrumented will be possible. Two methods can be used to achieve this. The first is using standard fluoroscopy to estimate the entry points from posteroanterior and lateral images taking care to align the fluoroscopy between each image so that a perfectly orthogonal view of the vertebra is obtained. Another method is to use 3D navigation to obtain a 3D reconstruction of the patient's spine in the intraoperative position and navigate the actual entry points prior to starting the procedure.

The surgical field is then sterilized and draped so that all entry points can be accessed. Care must be taken to drape widely so as to permit open thoracotomy if needed. The anesthesia team then isolates the right lung thus deflating the lung. A first portal is usually made in the anterior-axillary line in the T5–T6 intercostal space to provide access to the T5 vertebral body. A lower portal may be needed if the contemplated instrumentation starts lower than T5. This first portal is usually inserted in a blind fashion so care should be taken when entering the chest cavity to avoid injury to the lung. A 10-mm/45° scope is usually preferred for image quality. A second portal along the anterior-axillary line is made to allow for better visualization and manipulation of different instruments. This portal will also later be used for cable tensioning (Figure 10.3).

The pleura is then divided 1 cm anterior to the rib-head/vertebra junction over the entire length of the spine to be instrumented (Fig 10.4a, b). The pleuras are reflected off the anterior part of the vertebral body to allow exposure of the segmental vessels and to allow safe insertion of the screws. Using a harmonic scalpel, the segmental vessels are divided and cut. Bleeding is usually minimal. If bleeding occurs, dividing the vessels more anteriorly may provide control of

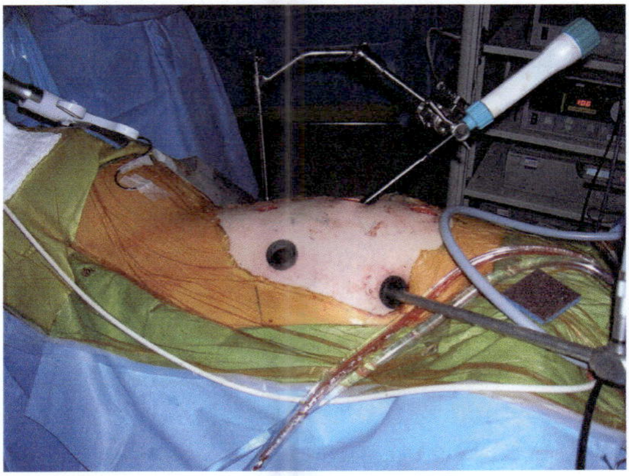

FIGURE 10.3 Portal placement for vertebral body tethering technique

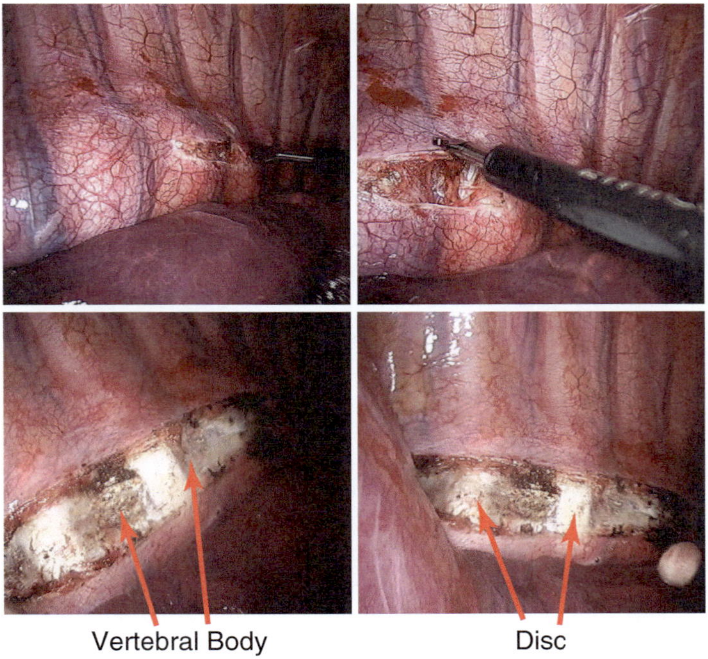

Figure 10.4 (**a**) Initial thoracoscopic view of the spine. (**b**) The pleura is then divided 1 cm anterior to the rib-head/vertebra junction over the entire length of the spine to be instrumented. (**c**) Vertebral bodies identified after pleural exposure. (**d**) Intervertebral discs identified after pleural exposure

the bleeding. Exposure from T4 to L2 is usually possible without having to use an open retroperitoneal approach although dissection distally may be blocked by the diaphragm attachments anteriorly to the spine. Retroperitoneal dissection is usually possible but a mini-open retroperitoneal approach may sometimes be needed to safely insert screws at levels distal to T12.

Once the spine is exposed, instrumentation can proceed (Fig 10.4c, d). Typically, two portals (sometimes three) are used to insert vertebral screws at each level. The portals are usually placed more posteriorly along the posterior-axillary line. The scapula may hinder direct access to the most proximal vertebral levels, and it may have to be retracted posteriorly (more commonly). A vertebral staple is inserted under fluoroscopic guidance and is secured into place. A vertebral tap is then used to prepare the screw trajectory. The screw path is then palpated to ensure intravertebral placement, and screw can then be placed. As the instrumentation used was not specifically designed for this indication, screws may need to be cut so as to accommodate the vertebral width available. Typically, screws in the upper thoracic spine have vertebral widths ranging between 25 and 30 mm. The position of the screws is assessed using fluoroscopy, and instrumentation proceeds distally to include all levels to be tethered anteriorly. Once all levels are instrumented, a cable is inserted through the distal instrumentation port and attached to the most proximal screw. The cable is then attached successively at each adjacent level while applying tension to partly correct the spinal deformity. The amount of tension applied to correct the deformity is still a subject of debate. Our preferred technique is to apply minimal tension at the extremities of the construct to prevent overcorrection and to apply more tension at the apex of the deformity to unload the asymmetrical forces on the vertebral end plates. We typically try to correct the disc wedging by applying enough tension to bring the end plates parallel. For very severe curves, overcorrection may be needed/achieved. Tension can be applied by a variety of methods. Some prefer to take the cable out of the chest cavity to apply tension using an external device connected to the vertebral screw. This technique is however cumbersome as the cable needs to be reintroduced in the chest cavity between each tightening. Another method is to grasp the cable with a non-traumatic forceps and to apply tension by rotating the forceps against the screw base with the inner locking screw in place. Once the desired tension is reached, the inner screw is tightened and secured.

The cable is then cut to length taking care to leave 2–3 cm of cable at each extremity in case there is overcorrection. Theoretically, one could release the proximal/distal tension in case of overcorrection (Figure 10.5).

The thoracic cavity is then rinsed and washed with normal saline. The lung is re-expanded under endoscopic view to make sure the different lobes are reinflated. A chest tube is installed through the distal instrumentation port, and the different ports are closed in anatomical layers.

The chest tube is placed under suction (−20 cm H_2O), and the patient is allowed to move as tolerated. The chest tube is removed 48–72 h post-op, and the patient is discharged home on day 3 or 4 post-op. Activities are restricted for the first 6 weeks with return to full activity thereafter.

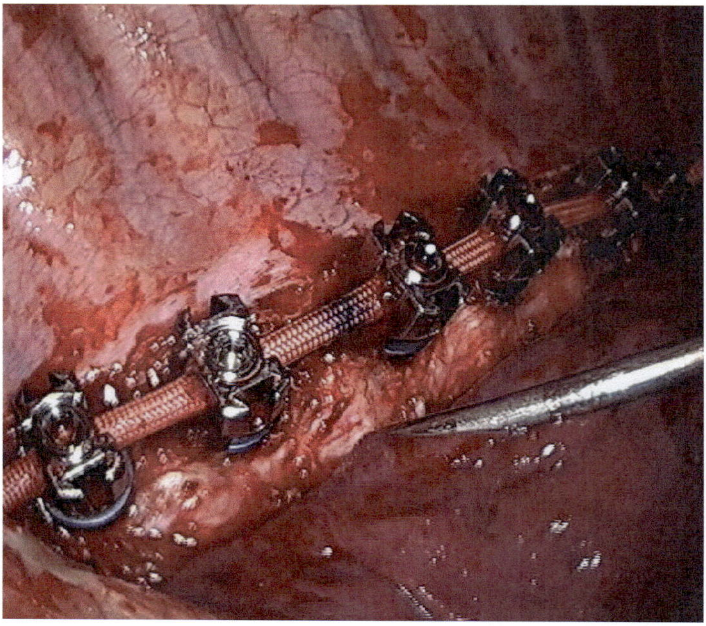

FIGURE 10.5 Final implants after tensioning the vertebral body tether

Tips and Tricks

- Proper identification of entry points/portals is key in insuring good screw trajectory.
- Screw starting point is usually just anterior to the rib head.
- Proper screw positioning is made easier by confirming staple position prior to using the vertebral tap.
- Cable tensioning should be done to avoid overtightening at the extremities of the construct.

Clinical Course and Outcome

At 24-month follow-up, the patient has had an excellent result with gradual correction of her deformity over time (Figure 10.6). Her sagittal T2–T12 profile was now 24°. She was now post-menarchal and a Risser 3. Her clinical exam showed she was nicely balanced coronally and sagittally

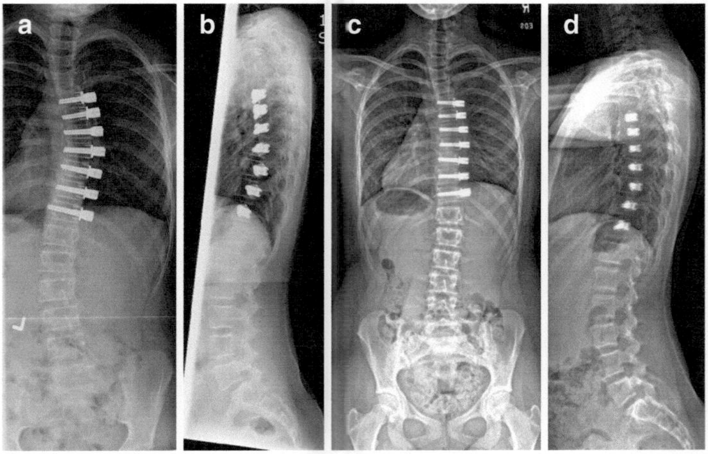

FIGURE 10.6 PA and lateral radiographs showing progressive correction of deformity over 24 months. PA (**a**) and lateral (**b**) X-rays at 6 weeks following surgery; PA (**c**) and lateral (**d**) X-rays at 24 months following surgery

with level shoulders and pelvis. Her rib prominence improved down to 3°. She was up to full activities at 3 months following surgery.

Clinical Pearls and Pitfalls

- Adequate single-lung ventilation is required, and CO_2 insufflation may aid in achieving this.
- Intraoperative fluoroscopy can help localize portals (in particular the posterior portals) for the placement of screws.
- Screw trajectory should be parallel to the vertebral end plates as much as possible.
- Segmental vessels need to be coagulated with a harmonic scalpel to help with exposure and screw placement.
- Localizing the rib head is an important landmark to guide placement of staple and screw in the anterior-posterior plane (avoid neural foramen/canal).
- Tensioning to get intraoperative correction to less than 20° is ideal.
- Consider leaving the ends of the tether approximately 1 inch longer than the screw tulip in the event of overcorrection.
- Preoperative flexibility of the curve is key, and *lack* of a *structural proximal thoracic* curve is also an important consideration for this procedure (Figure 10.7).
- Patient selection is fundamental to the success of this procedure.

Literature Review and Discussion

Spinal arthrodesis remains the gold standard in the management of progressive adolescent idiopathic scoliosis; however, concerns about the long-term effect of spinal fusion and decreased spinal mobility [1] have led to the development of growth modulation techniques that may allow correction of the deformity without fusion [2, 3]. Specific concerns with arthrodesis include halting vertebral growth over the fused

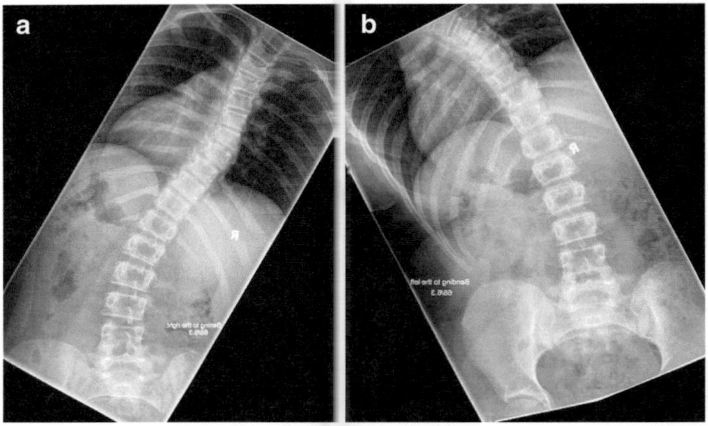

FIGURE 10.7 Right bend (**a**) X-ray showing flexibility of curve; left bend (**b**) X-ray showing no demonstrable lumbar curve

segments and the potential for disc degeneration of adjacent segments. VBS and AVBT are currently being investigated as potential fusionless treatment methods to manage progressive curves in the skeletally immature. The goal is to control the patient's remaining spinal growth to prevent further progression and achieve curve correction by exploiting the Heuter-Volkmann principle. The convex growth plates are compressed under tension, inhibiting their growth, while the concave growth plates continue to grow, hence straightening the spine.

The Heuter-Volkmann principle is thought to be intimately related to scoliosis progression. Compressive loads on the concavity decrease physeal growth leading to vertebral wedging, which induces more compressive inhibition of growth and curve progression. Distractive forces are felt to accelerate growth. This principle has been the impetus for a number of more recent animal studies showing the efficacy of anterior spinal growth modulation. Stokes [4] is credited with a classic rattail animal model, which demonstrated that the Heuter-Volkmann principle could predict vertebral body growth through mechanical modulation. Using external fixators, compression reduced rattail vertebral growth to 68% of normal, and distraction increased growth to 114%. The authors subsequently demonstrated that asymmetric loading of rattail vertebrae resulted in differential growth on the compression and tension sides enabling both the production of deformity and its subsequent correction [5, 6]. Others have also demonstrated spine deformity *creation* and subsequent control of its progression in experimental animal models using a variety of mechanical implants [7–13].

More recently, studies investigated the ability of anterior spinal growth modulation to *correct* experimental deformity. Braun et al. [14] noted tethering to be superior to staples in deformity correction in their caprine model. Chay et al. [18] reported a more favorable three-dimensional correction of their scoliosis porcine model using an anterior-based tether compared to a control group.

The authors of these experimental studies also reported on the health of the discs in the tethered segments and found no evidence of irreversible growth cartilage or disc injury [13, 15–18]. Decreased disc thickness, increased proteoglycan synthesis, and a change in collagen distribution between the concave and convex sides were reported; however there was no change in water and glycosaminoglycan content within the tethered discs. The clinical implications and reversibility of these changes remain unknown.

With advances in surgical techniques and implant technology, along with experimental studies showing the efficacy of anterior spinal growth modulation, there has been a renewed interest in fusionless techniques for the treatment of scoliosis.

Betz et al. [19, 20] have popularized VBS reporting on their initial clinical experience. Although the authors conclude that vertebral body stapling can be considered for patients with progressive scoliosis, a number of authors have noted limited if any significant efficacy of VBS in controlling curves. Betz and colleagues [21] found VBS to be 78% effective in thoracic curves ≤35° and 87% of thoracolumbar curves ≤35°. Others have also noted VBS to have a potential role in minor curves of ≤35° [21, 22]. Most treating surgeons however would consider skeletally immature patients with curves ≤35°.

Anterior vertebral body tethering has shown promise in particular for curves in skeletally immature patients in whom bracing is ineffective at halting progression. Although clinical data remains limited [23], there have been published reports on proof of concept [24] as well as emerging reports of patients with 2-year follow-up [25]. Samdani et al. [25] reported their first series of 11 skeletally immature patients with 2-year follow-up and found continued progressive correction of the tethered thoracic curve, the nonstructural lumbar curve, and the rib prominence. Patients had a mean age of 12.3 ± 1.6 years and mean Risser grade of 0.6 ± 1.1 with an average preoperative curve magnitude of 44.2° ± 9.0° which corrected to 20.3° ± 11° on the first erect X-ray, with continued improvement at 2 years to a mean 13.5° ± 11.6°. The authors noted a 70% correction of the curves with AVBT over 2-year follow-up.

Most recently, Samdani et al. [26] presented on 25 patients treated with AVBT who have now reached skeletal maturity. These patients' mean age was 12.5 ± 1.4 years with a mean Risser of 0.5 ± 1.0. The average preoperative Cobb was 40.9° ± 7.1° in this cohort which corrected to 20.1° ± 8.4° on the first erect X-ray with progressive improvement to skeletal maturity to a mean 14.0° ± 11.1°, noting a 66.1% correction over time. There were two patients who required subsequent surgery for overcorrection of their curves that required loosening of the tether. The authors did not report on any patient requiring a conversion to fusion surgery.

Newton and colleagues [27] presented their review of 17 patients treated with AVBT and highlighted some of the concerns that should caution treating surgeons using this technology. Their group of Risser 0 patients with a mean age of 11 years had a mean thoracic preoperative curve of 52° (40–67°). They defined clinical success as scoliosis reduction to <30° at most recent follow-up. Scoliosis at most recent follow-up was 23 ± 23° (−18–57°) with reduction due to growth modulation averaging 8 ± 17°. They found only nine patients with a clinical success and ten additional surgeries were undertaken in eight patients: four tether removals for overcorrection, one replaced broken tether, one contralateral lumber tether added, and one conversion to posterior fusion with three more planned. The authors concluded that, although the tether clearly affects spinal growth and avoided fusion in 13 of 17 patients, with current technology, it resulted in less than ideal outcome for 47% of patients.

Fusionless surgery for progressive idiopathic scoliosis has shown efficacy in animal models and more recently in its clinical application. AVBT has shown to be more effective than VBS in this setting; however ideal candidates and indications for AVBT continue to evolve. Currently, skeletally immature patients (Risser ≤2) with either isolated thoracic curves, thoracolumbar curves, or a double major pattern (Lenke 3/6) with Cobb angles between 40° and 65° may be considered. Caution should be exercised in extremely young, immature patients (open triradiate cartilage, age <10) for risk of overcorrection [21, 23, 24] and in very large curves (≥65°) for risk of tether failure [27]. The response of coronal correction may not equate to axial plane correction, and patients with a significant rib prominence deformity should also be warned. Finally, although thoracolumbar and lumbar curves can be considered, careful evaluation of the sagittal plane should be monitored, as anterior instrumentation is known to be kyphogenic. Although AVBT currently is gaining momentum for its clinical application in the surgical management for idiopathic scoliosis, data regarding its true effectiveness and long-term risk remain outstanding.

References

1. Marks M, Newton PO, Petcharaporn M, et al. Postoperative segmental motion of the unfused spine distal to the fusion in 100 patients with adolescent idiopathic scoliosis. Spine (Phila Pa 1976). 2012;37(10):826–32. https://doi.org/10.1097/BRS.0b013e31823b4eab.

2. Nachlas IW, Borden JN. The cure of experimental scoliosis directed growth control. J Bone Joint Surg Am. 1951;33(1):24–34.
3. Smith AD, von Lackum HL, Wylie R. An operation for stapling vertebral bodies in congenital scoliosis. J Bone Joint Surg Am. 1954;36(2):342–8.
4. Stokes IAF, Spence H, Aronson DD, Kilmer N. Mechanical modulation of vertebral body growth. Implications for scoliosis progression. Spine. 1996;21(10):1162–7.
5. Stokes IAF, Aronsson DD, Spence H, Iatridis JC. Mechanical modulation of intervertebral disc thickness in growing rat tails. J Spinal Disord. 1998;11(3):261–5.
6. Mente PL, Aronsson DD, Stokes IA, Iatridis JC. Mechanical modulation of growth for the correction of vertebral wedge deformities. J Orthop Res. 1999;17(4):518–24.
7. Braun JT, Ogilvie JW, Akyuz E, et al. Fusionless scoliosis correction using a shape memory alloy staple in the anterior thoracic spine of the immature goat. Spine. 2004;29:1980–9.
8. Braun JT, Ogilvie JW, Akyuz E, Brodke DS, Bachus KN, Stefko RM. Experimental scoliosis in an immature goat model: a method that creates idiopathic-type deformity with minimal violation of the spinal elements along the curve. Spine. 2003;28(19):2198–203.
9. Wall EJ, Bylski-Austrow DI, Kolata RJ, Crawford AH. Endoscopic mechanical spinal hemiepiphysiodesis modifies spine growth. Spine. 2005;30(10):1148–53.
10. Newton PO, Fricka KB, Lee SS, Farnsworth CL, Cox TG, Mahar AT. Asymmetrical flexible tethering of spine growth in an immature bovine model. Spine. 2002;27(7):689–93.
11. Newton PO, Upasani VV, Farnsworth CL, et al. Spinal growth modulation with use of a tether in an immature porcine model. J Bone Joint Surg Am. 2008;90(12):2695–706.
12. Braun JT, Ogilvie JW, Akyuz E, Brodke DS, Bachus KN. Creation of an experimental idiopathic-type scoliosis in an immature goat model using a flexible posterior asymmetric tether. Spine. 2006;31(13):1410–4.
13. Hunt KJ, Braun JT, Christensen BA. The effect of two clinically relevant fusionless scoliosis implant strategies on the health of the intervertebral disc. Spine. 2010;35:371.
14. Braun JT, Hoffman M, Akyuz E, et al. Mechanical modulation of vertebral growth in the fusionless treatment of progressive scoliosis in an experimental model. Spine. 2006;31:1314–20.

15. Upasani VV, Farnsworth CL, Chambers RC, et al. Intervertebral disc health preservation after six months of spinal growth modulation. J Bone Joint Surg Am. 2011;93(15):1408–16.
16. Newton PO, Farnsworth CL, Upasani VV, Chambers RC, Varley E, Tsutsui S. Effects of intraoperative tensioning of an anterolateral spinal tether on spinal growth modulation in a porcine model. Spine. 2011;36(2):109–17.
17. Newton PO, Farnsworth CL, Faro FD, et al. Spinal growth modulation with an anterolateral flexible tether in an immature bovine model: disc health and motion preservation. Spine. 2008;33(7):724–33.
18. Chay E, Patel A, Ungar B, et al. Impact of unilateral corrective tethering on the histology of the growth plate in an established porcine model for thoracic scoliosis. Spine. 2012;37(15):E883–9.
19. Betz RR, Kim J, D'andrea LP, Mulcahey MJ, Balsara RK, Clements DH. An innovative technique of vertebral body stapling for the treatment of patients with adolescent idiopathic scoliosis: a feasibility, safety, and utility study. Spine. 2003;28(20S):S255–65.
20. Betz RR, Ranade A, Samdani AF, et al. Vertebral body stapling: a fusionless treatment option for a growing child with moderate idiopathic scoliosis. Spine. 2010;35(2):169–76.
21. Bumpass DB, Fuhrhop SK, Schootman M, Smith JC, Luhmann SJ. Vertebral body stapling for moderate juvenile and early adolescent idiopathic scoliosis: cautions and patient selection criteria. Spine. 2015;40(24):E1305–14.
22. Cuddihy L, Danielsson A, Cahill PJ, et al. Vertebral body stapling vs. bracing for patients with high-risk moderate idiopathic scoliosis. Biomed Res Int. 2015. https://doi.org/10.1155/2015/438452.
23. Samdani AF, Ames RJ, Kimball JS, et al. Anterior vertebral body tethering for immature adolescent idiopathic scoliosis: one-year results on the first 32 patients. Eur Spine J. 2015;24(7):1533–9.
24. Crawford CH, Lenke LG. Growth modulation by means of anterior tethering resulting in progressive correction of juvenile idiopathic scoliosis. J Bone Joint Surg Am. 2010;92(1):202–9.
25. Samdani AF, Ames RJ, Kimball JS, et al. Anterior vertebral body tethering for idiopathic scoliosis: two-year results. Spine. 2014;39(20):1688–93.
26. Samdani AF, Ames RJ, Pahys JM et al. Anterior vertebral body tethering for immature idiopathic scoliosis: results of patients reaching skeletal maturity. Paper presented at 50th SRS Annual Meeting; September–October 2015; Minneapolis, MN. https://

www.srs.org/UserFiles/file/meetings/am15/AM15_Abstracts_Web.pdf.

27. Newton PO, Saito W, Yaszay B, Bartley C, Bastrom T. Successes and failures following spinal growth tethering for scoliosis—a retrospective look 2 to 4 years later. Paper presented at 51st SRS Annual Meeting; September 2016; Prague, Czech Republic. https://www.srs.org/UserFiles/file/am16FP-book-WEB-v9sm2.pdf.

Chapter 11
Anterior Vertebral Body Stapling for the Treatment of Idiopathic Scoliosis

James T. Bennett, Amer F. Samdani, Robert J. Ames, and Randal R. Betz

Case Presentation

We present a 9-year-old girl (Risser 0) with juvenile idiopathic scoliosis with a 25° progressive thoracic curve and a 22° compensatory lumbar curve with 10° of kyphosis from T5 to T12 (Fig. 11.1). The curve had continued to progress despite attempted bracing. The family was interested in alternative treatment options including growth modulation with VBS.

J.T. Bennett, MD • R.J. Ames, MD
Temple University Hospital, Philadelphia, PA, USA
Shriners Hospitals for Children, Philadelphia, PA, USA
e-mail: james.t.bennett@gmail.com

A.F. Samdani, MD
Shriners Hospitals for Children, Philadelphia, PA, USA
e-mail: amersamdani@gmail.com

R.R. Betz, MD (✉)
The Institute for Spine and Scoliosis, Lawrenceville, NJ, USA
e-mail: randalrbetz@gmail.com

R. El-Hawary, C.P. Eberson (eds.), *Early Onset Scoliosis*,
https://doi.org/10.1007/978-3-319-71580-3_11

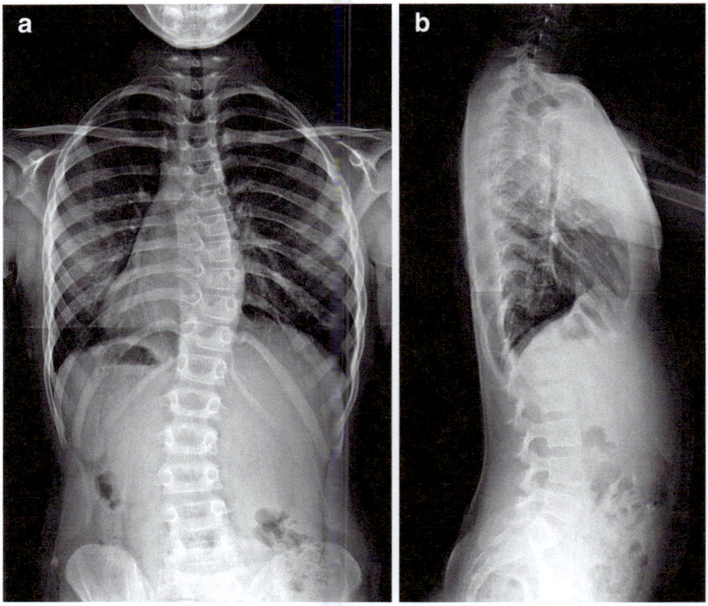

FIGURE 11.1 (**a**, **b**) Posteroanterior and lateral radiographs of a 9-year-old girl with juvenile idiopathic scoliosis (Risser 0), who presented with a right-sided thoracic curve measuring 25°, a compensatory lumbar curve measuring 22°, and 10° of kyphosis (T5–T12)

History and Physical Examination

The patient had a normal birth and developmental history with no other medical problems and no family history of scoliosis. She had no reported hypersensitivity to nickel and did not have any respiratory disease such as uncontrolled asthma that would prevent her from receiving general anesthesia with single-lung ventilation.

On physical exam, she had a 7° right thoracic rib prominence with Adams forward bend test that corrected with side bending. She had level shoulders and hips with no significant trunk shift. She had a normal neurologic exam. There were no cutaneous lesions or other abnormalities noted.

Diagnostic Studies

The patient had standing posteroanterior (PA), bending, and lateral spine radiographs documenting progression of her curve. An MRI was obtained that showed no intraspinal anomalies. Prior to surgery, the patient was immature (Risser 0) with a flexible right-sided thoracic curve measuring 25° and a compensatory lumbar curve measuring 22°.

Management Chosen

After the risks, benefits, and alternatives were discussed with the patient and family, they elected to proceed with an anterior VBS of her thoracic curve from T6 to T12. They were interested in growth modulation treatment due to progression of the curve despite compliance with bracing and wanted to avoid a spinal fusion. They understood that the staples do not have FDA approval for this indication.

Surgical Procedure

The patient underwent general anesthesia and intubation with a double-lumen endotracheal tube. She was positioned on the operating room table in the lateral decubitus position with the convexity (right side) of the curve facing upwards. An axillary roll and padding of all bony prominences were placed for passive gravity-assisted curve correction. Neuromonitoring was utilized, as it is a helpful adjunct if a segmental vessel requires ligation. Fluoroscopy was used to confirm the levels to be stapled (each curve should be stapled from the upper end vertebra to the lower end vertebra), in this case T6–T12, and to center the thoracoscopic ports over the midportion of the vertebral bodies. The patient was prepped and draped similar to a thoracotomy, in case conversion to an open procedure was needed secondary to any complications. Single-lung ventilation of the dependent lung was utilized for visualization of the vertebrae.

The first port was made at the sixth intercostal space along the anterior axillary line (we typically place the port between the fifth and seventh intercostal spaces depending on the size of curve and patient's body habitus) for placement of the scope. Visualization was aided by carbon dioxide gas insufflation. Additional working ports were placed in the posterior axillary line for staple insertion (generally two to three staples can be placed through each incision). Of note, the lumbar vertebrae can be accessed by a mini-open retroperitoneal approach through a small lateral oblique incision with blunt retroperitoneal dissection and posterior retraction of the psoas muscle (a transpsoas approach using a tube system similar to lateral lumbar interbody fusion [XLIF] can also be used).

A radiopaque trial instrument was used to determine the size of each Nitinol memory shape alloy staple (Medtronic; Memphis, TN) that ranged in size from 3 to 8 mm. Four-prong staples were used as they decrease surgical time by placing a single staple versus two double-prong staples (although occasionally a single double-prong staple is required for the smaller upper thoracic vertebrae). The staple size was determined with the trial instrument by selecting the smallest staple that spanned each disc space. The parietal pleura and segmental vessels were preserved. The appropriately sized trial was then used to create pilot holes for the staple, and the staple was then malleted in place. Prior to insertion the staples were chilled in a basin of sterile ice to keep the prongs straight, since they bend into their original "C" shape for secure fixation in the vertebrae when they reach body temperature, which occurs within approximately 30 s.

Fluoroscopy was used to obtain anteroposterior images to determine proper staple position across the disc space, which was aided by direct visualization with the thoracoscope through the first port to place the staple directly lateral on the vertebral body and just anterior to the rib head in the thoracic spine. In the lumbar spine, the correct position is in the posterior half of the vertebral body to prevent kyphosis at those levels. The entirety of the thoracic curve from the upper end vertebra (T6) to the lower end vertebra (T12) was stapled using the previously described steps. Final fluoroscopic images were obtained to ensure that the staples were in the appropriate position. A chest tube was placed through the anterior port to prevent a pneumothorax and to drain any potential effusion. Intercostal blocks at the surgical levels were performed prior to closure of the ports to assist with pain control.

Clinical Course and Outcome

Postoperatively, the patient went to the intensive care unit per standard protocol. On postoperative day 1, she was transferred to the floor and ambulated with minimal pain controlled with opioid analgesia and Ketorolac. She required nighttime bracing as her thoracic curve was >20° (22°) on her first erect radiograph (Fig. 11.2). The chest tube was removed on postoperative day 1 with an output of <100 mL over 24 h. The patient

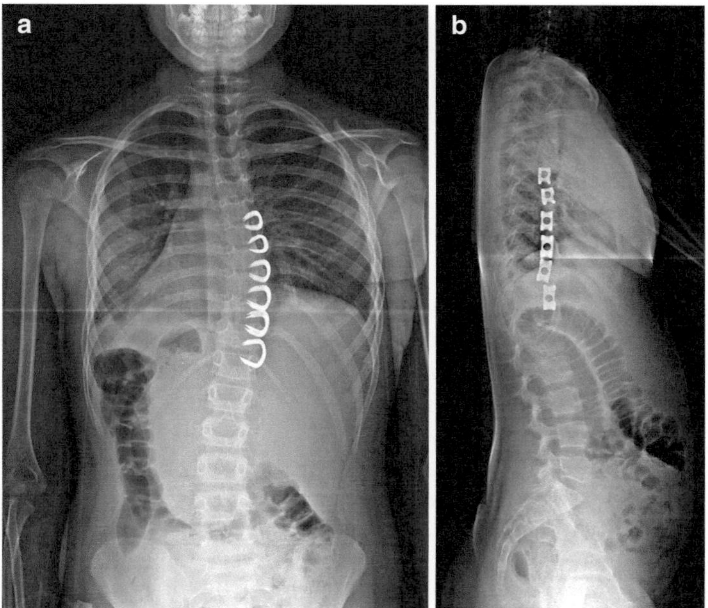

FIGURE 11.2 (**a**, **b**) First erect posteroanterior and lateral radiographs after thoracic vertebral body stapling from T6 to T12, with main thoracic curve correction to 22° and lumbar curve correction to 16°

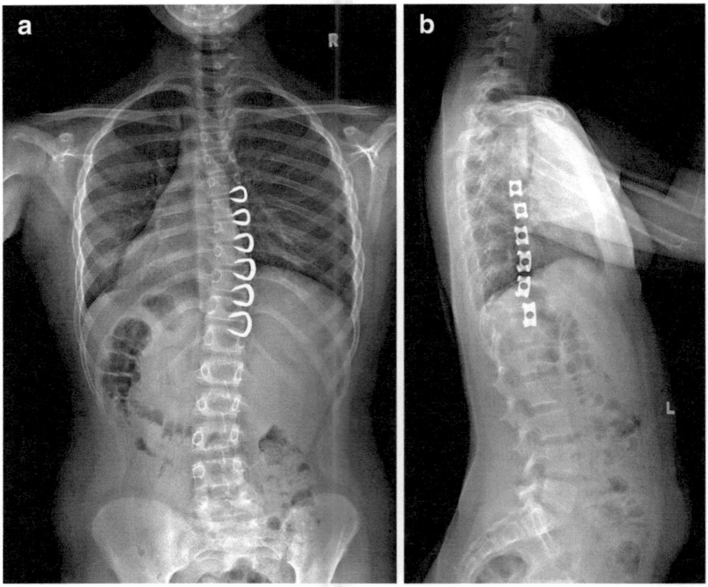

FIGURE 11.3 (**a**, **b**) One-year posteroanterior and lateral radiographs demonstrating thoracic curve correction to 14° and lumbar curve correction to 17°

was discharged on postoperative day 4 with her brace and returned at 3 and 6 weeks for a wound check. At 6 weeks she was allowed to return to all activities as tolerated. She returned again for follow-up at 6-month intervals to monitor curve correction; when her thoracic curve measured <20° at 1-year follow-up, her nighttime brace was discontinued. At 1 year her thoracic curve had corrected to 14° and her lumbar curve measured 17° (Fig. 11.3). At her most recent follow-up 4.5 years after surgery, she had matured (Risser stage 4), with continued correction of her thoracic and lumbar curves to 13° and 9°, respectively, and a thoracic kyphosis of 20° (Fig. 11.4).

Clinical Pearls and Pitfalls

- Although most surgeons with experience in anterior spine surgery and minimally invasive techniques are comfortable

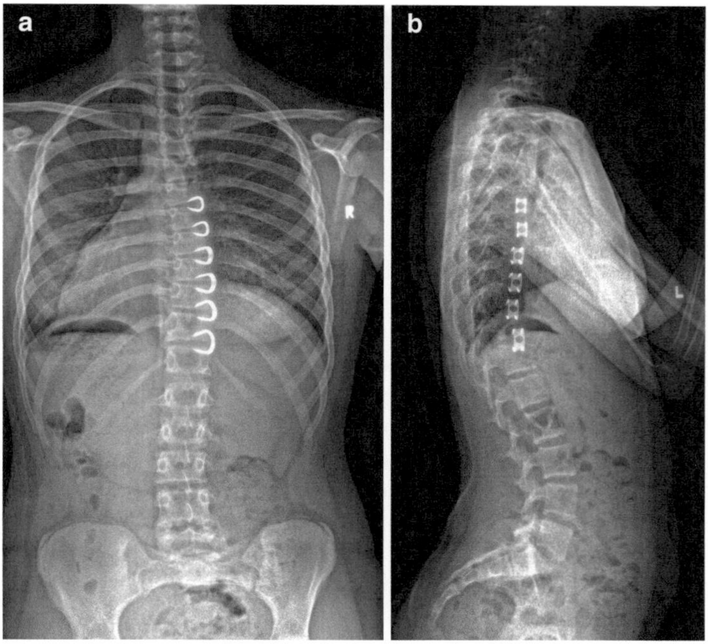

FIGURE 11.4 (**a**, **b**) Posteroanterior and lateral radiographs at most recent follow-up 4.5 years after surgery showing maturation of the patient (Risser 4) with improved correction of her thoracic and lumbar curves to 13° and 9°, respectively, with a kyphosis (T5–T12) of 20°

performing this procedure, it may be helpful to ask general or thoracic surgeon to assist with the approach.

- Staples that cross the thoracolumbar junction require partial reflection of the diaphragm in front of the spine. We try to avoid stapling across the L3–L4 disc due to the risk of nerve root injury from retraction of the psoas or from a transpsoas approach. When positioning, it is helpful to slightly flex the up leg to relieve tension on the psoas muscle.
- Each curve should be stapled from the upper end vertebra to the lower end vertebra. If the patient has two curves >25°, then both curves should be stapled, which will require intraoperative repositioning.

- Maximizing correction on the operating room table is important, as the best results are obtained when the first erect radiograph results in a curve <20°. This can be achieved by corrective positioning of the patient with gravity-assisted curve correction (aided by placing the axillary roll slightly more caudad at the apex of the proximal thoracic curve) and applying pressure to the spinal segment prior to staple insertion, with the inserter placed in the previously implanted staple.
- If the thoracic curve is >20° on the first erect radiograph, the patient should wear a nighttime brace until the curve is below <20° out of the brace. We recommend placing patients with lumbar curves treated with stapling in a soft corset for 4 weeks due to increased mobility of this region of the spine and to wear a nighttime brace if they are aiming for complete resolution of the deformity.
- In patients with significant hypokyphosis (<10°), consider placing thoracic staples more anteriorly to impart more kyphosis or adding a two-prong staple more anteriorly. In contrast, kyphosis >40° is a relative contraindication to stapling due to the propensity for hyperkyphosis from the anterior procedure. One should obtain a Stagnara true lateral X-ray of the spine or a 3-D reconstruction of the spine or review the sagittal cuts of the MRI to confirm a true kyphosis before excluding the patient from consideration for the procedure. Lumbar staples should be placed in the posterior half of the vertebral body to maintain normal lordosis.
- Segmental vessel injury resulting in increased blood loss may require conversion of the thoracoscopic port to a mini-open incision with ligation of the vessel (this happened only once to the senior author in his first series of 39 patients). In addition, if one encounters problems with single-lung ventilation, two mini-thoracotomies centered at T4–T5 and T9–T10 may be utilized for access.
- We recommend follow-up every 6 months until skeletal maturity with standing PA and lateral radiographs to monitor for overcorrection. We are aware of four patients

who have experienced overcorrection of a stapled curve (two thoracic curves and two lumbar curves). Three of the four patients underwent staple removal between 1 and 4 years after the initial stapling procedure. As a result, we recommend delaying stapling until 8 years of age to minimize this risk as well as removing the stapling if >10° of overcorrection is noted.

Literature Review and Discussion

In 2003, the senior author showed that stapling is a safe and effective treatment alternative to bracing for moderate idiopathic scoliosis in a subset of patients with significant growth remaining [1]. Later, the authors retrospectively reviewed 28 of 29 patients (26 thoracic and 15 lumbar curves) with idiopathic scoliosis treated with VBS followed for a minimum of 2 years and found that in those patients with a preoperative thoracic curve <35°, the success rate was 77.7% [2–4]. This success rate improved to 85.7% when those curves were ≤20° on their first erect radiograph. These findings are why we aim to get maximum intraoperative correction and recommend nighttime bracing for those patients with thoracic curves that are >20° on their first erect radiograph.

Additionally, patients with lumbar curves between 20° and 45° had a success rate of 86.7%. These results are considered much better than the natural history of patients in the study by Dimeglio et alstudy [5] where progression to fusion occurred in 75–100% of patients in this age and curve size. The procedure was considered a success when the curves stayed within 10° of preoperative measurement or improved more than 10°.

In those patients with thoracic curves >35°, the failure rate was 75%, with continued progression beyond 50° resulting in a fusion. Of note, curve correction, surgical time, and blood loss for those fusions following failed stapling were comparable to primary spinal fusions. There was no need for staple removal in order to do the posterior spinal fusion, and at the time of surgery, the spine was noted to still be correctable.

Recently, Cuddihy et al. [6] compared a cohort of 42 patients treated with VBS to a matched bracing cohort of 129 consecutive patients with moderate idiopathic scoliosis from the Göteborg bracing database. They found that for thoracic curves <35°, VBS had a success rate of 81% compared to 61% for bracing, although this was not statistically significant ($p = 0.16$). Thoracic curves between 35° and 44° had poor success rates for both VBS and bracing. Lumbar curves measuring <35° had similar success rates (80%) in both groups. This study suggested that in high-risk patients with thoracic curves 25°–34°, VBS may provide better results compared to bracing.

Because all studies suggest that both stapling and bracing may be ineffective for thoracic curves >35°, we recommend either adding hybrid instrumentation with rib to spine distraction rods in the concavity of the curve or using a more powerful growth modulation option such as vertebral body tethering for larger thoracic curves that are 35°–75°.

In 2015, Bumpass et al. [7] published their results on VBS in patients with moderate idiopathic scoliosis (25°–40° curves) with 4 years of follow-up. They found that thoracic curves <35° had a sucess rate of 79%, similar to that reported by Betz et al. [4], but thoracolumbar curves <35° achieved a sucess rate of only 70% compared to the 86.7% reported by Betz et al. This difference is likely due to either failure to brace if the curves are >20° on the first erect radiograph or possibly the longer follow-up in the Bumpass study.

There are very few complications related to VBS, with the majority related to the approach. We are aware of five cases in which a staple loosened or backed out, four of which were seen within 2 months of the initial procedure. Loosening was asymptomatic in three of the five patients, two of whom underwent revision stapling. One patient experienced pain with a loose staple 2.5 years after the initial procedure and had removal of the staple with complete relief of pain. Four broken staples have been reported, all in the lumbar spine and all within 6–12 months of the initial procedure. Two of the four patients experienced pain, one of which had removal of the broken staple with complete pain relief. This is one of the reasons we recommend using a soft corset for these lumbar curves postoperatively, even though none of these curves progressed with further follow-up.

Other complications we have encountered include a rupture of a pre-existing unrecognized congenital diaphragmatic hernia requiring repair, injury to a segmental spinal vein requiring conversion to a mini-open thoracotomy to ligate the vein, damage to the thoracic duct resulting in a chylothorax treated with total parenteral nutrition and a chest tube, mild pancreatitis that resolved with a low-fat diet, and clinically significant atelectasis treated conservatively in two patients [1, 8]. To our knowledge, there have been no reported instances of damage to the great vessels, lung parenchyma, heart, abdominal organs, or kidneys with VBS.

Some authors suggest that VBS may be detrimental to the disc space over the long-term. However, recent animal models have shown that hemi-staples across the disc may decrease the growth plate hypertrophic zone and cell height while showing positive signs of disc health sustainability [9]. Biomechanical studies suggest that although stapling does reduce motion particularly in the axial plane, it is much less than that seen with fusion [10]. In addition, staple fixation does not result in consistently elevated adjacent segment motion. We have also noted that on postoperative radiographs, there is micro motion seen between the staple and bone as demonstrated by a "halo effect" around the staple prongs, suggesting that there is no rigid fixation, and motion preservation throughout the disc space is likely preserved. In addition, MRIs obtained postoperatively for various reasons do not show disc degeneration. Furthermore, in the patients requiring posterior spinal fusion after stapling, we have not seen any evidence of spontaneous fusion, nor have we encountered decreased curve correction. As a result, we feel that VBS does not appear to have any detrimental effect to the disc space, although more long-term clinical studies are needed.

Based on our experience, the current indications for VBS are age less than 13 years for girls and less than 15 years for boys with at least 1 year of growth remaining (Risser 0–1, Sanders digital stage ≤4). In addition, we recommend waiting until the child is at least 8 years of age to decrease the risk of overcorrection. Thoracic curves should be 25°–35° and lumbar curves should be 25°–45°. For best results, the curves should be flexible, bending to <20° with minimal rotation, and kyphosis should measure <40°.

References

1. Betz RR, Kim J, D'Andrea LP, Mulcahey MJ, Balsara RK, Clements DH. An innovative technique of vertebral body stapling for the treatment of patients with adolescent idiopathic scoliosis: a feasibility, safety, and utility study. Spine (Phila Pa 1976). 2003;28(20S):S255–65.
2. Trobisch PD, Samdani A, Cahill P, Betz RR. Vertebral body stapling as an alternative in the treatment of idiopathic scoliosis. Oper Orthop Traumatol. 2011;23(3):227–31.
3. Lavelle WF, Samdani AF, Cahill PJ, Betz RR. Clinical outcomes of nitinol staples for preventing curve progression in idiopathic scoliosis. J Pediatr Orthop. 2011;31(1 Suppl):S107–13.
4. Betz RR, Ranade A, Samdani AF, et al. Vertebral body stapling: a fusionless treatment option for a growing child with moderate idiopathic scoliosis. Spine (Phila Pa 1976). 2010;35(2):169–76.
5. Dimeglio A, Canavese F, Charles YP. Growth and adolescent idiopathic scoliosis: when and how much? J Pediatr Orthop. 2011;31(1 Suppl):S28–36.
6. Cuddihy L, Danielsson AJ, Cahill PJ, et al. Vertebral body stapling versus bracing for patients with high-risk moderate idiopathic scoliosis. Biomed Res Int. 2015;2015:438452.
7. Bumpass DB, Fuhrhop SK, Schootman M, Smith JC, Luhmann SJ. Vertebral body stapling for moderate juvenile and early adolescent idiopathic scoliosis: cautions and patient selection criteria. Spine (Phila Pa 1976). 2015;40(24):E1305–14.
8. Betz RR, D'Andrea LP, Mulcahey MJ, Chafetz RS. Vertebral body stapling procedure for the treatment of scoliosis in the growing child. Clin Orthop Relat Res. 2005;(434):55–60.

9. Driscoll M, Aubin CE, Moreau A, Wakula Y, Amini S, Parent S. Novel hemi-staple for the fusionless correction of pediatric scoliosis: influence on intervertebral disks and growth plates in a porcine model. Clin Spine Surg. 2016;29(9):457–64.
10. Puttlitz CM, Masaru F, Barkley A, Diab M, Acaroglu EA. Biomechanical assessment of thoracic spine stapling. Spine (Phila Pa 1976). 2007;32(7):766–71.

Chapter 12
Congenital Resection for Early-Onset Scoliosis

Michael Glotzbecker and John Emans

Case Presentation

An otherwise healthy 3-year-old child was noted by her mother to have a prominent area in the lumbar spine while bathing. Plain X-rays showed a lumbar hemivertebra with significant torso imbalance (Fig. 12.1). Screening MRI was normal. Brace treatment was suggested at another institution. The child walked normally at age 14 months and at age 3 was toilet trained.

History and Physical Examination

Gestation, birth, and delivery were unremarkable. There was no family history of congenital anomalies and no history of maternal diabetes or exposure to valproic acid or carbon monoxide.

Examination showed a healthy, vigorous child with normal gait and normal extremities. The waist was asymmetric with prominence of the right hip relative to the left and a slight left

M. Glotzbecker, MD • J. Emans, MD (✉)
Department of Orthopedic Surgery, Boston Children's Hospital and Harvard Medical School, Boston, MA, USA
e-mail: michael.glotzbecker@childrens.harvard.edu; john.emans@childrens.harvard.edu

R. El-Hawary, C.P. Eberson (eds.), *Early Onset Scoliosis*, https://doi.org/10.1007/978-3-319-71580-3_12

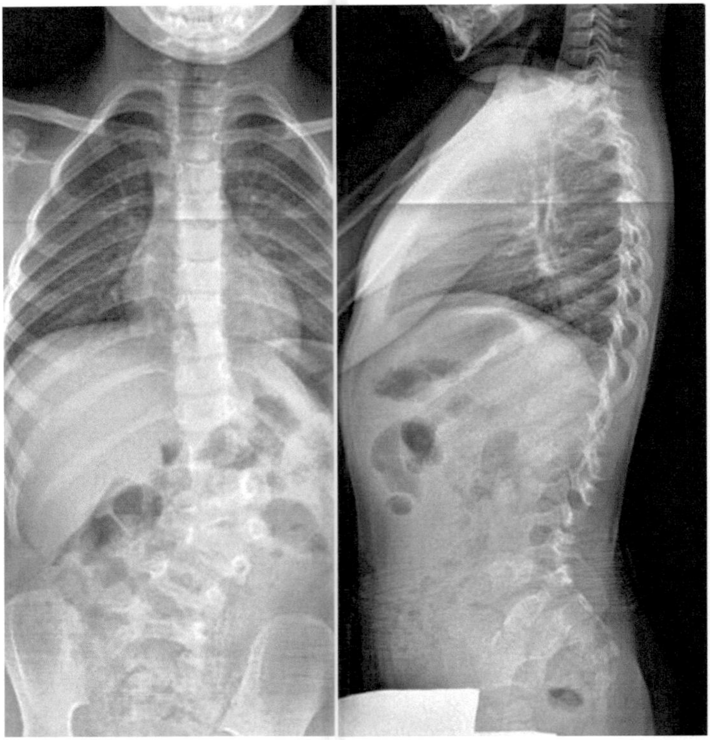

Figure 12.1 Upright radiograph shows the upper lumbar hemivertebra with a significant left torso shift and curvature below. Lateral X-ray shows slight focal kyphosis at the level of the hemivertebra. The left pelvis is slightly lower, indicating a minimal leg length discrepancy

leg length discrepancy. The left lumbar prominence was visible on forward bending with an inclinometer reading of 7°. Reflexes were symmetric including abdominal reflexes. No sacral skin dimple was present.

Diagnostic Studies

An MRI had already been done, but could have been deferred until before surgery as the child had no clinical signs of tethered spinal cord. If identified at a young age (patients under age 6–8 weeks), a screening ultrasound may replace the need for a sedated MRI at a later date. If there are no neurologic findings to suggest spinal cord pathology, the MRI can be deferred until immediately preoperatively to avoid early anesthetic exposure. A screening renal US was also obtained as it is recommended in the presence of congenital spinal anomalies. CT scan of the lumbar spine was done preoperatively and included coronal and sagittal reformatting and a three-dimensional reconstruction (Fig. 12.2). The CT

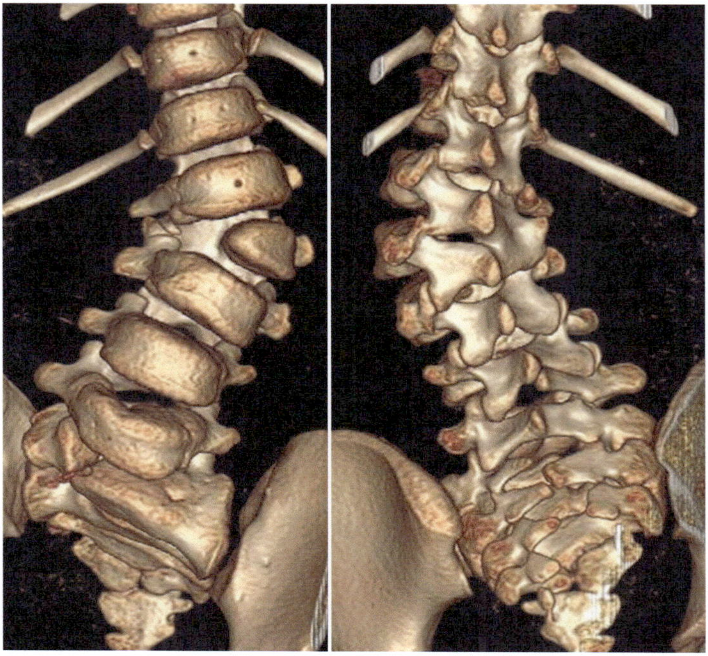

FIGURE 12.2 3D reconstruction is critical in preoperative planning, as there may be non-concordance of the vertebral body anatomy and laminar anomalies. In this patient the hemivertebra is fully segmented and the hemi-lamina is at the same level. Axial images show the concave pedicles to be medially oriented. The CT also reveals other anomalies at the lumbosacral junction not immediately apparent on plain X-ray

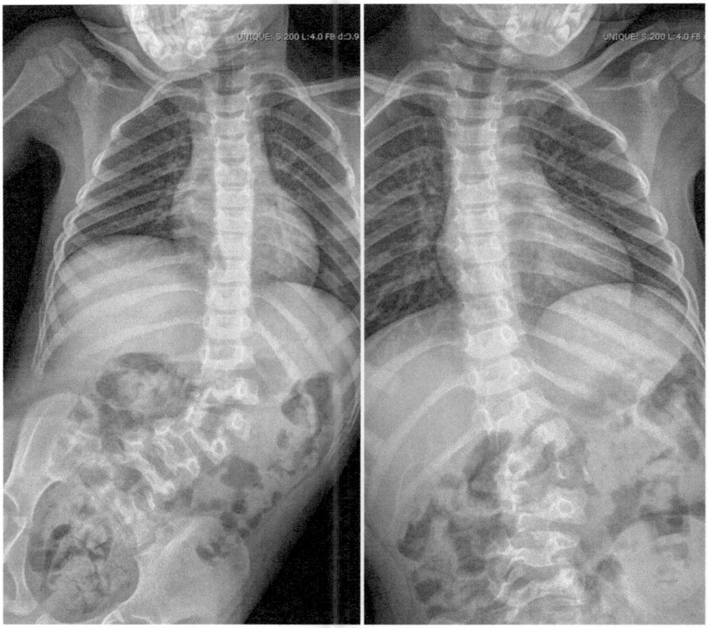

Figure 12.3 Supine bending X-rays show the curves above and below the hemivertebra to be flexible, implying that they will resolve when the angular deformity of the hemivertebra is removed. The right bending X-ray suggests fixed lumbosacral obliquity which will likely persist

scan confirmed a fully segmented hemivertebra and hemilamina at the same level, partly fused to the lamina above. Partial sacralization of L5 and a right-sided L4-L5 hemilamina was also noted. In addition to repeat standing PA and lateral entire spine X-rays, AP supine bending X-rays (Fig. 12.3) were done to assess flexibility of the normally segmented spine above and below.

Management Chosen

Brace treatment was suggested at the first institution. Although bracing may improve torso imbalance and may be useful in long flexible congenital deformities involving a long section of the spine, bracing is unlikely to affect the local deformity caused by the hemivertebra [1]. Surgical options include *in situ* fusion, convex hemi-epiphysiodesis, and hemivertebra excision [2–12]. The hemivertebra involves a very short segment of the spine yet causes significant torso imbalance and large compensating curves above and below. Fusion *in situ* would stop the local curve progression but leave residual deformity above and below. Convex instrumented hemi-epiphysiodesis is a viable option and easily performed and carries little risk of neurologic injury, but does not quickly or reliably correct deformity, relying on continued asymmetric growth to achieve correction [1, 12]. If the global deformity surrounding a hemivertebra is minimal, or if the deformity is in area where resection is more challenging, hemi-epiphysiodesis is a good option. Hemivertebra excision however can achieve immediate correction of the local deformity and depending on preoperative bending X-rays will correct the normally segmented flexible curves above and below. Hemivertebra excision does entail some risk of neurologic injury, blood loss, and loss of fixation. Hemivertebra excision can be done successfully as posterior-only or anteroposterior approaches [2–9, 13]. Posterior-only hemivertebra excision has the advantage of a single incision and is most easily performed when there is a kyphotic deformity. Anterior and posterior hemivertebra excision may be preferable in a severely lordotic deformity or in a patient in whom excessive bleeding would not be tolerated. Generally, hemivertebra excision is most satisfactory at the thoracolumbar junction, the lumbar spine, and the lumbosacral junction. Although surgically challenging, it is also useful at the cervicothoracic junction. Hemivertebra excisions in the mid-thoracic spine seem to achieve less correction and are prone to recurrent deformity.

Hemivertebra excision was chosen with a posterior-only approach. Posterior-only hemivertebra excision was felt to be feasible in this child, and immediate correction of the torso imbalance and curves above and below was desired. Waiting until age 4–6 was suggested to allow for more vertebral maturity and permit more certain implant fixation.

We arbitrarily choose this age as the time at which the vertebral structures are large enough to permit reliable fixation, yet the neural structures are still young enough to best tolerate manipulation without injury. In this child follow-up at age 4 years showed that the torso imbalance had worsened; therefore, we proceeded with a posterior hemivertebra excision [3].

Surgical Procedure

Preparation

Posterior-only hemivertebra excision was performed using routine general anesthesia, somatosensory-evoked and transcranial motor-evoked potential monitoring, as well as free-running EMGs. Tranexamic acid was used. Positioning was prone on a pediatric scoliosis frame with the hemivertebra side tipped slightly upward. Location of the hemivertebra was confirmed fluoroscopically and the skin marked with the location of the hemivertebra pedicle before the incision.

Exposure

The skin incision was made slightly off midline toward the side of the hemivertebra to facilitate retraction. Subperiosteal exposure of only the lamina above and lamina below the hemivertebra was made. Access to the pedicles of the vertebra above was made by continuing the midline incision cephalad as a bilateral muscle-splitting incision, taking care to remain extra-periosteal to reach the lateral aspect of the superior articular facet and pedicle entry point of the lamina above the hemivertebra. Inadvertent exposure of laminae at this age will result in unintended posterior fusion with undesired loss of mobility and possible crankshaft. Therefore, great care is taken to expose only that portion of the posterior spine which will be used (Fig. 12.4).

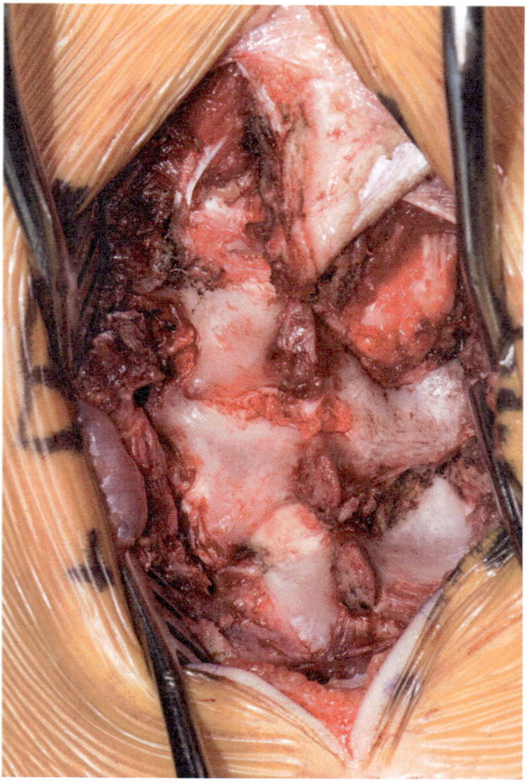

FIGURE 12.4 Only the desired laminae for fusion are exposed. All else remains covered with muscle and periosteum. A bilateral muscle-splitting incision above allows access to the pedicles of the superior vertebra to be fused

Fixation

A 3.5 mm titanium rod system is usually sufficient fixation except in larger children. Pedicle screws were placed in the vertebra above and below and a supra-laminar and infra-laminar hook placed as in the "three-rod technique" described by Hedequist (Figs. 12.5 and 12.6). Levels were

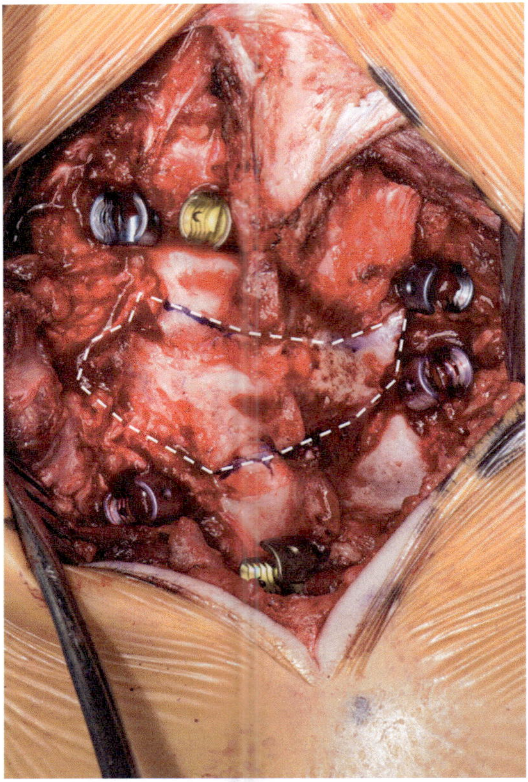

FIGURE 12.5 Pedicle screws and supra- and infra-laminar hooks are shown in place before hemivertebra excision. Dotted area shows laminae to be excised

confirmed radiographically before placing fixation points. Study of the preoperative CT showed that the concave pedicle trajectories were more medial than normal, and this information was used to assist freehand placement of screws. Screws were stimulated and were below threshold criteria and were imaged fluoroscopically to assure appropriate placement.

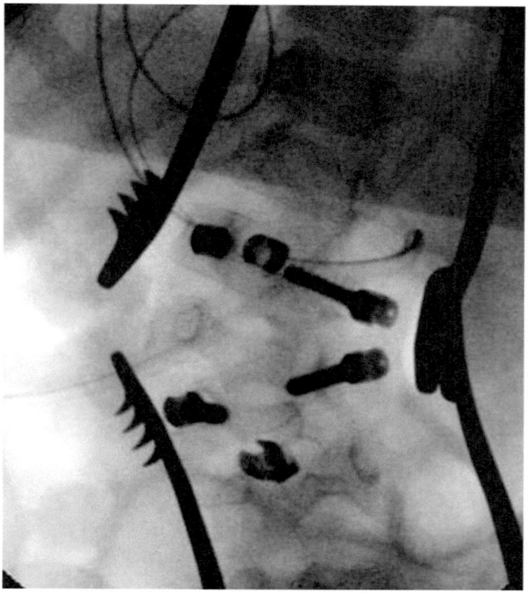

FIGURE 12.6 Pedicle screw position was confirmed by fluoroscopic imaging. The concave pedicle screws appear medial in placement, but this trajectory was expected from the pre-op CT

Hemivertebra Excision

The hemivertebra was excised in stages. First the hemi-lamina corresponding to the hemivertebra body was excised with rongeurs. In this patient, the hemi-lamina was congenitally fused to the lamina above so that a cut was made between the hemi-lamina and the lamina above. Sometimes the lamina corresponding to the hemivertebra has a very different shape or connection to adjacent laminae. Reference to the three-dimensional CT reconstruction will help define the posterior elements to be removed as there may be discordance between the anterior and posterior congenital malformations. While in the simple hemivertebrae excision it is generally not needed, anecdotally, with the advance of 3D printing capabilities, more complex deformities can be assessed preoperatively to help to create a surgical plan. Where possible the laminar excision should be done such that the remaining lamina will contact each other encouraging bony union and stability. If too much is excised, a laminar gap will remain. If too little is excised, closing the deformity will be obstructed by the laminar contact (Fig. 12.7). After removing the lamina, the nerve root

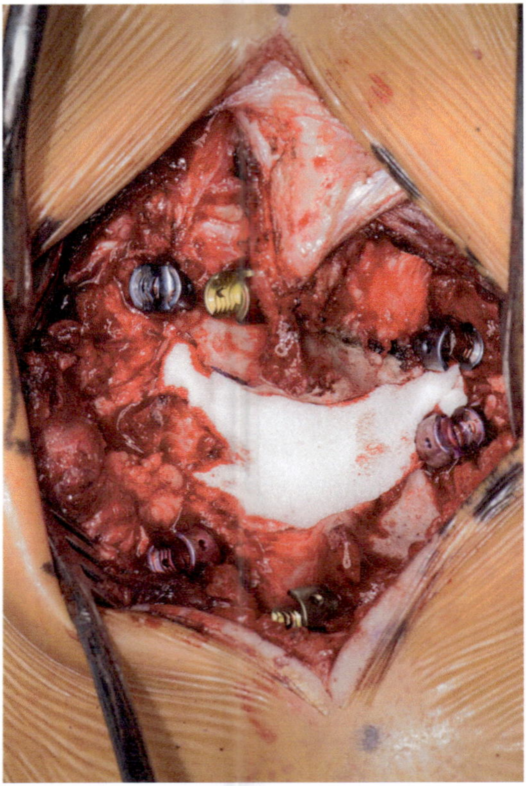

FIGURE 12.7 The hemi-lamina has been removed, leaving pedicle and transverse process. White gelatin foam temporarily covers and marks the excision. The remaining laminae above and below have been trimmed to fit together when the deformity is corrected

above and below the pedicle of the hemivertebra was identified and freed from any significant fibrous tissue. These two nerve roots must be free enough so that when the hemivertebra is removed, the two nerve roots can easily occupy one newly created neural foramen.

Next the transverse process corresponding to the hemivertebra was removed. If the hemivertebra is opposite a rib, then a several centimeter portion of the medial rib and rib head should also be excised. Dissection was then carried down the lateral aspect of the hemivertebra body and curved to follow the vertebra ventrally. This can be done either subperiosteally or, in this patient, was done extra-periosteally. The first is easiest but the latter allows easier access to the disk above and below. Either must be done with care to avoid inadvertent injury to the structures anterior to the spine. Using curettes and a high-speed diamond burr, the interior of the pedicle and hemivertebra were then excised. Use of large curettes allows harvesting the hemivertebra cancellous bone as autograft. The medial wall of the pedicle and the dorsal wall of the hemivertebra were retained at this stage. The disk above and below the hemivertebra including the cartilaginous end plates and the disk contralateral to the hemivertebra to the annulus are then excised. This is the most challenging portion of the procedure, since in children the rubbery disk and cartilaginous material is much stronger than the adjacent bone. Curettes, thin elevators, and a high-speed burr were used to excise disk material without damaging the vertebral bony endplates above and below. If the end plate above or below is peaked in shape, then it may need to be trimmed to allow closure of the wedge. Excising the hemivertebra bone alone is not enough; rather one must excise a wedge consisting of hemivertebra, disk, and if necessary some of the endplate above or below (Fig. 12.8).

Lastly, the medial wall of the pedicle and dorsal wall of the vertebral body were excised using rongeurs and back-angled curettes (Fig. 12.9). Often this stage of the procedure is accompanied by significant epidural bleeding which can be

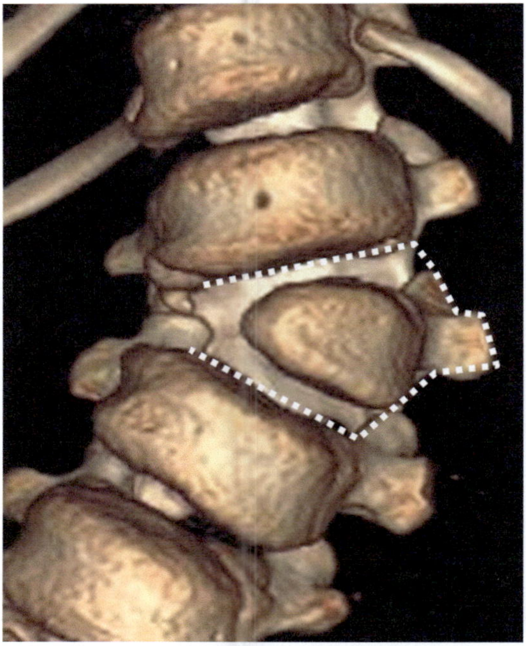

Figure 12.8 Excising the bony hemivertebra is not enough to achieve complete correction. Excision should include the disc above and below and disc opposite the hemivertebra. This is best thought of as a "wedge" excision rather than a hemivertebra excision

controlled by bipolar cautery. Retraction of the dura is usually necessary to see and remove the posterior wall of the vertebral body and its entirety. Dural retraction can be with nerve root retractors but must be gentle. Available morcellized autograft from the excised lamina and vertebral body was then placed anteriorly between the two residual vertebral bodies to facilitate anterior fusion. Anterior structural graft or a cage is in our experience not needed. In contrast to a vertebral column resection, the spine remains stable during the resection, and temporary rods are generally not required.

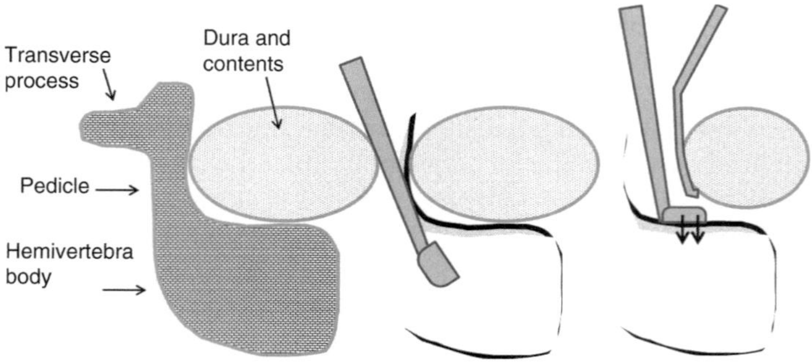

FIGURE 12.9 Left to right—stepwise removal of the hemivertebra. First the transverse process, lateral pedicle, and vertebral body and discs are removed, leaving the medial pedicle wall and dorsal vertebral body shell. Second the medial pedicle and dorsal cortex are removed with a back-angled curette while protecting the dura. This latter stage is often accompanied by epidural bleeding requiring bipolar cautery control

Correction

Rods were then placed between the pedicles screws but not tightened and a third rod placed joining the hooks. Correction was achieved by compressing the hooks toward each other. The rods joining the pedicles were left loose, guiding the correction. All the force of correction was borne by the hooks and joining rod and lamina. Pedicle screws and joining rods were then tightened. Often the rods must be exchanged for shorter rods after correction. Any exposed dura or epidural fat is covered with a shaped piece of gel foam to keep bone graft out of the spinal canal. Correction was assessed in the coronal and sagittal plane by fluoroscopy (Fig. 12.10). Sometimes it is necessary to distract on the concave and compress slightly more on the convex side to achieve the appropriate correction. In the lateral view there should not be residual abnormal kyphosis or lordosis. A common error is to not excise completely enough anteriorly such that when the posterior structures are compressed and undesired segmental lordosis occurs. The tendency to create undesired lordosis at the level of the resection can be avoided by thorough anterior excision and is probably facilitated by use of fixed-angle screws rather than multiaxial screws. Available surfaces were then lightly decorticated and the remaining autograft supplemented by crushed cancellous bone mixed with vancomycin powder to facilitate the posterior one-level fusion. Closure was routine with a waterproof dressing left in place for 12 days postoperatively. A postoperative brace was measured while the patient was still anesthetized. SSEP and MEP potentials remained normal throughout. Blood loss was 75 mL.

Clinical Course and Outcome

The patient was managed postoperatively on the orthopedic surgical floor. Urinary catheter was removed on post-op day 1 and ambulation began on day 2. The postoperative brace was introduced on the third postoperative day but was not tolerated all day until 2 weeks later. Patient was discharged on the fourth postoperative day. An upright postoperative X-ray was obtained before discharge and 1 month, 3 months, 6 months, and 1 year (Fig. 12.10). The brace was used during the day but not for sleeping for 3 months. For the first 3 months, activity was restricted to exclude recess and other high-impact activities. Thereafter activity was not restricted. The patient remained visually symmetric and pain-free. Radiographs showed spontaneous improvement in the curves above and below (Fig. 12.11).

Clinical Pearls and Pitfalls

- A three-dimensional CT scan preoperatively helps in surgical planning and may identify a mismatch between the hemi-vertebral body and laminar anomalies. Recognizing this preoperatively is critical [14].
- Think of the procedure as a "wedge" resection of hemivertebra and adjacent disc extending nearly all the way to the contralateral annulus. Just excising the hemivertebra bone

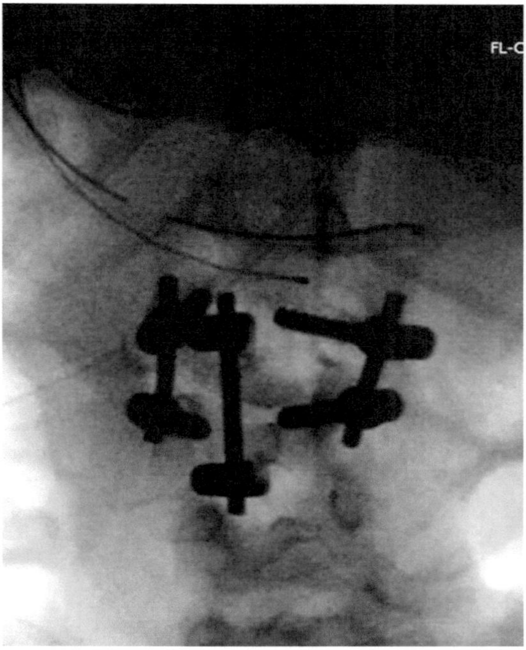

FIGURE 12.10 Intraoperative assessment of correction. In this patient a slight residual angulation was allowed to counterbalance the fixed lumbosacral obliquity and anomalies below

without the rest of the "wedge" will limit correction and may cause inadvertent segmental lordosis.

- Use the third rod connecting laminar hooks to generate all the force of correction [3]. This will spare the pedicle screws excessive force and preclude loss of pedicle screw fixation and the need for extension of the fixation to a vertebra above or below.

Literature Review and Discussion

Traditionally, hemivertebra excision was performed by a combined anterior/posterior approach, but more contemporary posterior-only approaches have demonstrated similar

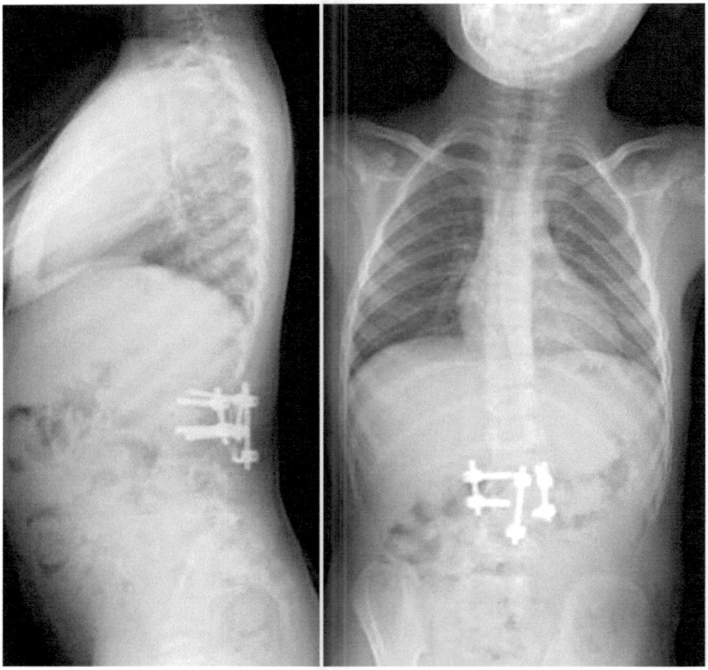

FIGURE 12.11 Standing radiographs at 1 year postoperatively show the curves above and below the hemivertebra are resolved, with slight residual fixed lumbosacral obliquity below

results with regard to complication rates and ability to correct the deformity [4–9, 13, 15].

While the historical complication rate and risk may be slightly higher with hemivertebra excision when compared to *in situ* fusion or convex growth arrest, the ability to correct deformity is greater with resection [10–12, 15]. In a multicenter comparative study of 76 patients with a minimum of a 2-year follow-up, patients treated with resection had better percent correction, shorter fusion, and less blood loss but did demonstrate a higher complication rate [15]. However, complications of implant failure and pedicle screws cutting out [6, 9] may be avoided by using a three-rod technique that compresses across the lamina rather than stressing the pedicles [3]. Posterior-only hemivertebra excision using a three-rod technique is a safe, reliable method to achieve deformity correction in patients requiring hemivertebrae excision.

References

1. Winter RB, et al. The Milwaukee brace in the nonoperative treatment of congenital scoliosis. Spine. 1976;1(2):85–96.
2. Atici Y, et al. The results of closing wedge osteotomy with posterior instrumented fusion for the surgical treatment of congenital kyphosis. Eur Spine J. 2013;22(6):1368–74.
3. Hedequist D, Emans J, Proctor M. Three rod technique facilitates hemivertebra wedge excision in young children through a posterior only approach. Spine (Phila Pa 1976). 2009;34(6):E225–9.
4. Mladenov K, Kunkel P, Stuecker R. Hemivertebra resection in children, results after single posterior approach and after combined anterior and posterior approach: a comparative study. Eur Spine J. 2012;21(3):506–13.
5. Ruf M, Harms J. Hemivertebra resection by a posterior approach: innovative operative technique and first results. Spine (Phila Pa 1976). 2002;27(10):1116–23.
6. Ruf M, Harms J. Posterior hemivertebra resection with transpedicular instrumentation: early correction in children aged 1 to 6 years. Spine (Phila Pa 1976). 2003;28(18):2132–8.
7. Wang S, et al. Posterior hemivertebra resection with bisegmental fusion for congenital scoliosis: more than 3 year outcomes and analysis of unanticipated surgeries. Eur Spine J. 2013;22(2):387–93.
8. Zhang J, et al. The efficacy and complications of posterior hemivertebra resection. Eur Spine J. 2011;20(10):1692–702.
9. Zhu X, et al. Posterior hemivertebra resection and monosegmental fusion in the treatment of congenital scoliosis. Ann R Coll Surg Engl. 2014;96(1):41–4.
10. Uzumcugil A, et al. Convex growth arrest in the treatment of congenital spinal deformities, revisited. J Pediatr Orthop. 2004;24(6):658–66.
11. Winter RB, et al. Convex growth arrest for progressive congenital scoliosis due to hemivertebrae. J Pediatr Orthop. 1988;8(6):633–8.

12. Winter RB, Moe JH. The results of spinal arthrodesis for congenital spinal deformity in patients younger than five years old. J Bone Joint Surg Am. 1982;64(3):419–32.
13. Bradford DS, Boachie-Adjei O. One-stage anterior and posterior hemivertebral resection and arthrodesis for congenital scoliosis. J Bone Joint Surg Am. 1990;72(4):536–40.
14. Hedequist DJ, Emans JB. The correlation of preoperative three-dimensional computed tomography reconstructions with operative findings in congenital scoliosis. Spine (Phila Pa 1976). 2003;28(22):2531–4. discussion 1
15. Yaszay B, et al. Efficacy of hemivertebra resection for congenital scoliosis: a multicenter retrospective comparison of three surgical techniques. Spine (Phila Pa 1976). 2011;36(24):2052–60.

Chapter 13
The Vertical Expandable Prosthetic Titanium Rib (VEPTR) for Congenital Scoliosis

Daniel J. Miller, Michael R. Eby, Robert M. Campbell, and Patrick J. Cahill

Case Presentation

History and Physical Examination

The patient presented as a 14-month-old boy who was referred for consultation from another center for congenital scoliosis with fused ribs in the setting of VACTERL association (a condition characterized by the presence of three or more of the following: vertebral defects, anal atresia, cardiac defects, tracheoesophageal fistula, renal anomalies, or limb abnormalities). The spinal deformity was diagnosed on prenatal ultrasound and, per the parents, had progressed visibly since delivery.

Past medical history revealed that the patient was born prematurely at 33 weeks via cesarean section. Following

D.J. Miller, MD • M.R. Eby, MD • R.M. Campbell, MD (✉)
P.J. Cahill, MD
Division of Orthopedic Surgery, The Children's Hospital of Philadelphia, Philadelphia, PA, USA
e-mail: ebym@email.chop.edu; CampbellRM@email.chop.edu; cahillp1@email.chop.edu

R. El-Hawary, C.P. Eberson (eds.), *Early Onset Scoliosis*,
https://doi.org/10.1007/978-3-319-71580-3_13

birth, he spent 7 weeks in the neonatal intensive care unit (NICU) for low birth weight (3 pounds, 11 ounces) with his hospital course complicated by necrotizing enterocolitis. Past medical history was otherwise remarkable for gastroesophageal reflux, tracheomalacia, a solitary left kidney, a hypoplastic left thumb, and severe obstructive sleep apnea necessitating supplemental oxygen and apnea monitoring at night.

Since birth, the patient had experienced multiple respiratory illnesses requiring hospitalization. His parents noted that he became tachypneic with crying but had no apparent dyspnea at rest.

Past surgical history included a gastrostomy tube placement at 10 months of age for feeding support secondary to poor swallow function. There was no family history of spinal deformity. Developmentally, he began sitting at age 9 months and was crawling at 11 months.

At our initial evaluation, the patient was a pleasant and alert infant. Resting respiratory rate was mildly elevated at 40 breaths per minute with an oxygen saturation of 98% on room air. His weight was 8.2 kg, below the fifth percentile for age.

He was normocephalic with normal facies. On cardiac exam, his heart was on regular rate and rhythm with no murmurs and good perfusion. He demonstrated severe hypoplasia of the left hemithorax with depression of the left shoulder. On respiratory exam, he had greater aeration in his right lung fields relative to the left side. Thumb excursion test was +0 bilaterally. There was no tenderness on palpation of the spine. There were no hairy patches, sacral dimples, café au lait spots, or other cutaneous abnormalities about the spine. Muscle bulk, range of motion, and tone were normal throughout bilateral upper and lower extremities. The left thumb was completely absent. The patient was able to sit and crawl independently in a coordinated fashion.

Diagnostic Studies

Radiographic evaluation demonstrated a right thoracic curve measuring 89° with multiple congenital vertebral anomalies and multiple areas of rib fusion on the left concave side (Fig. 13.1). Review of previously obtained radiographs showed evidence of significant curve progression over the previous 9 months (Fig. 13.2). Previous spinal MRI demonstrated no neuraxial lesions.

The patient was referred for further testing and an evaluation by a multidisciplinary team at our Center for Thoracic Insufficiency (CTIS). A dynamic MRI of the chest and thorax demonstrated posterior obstruction blockade on the left side of the diaphragm. A CT scan of the chest and spine revealed multiple hemivertebrae and block vertebra throughout the thoracic spine with associated left-sided rib fusions (Fig. 13.3). Infant pulmonary function testing, specifically designed to

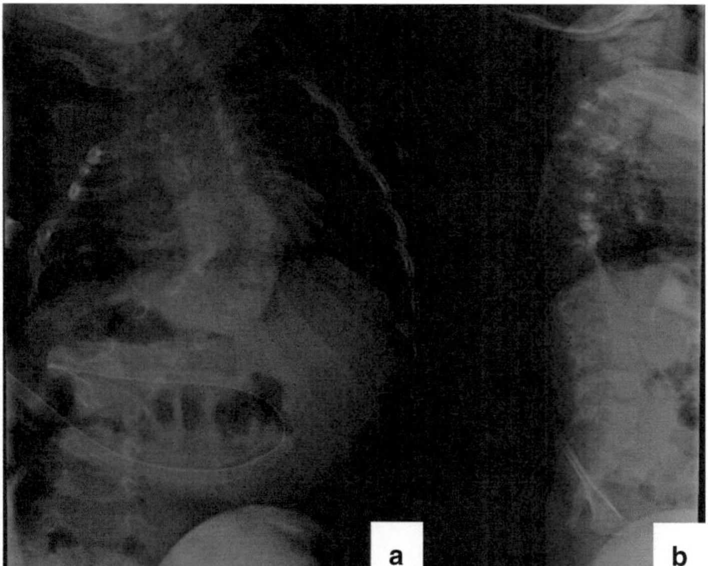

FIGURE 13.1 PA (**a**) and lateral (**b**) radiograph at time of evaluation demonstrating a right thoracic curve measuring 89° with multiple congenital vertebral anomalies and multiple areas of rib fusion on the left concave side

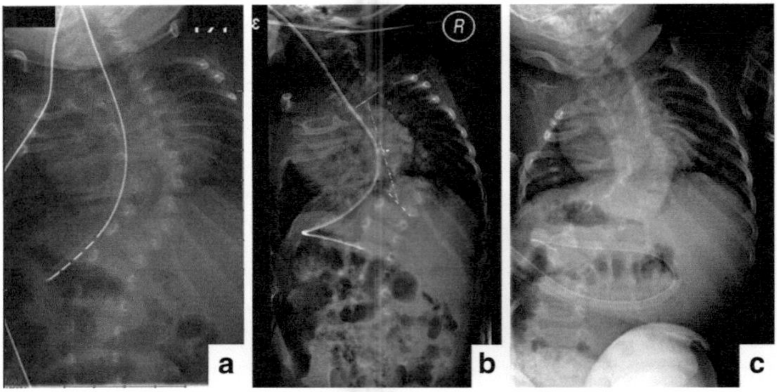

FIGURE 13.2 PA radiographs taken at 1 month of age (**a**), 3 months of age (**b**), and 10 months of age (**c**) demonstrate evidence of curve progression from 74° to 89°

incorporate the physiologic and cognitive development of young children, demonstrated decreased vital capacity, decreased forced expiratory flow, decreased total lung capacity, and decreased chest wall compliance consistent with restrictive lung disease pattern [1].

Management Chosen

Given the degree of chest wall deformity, congenital scoliosis, restrictive lung disease, and evidence of deformity progression, surgery was recommended. The decision was made to proceed with a unilateral, left-sided opening wedge thoracostomy with implantation of rib-to-rib and rib-to-spine VEPTR (DePuy Synthes Spine, Raynham, MA) constructs.

Surgical Procedure

VEPTR Insertion

The patient was positioned prone on gel rolls on a Jackson frame (Mizuho OSI, Union City, CA) after induction of

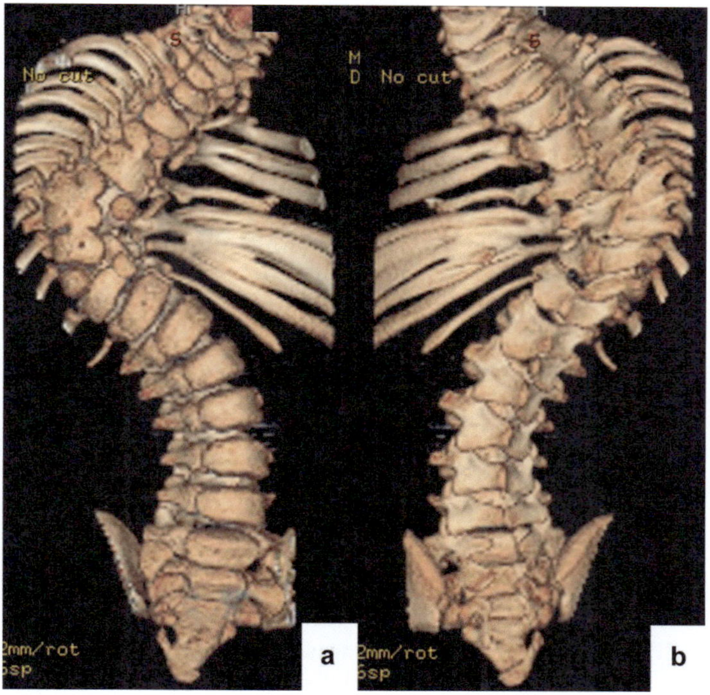

FIGURE 13.3 Anterior (**a**) and posterior (**b**) views of CT three-dimensional reconstructions reveal multiple hemivertebrae and block vertebra throughout the thoracic spine with associated left-sided rib fusions

anesthesia and neuromonitoring. A curvilinear incision was made between the spine and the medial border of the left scapula. The trapezius and rhomboids were split in line with the incision. The paraspinal muscles were elevated lateral to medial to the tips of the transverse processes.

The broad, fused bones of ribs 3 and 4 were subperiosteally exposed, and a proximal VEPTR cradle was placed around these ribs. A lamina spreader was used to distract open the intercostal space caudal to the fourth rib with partial correction of the tilt of the spine. Care was taken to avoid violating the pleura. A second opening wedge thoracostomy was made between ribs 10 and 11. A Kerrison rongeur was used to remove areas of bone fusion between these ribs from anterior to posterior with care and was taken to avoid violating the diaphragm. A rib spreader was utilized to distract open this second thoracotomy with improved spinal correction.

A second incision was made over the planned distal lumbar spine anchor sites. The subcutatneous tissues were dissected and the left-sided paraspinal muscles of the L3 and L4 vertebrae were carefully elevted. A rongeur was used to create an opening in the ligamentum flavum and the channel for the downgoing laminar hooks. These hooks were placed at the L3 and L4 levels.

A 220 mm radius VEPTR lumbar extension rod and rib support construct was sized, cut, and based on the distance between the proximal anchors and the caudal rib cage (in this case size 7). The distal (rod) portion was contoured with valgus and slight lordosis. A Kelly clamp was used to create a subfascial tunnel, and a chest tube was used to shuttle the VEPTR device. The VEPTR was subsequently engaged in the cradle proximally and hooks distally. Distraction was imparted distally to tension the laminar hooks and to further correct the spinal deformity.

At this point, spinal cord monitoring indicated loss of signals from the left upper extremity. In light of these changes, distraction was ceased and the patient's blood pressure was raised. Within 5 min, all signals returned to the left upper extremity.

At this point, it was felt that complete acute correction would not be safely possible, so gentle distraction was reapplied with a goal of achieving approximately 75% of expected correction.

A second VEPTR cradle was placed laterally around the fused bones of ribs 3 and 4. The 11th rib was subperiosteally exposed and prepared for anchor insertion. This rib was chosen because it was thought to be the most distal rib suitable for anchor fixation based on its size and horizontal orientation. A

VEPTR cradle was placed laterally around the 11th rib. 220 mm radius VEPTR proximal and distal extensions were chosen based on the distance between the proximal and distal rib anchors (in this case size 5). These extensions were mated together and inserted into the proximal and distal rib anchors. To prevent a large intercostal gap and associated flail chest at the site of the opening wedge thoracostomy, the middle segment of ribs were centralized and held in place with zero Prolene nonabsorbable suture (Ethicon, Bridgewater, NJ).

After final tightening, the wounds were irrigated copiously. Bone graft was placed over the transverse processes of ribs of attachment, the third and fourth rib, and also over the distal lumbar unilaterally at L3–L4. Skin flaps were gently stretched, and the wounds were closed in layers over drains. Postoperative images are provided in Fig. 13.4. No postoperative complications occurred, and patient had no evidence of neurologic compromise on postoperative examination. He was discharged home on postoperative day 7.

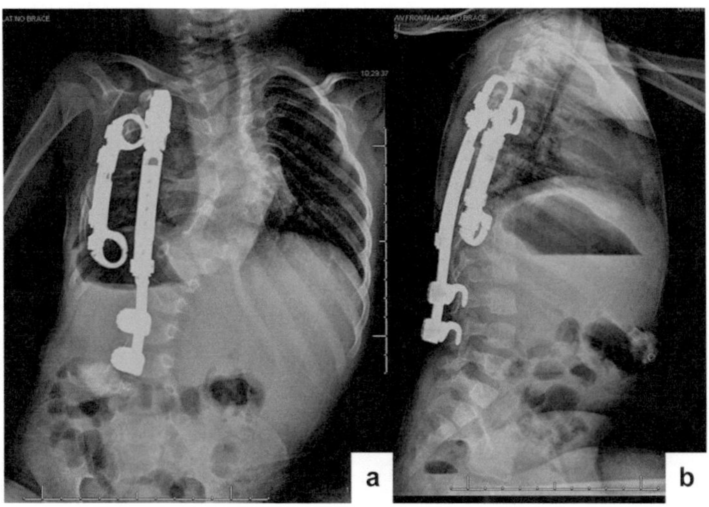

FIGURE 13.4 PA (**a**) and lateral (**b**) radiographs taken days following initial opening wedge thoracostomy and VEPTR implantation

VEPTR Lengthening

Four months after the index implantation procedure, the VEPTR construct was distracted to allow for thoracic growth and continued control of spinal deformity. A repeat lengthening procedure occurred 5 months later. During each lengthening procedure, distraction of 1.0–2.0 cm was accomplished (Fig. 13.5).

VEPTR Exchange

After two lengthening procedures, the initial implants reached full excursion and was scheduled for an exchange of implants.

A longitudinal incision was made through an existing scar over the distal lumbar anchors of the hybrid VEPTR, and both hooks were visualized and loosened. A second incision was made over the distal aspect of the expandable portion of the device. The distraction lock was removed, and then the lumbar extension was uncoupled from the proximal extension and removed. A new, longer distal extension was measured, cut, contoured, and reinserted into the proximal extension sleeve and distal hooks. The distal lumbar hooks tightened into place after distraction was performed.

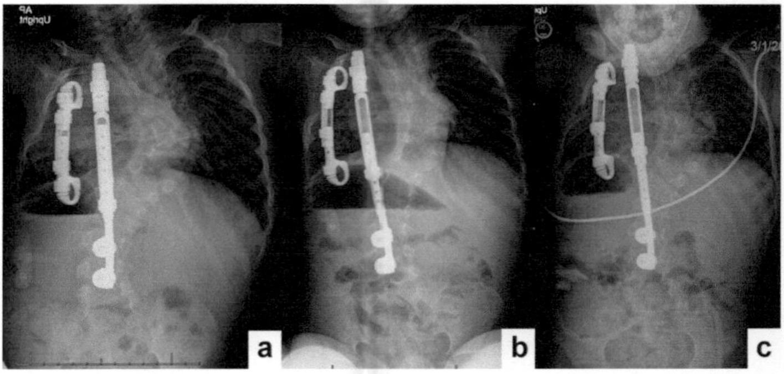

FIGURE 13.5 PA radiographs from before the first distraction (**a**, 4 months following initial surgery), after the first distraction (**b**, 4 months following initial surgery), and after the second distraction (**c**, 9 months following initial surgery)

Next the left rib-to-rib VEPTR was addressed. The device was visualized through the thoracotomy incision, and the distal extension portion was removed and exchanged for a longer, size 7, distal component. Proximal and distal anchors were stable and were unchanged during the revision. The patient tolerated the exchange without complication and was discharged home on postoperative day 4. Postoperative images are provided in Fig. 13.6.

VEPTR Lengthening

Four months after the VEPTR exchange, subsequent lengthening procedures resumed at intervals of every 4–6 months. During each lengthening procedure, distraction of ~0.5 cm

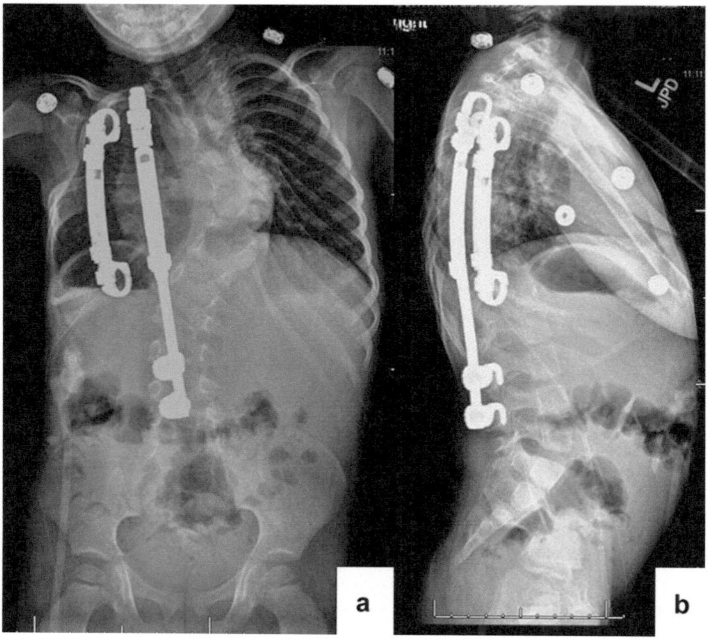

FIGURE 13.6 PA (**a**) and lateral (**b**) radiographs taken following VEPTR device exchange

was accomplished. Average length of stay for lengthening procedures was one night.

Clinical Course and Outcome

The patient tolerated the course of treatment well without any complications or unexpected hospitalizations. Over the course of treatment, the parents noted a subjective improvement in pulmonary function characterized by decreased episodes of tachypnea and a curtailed need for supplemental oxygen.

Radiographs demonstrate interval correction and maintenance of alignment over 5 years of follow-up (Fig. 13.7).

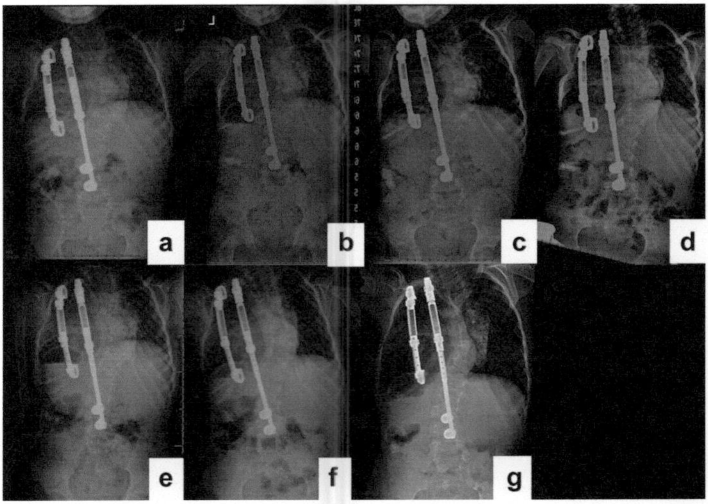

FIGURE 13.7 PA radiographs from before the third distraction (**a**, 19 months following initial surgery), after the fourth distraction (**b**, radiograph taken 26 months following initial surgery), after the fifth distraction (**c**, radiograph taken 32 months following initial surgery), after sixth distraction (**d**, radiograph taken 38 months following initial surgery), after seventh distraction (**e**, radiograph taken 44 months following initial surgery). After eighth distraction (**f**, radiograph taken 50 months following initial surgery), after ninth distraction (**g**, radiograph taken 56 months following initial surgery)

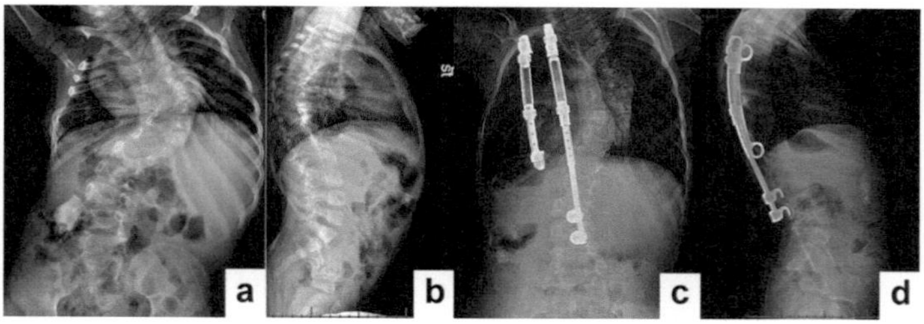

FIGURE 13.8 Preoperative PA (**a**) and lateral radiographs (**b**); PA (**c**) and lateral radiographs (**d**) at most recent follow-up 5 years after initial opening wedge thoracostomy and VEPTR implantation. A total of 7.3 cm in T1–S1 height was gained from pre-initial surgery to most recent follow-up

During the course of treatment and subsequent follow-up, no complications have been noted. At most recent follow-up, a 49° right-sided curve from T2 to T12 and a 23° left-sided curve from T12 to L4 were present.

T1–S1 height gained from pre-initial to final was 7.3 cm (Fig. 13.8), with 6.6 cm gained from post-initial to most recent follow-up. His care plan moving forward will include a planned device removal and reinsertion of new VEPTR devices because he has currently reached the length of his VEPTR implants with no further expansions available. Following device exchange, he will resume continued serial lengthening every 6–9 months with an eventual instrumented fusion near skeletal maturity.

Clinical Pearls and Pitfalls

- Thoracic insufficiency syndrome is the inability of the thorax to support normal or lung growth or respiration.
- Congenital thoracic scoliosis associated with fused ribs may adversely affect thoracic function and growth.
- The goals of treatment in patients with thoracic insufficiency syndrome secondary to congenital chest wall and/or spinal deformities include maximizing thoracic growth,

optimizing pulmonary function, and controlling deformity while minimizing complications.

- Opening wedge thoracostomy lengthens the constricted section of rib cage and hemithorax.
- A rib-to-rib VEPTR device can stabilize an opening wedge thoracostomy.
- A rib-to-spine VEPTR construct is effective in controlling spinal deformity.
- In order to accommodate growth and preserve deformity correction, multiple surgeries, including revisions, are required when VEPTR implantation is performed at a young age.

Literature Review and Discussion

Congenital scoliosis results from developmental defects in vertebral formation. The currently accepted classification system stratifies patients broadly based on the mechanism causing the developmental anomalies (e.g., failure of segmentation, failure of formation, or both) and the morphology of the abnormal vertebrae [2]. Another important factor in congenital scoliosis is the presence or absence of rib abnormalities, in particular fused ribs. More than half of patients with congenital scoliosis have some form of rib abnormalities, and up to 41% have fused ribs [3]. In patients with rib anomalies, the spinal deformity cannot be viewed in isolation; rather attention must be paid to the thorax as a whole.

Thoracic insufficiency syndrome (TIS) is the inability of the thorax to support normal respiration or lung growth and is frequently seen in patients with severe congenital scoliosis and chest wall deformities. Normal respiration requires a minimum volume as well as compliance of the thoracic cavity in order to allow for development of adequate lung tissue and to generate air exchange, respectively. The vertical height of the spine directly affects the volume of the thorax, and allowing for vertical growth of the spine is essential to expanding thoracic volume over time to support growth of normal lung parenchyma. Fused ribs also restrict the width and depth of the thoracic cavity and prevent the chest wall from expanding appropriately. Further reduction in thoracic volume and rib motion can be attributed to the three-dimensional rotational deformity seen in congenital scoliosis with rib anomalies termed as "windswept thorax," contributing to the pattern of extrinsic restrictive lung disease [4].

The developmental disturbances that cause congenital scoliosis occur during weeks 4–6 of gestation. This period is a pivotal time for the development of many organ systems, which helps to explain the numerous developmental abnormalities and associated syndromes common to congenital scoliosis [5]. Thorough examination of patients for extra spinal abnormalities is essential [6]. MRI evaluation of the spine is recommended in patients with congenital scoliosis of the high prevalence of neural axis abnormalities (approximately 21–35%) [3, 7].

As with all forms of scoliosis, the most important factor that will guide treatment is the rate of curve progression. Progression of curves accelerates in a bimodal pattern, with the highest rate of progression before the age of 5 and then again peaking during adolescent growth [8]. In congenital scoliosis, the various morphologies can provide some prognostic information. The spine grows collectively from the individual growth at the superior and inferior end plates of each vertebra [9]. Therefore, anomalies that asymmetrically disturb the formation of a discrete disk complex surrounded by two end plates provide asymmetric growth potential to allow for rapid curve progression. This is best understood by examining the morphology of the congenital scoliosis pattern with the highest rate of progression, a unilateral unsegmented bar with contralateral hemivertebrae [10]. The unilateral bar functions as a focal tether to one side of the spine, while a hemivertebra with two intact end plates has significant potential for growth, causing contralateral convex overgrowth at a high rate. In a similar fashion, fused ribs increase the likelihood of curve progression as they create a lateral tether that anchors two or more levels of the spine providing a rotational point for the contralateral spine and thorax to grow about [4].

Current treatment options include bracing, casting, hemivertebra excision, wedge resection, convex hemiepiphysiodesis, fusionless growing constructs, or fusion [11]. There is no evidence that bracing provides any effective treatment to prevent curve progression in congenital scoliosis as the curves are typically inflexible [5]. Early casting has been shown to effectively delay surgery in patients without chest wall abnormalities and is an alternative to growing instrumentation as a practice to prevent curve progression and delay definitive fusion to allow for longitudinal spine growth. Demirkiran et al. showed in one case series that serial derotational casting was able to delay surgical intervention by 26.3 months in patients with congenital scoliosis without rib abnormalities [12].

Indications for opening thoracostomy and VEPTR in congenital scoliosis include fused ribs or severe thoracic deformity in patients with significant growth remaining. This provides added benefit over spinal instrumentation alone as it allows for expansion of the thoracic cavity, and osteotomy of the fused ribs allows for more correction of the scoliotic deformity [13]. VEPTR placement allows for surgical lengthening of the concave hemithorax which allows for expansion of that constricted hemithorax while also indirectly correcting the scoliotic deformity.

In patients with congenital scoliosis and fused ribs, Campbell has shown continued growth averaging 7.1–7.9 mm per year of the thoracic spine after VEPTR implantation with opening wedge thoracostomy [14, 15]. The percentage of predicted normal vital capacity was also improved and more pronounced in patients who underwent implantation before the age of 2. Prognostication of future respiratory failure in adulthood based off postoperative predicted normal vital capacity in young patients is confounded by many direct and indirect variables, which makes translation of the improved measures into improved outcomes difficult. In addition, an average scoliotic deformity correction of 25° was achieved in this case study.

Implantation of VEPTR at an earlier age is shown to achieve more growth and improved pulmonary function values. Improved results of early intervention are even more pronounced in patients with severe chest wall deformity, which becomes increasingly difficult to reverse with expansion thoracostomy as it progresses. Early implantation may also prevent a compensatory lumbar curve from developing and ultimately shorten the total number of levels that need eventual fusion [15].

Complication rates are very high in surgical management of congenital scoliosis patients, and this is exacerbated by the numerous lengthening and revision surgeries required. Commonly reported complications include migration of the superior cradle through the first rib, acute thoracic outlet syndrome, brachial plexus injury, soft tissue coverage, and wound infections [15]. Despite the high incidence of complications, early opening wedge thoracostomy and VEPTR implantation remain our preferred treatment for patients with congenital scoliosis and associated fused ribs in order to restore thoracic volume and correct spinal deformity while preserving growth.

References

1. Seed L, Wilson D, Coates AL. Children should not be treated like little adults in the PFT lab. Respir Care. 2012;57(1):61–70; discussion 71-74.
2. McMaster MJ, Ohtsuka K. The natural history of congenital scoliosis. A study of two hundred and fifty-one patients. J Bone Joint Surg Am. 1982;64(8):1128–47.
3. Ghandhari H, et al. Vertebral, rib, and intraspinal anomalies in congenital scoliosis: a study on 202 Caucasians. Eur Spine J. 2015;24(7):1510–21.
4. Campbell RM Jr, et al. The characteristics of thoracic insufficiency syndrome associated with fused ribs and congenital scoliosis. J Bone Joint Surg Am. 2003;85-A(3):399–408.
5. Hedequist D, Emans J. Congenital scoliosis. J Am Acad Orthop Surg. 2004;12(4):266–75.

6. Liu YT, et al. A retrospective study of congenital scoliosis and associated cardiac and intraspinal abnormities in a Chinese population. Eur Spine J. 2011;20(12):2111–4.
7. Prahinski JR, et al. Occult intraspinal anomalies in congenital scoliosis. J Pediatr Orthop. 2000;20(1):59–63.
8. Dimeglio A. Growth in pediatric orthopaedics. J Pediatr Orthop. 2001;21(4):549–55.
9. Bick EM, Copel JW. Longitudinal growth of the human vertebra; a contribution to human osteogeny. J Bone Joint Surg Am. 1950;32 A(4):803–14.
10. McMaster MJ. Congenital scoliosis caused by a unilateral failure of vertebral segmentation with contralateral hemivertebrae. Spine (Phila Pa 1976). 1998;23(9):998–1005.
11. Hedequist D, Emans J. Congenital scoliosis: a review and update. J Pediatr Orthop. 2007;27(1):106–16.
12. Demirkiran HG, et al. Serial derotational casting in congenital scoliosis as a time-buying strategy. J Pediatr Orthop. 2015;35(1):43–9.
13. Yazici M, Emans J. Fusionless instrumentation systems for congenital scoliosis: expandable spinal rods and vertical expandable prosthetic titanium rib in the management of congenital spine deformities in the growing child. Spine (Phila Pa 1976). 2009;34(17):1800–7.
14. Campbell RM Jr, Hell-Vocke AK. Growth of the thoracic spine in congenital scoliosis after expansion thoracoplasty. J Bone Joint Surg Am. 2003;85-A(3):409–20.
15. Campbell RM Jr, et al. The effect of opening wedge thoracostomy on thoracic insufficiency syndrome associated with fused ribs and congenital scoliosis. J Bone Joint Surg Am. 2004;86-A(8):1659–74.

Chapter 14 Hemiepiphysiodesis for the Treatment of Congenital Scoliosis

Senol Bekmez and Muharrem Yazici

Case Presentation

History and Physical Examination

This 3.5-year-old female patient presented to the authors' spine clinic with complaints of spine deformity and trunk imbalance. These symptoms were detected soon after she started to ambulate and were noted by her parents to progress within months. According to her mother, she was easily exhausted with physical activity and appeared to be more prone to respiratory tract infections than her peers. Her previous medical history included a spine detethering procedure, performed at age 2 years, due to low conus and tethered cord.

S. Bekmez, MD • M. Yazici, MD (✉)
Department of orthopedics and Traumatology, Cankaya Hospital, Ankara, Turkey
Department of orthopedics and Traumatology, Hacettepe University School of Medicine, Ankara, Turkey
e-mail: drsenolbekmez@gmail.com; mimyazici@gmail.com

R. El-Hawary, C.P. Eberson (eds.), *Early Onset Scoliosis*,
https://doi.org/10.1007/978-3-319-71580-3_14

- Independent ambulator with marked trunk imbalance
- No hairy patch or epidermal lesion over the skin of the posterior lumbar spine
- Left thoracic prominence with elevated left shoulder
- Decreased chest wall compliance greater on the concave side as determined with the thumb excursion test
- Neurologically intact with symmetrical abdominal reflexes, no pathological reflexes, and no spasticity

Diagnostic Studies

- Standing posteroanterior and lateral radiographs demonstrated left thoracic scoliosis with multiple anomalies of formation and segmentation in the thoracic vertebrae. In addition, multiple rib anomalies including rib fusions were detected (Fig. 14.1).
- The magnitude of the main curve (T5–T11 Cobb angle) was 57°.
- T2–T12 kyphosis angle was 32°. A local hypokyphosis of 8° was noted between T5 and T10.
- Computed tomography with 3D reconstruction of the entire spine revealed multiple anomalies of formation and segmentation with multiple rib anomalies between T1 and T12. An unsegmented bar was also noted in the concave side (Fig. 14.2).
- A low conus medullaris was reported on magnetic resonance imaging (MRI) of the spine (Fig. 14.3).
- Echocardiography and ultrasound examination of the urogenital systems were both unremarkable for associated congenital anomalies.

Management Chosen

Although bracing has not been found to be reliably effective in congenital scoliosis, it was utilized as a first step in treatment, with hopes to achieve a delay in surgery. As there was a 15° increase in deformity within 1 year, bracing treatment was abandoned (Fig. 14.1). At this time, the

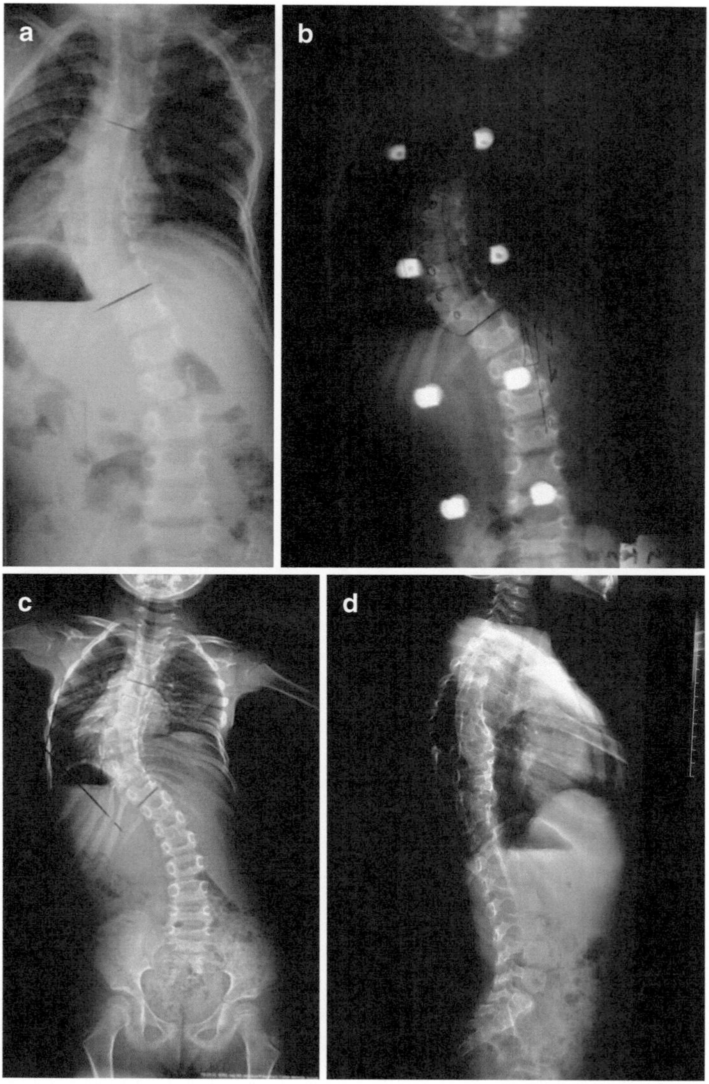

FIGURE 14.1 Standing posteroanterior radiograph revealed congenital scoliosis with multiple formation and segmentation anomalies (**a**). Bracing treatment was attempted (**b**), but it was then abandoned after 1 year, as a 15° increase in deformity magnitude was documented (**c**). Preoperative lateral radiograph (**d**)

patient met indications for surgical treatment due to marked deformity progression with associated trunk imbalance that could in the future diminish cardiopulmonary function.

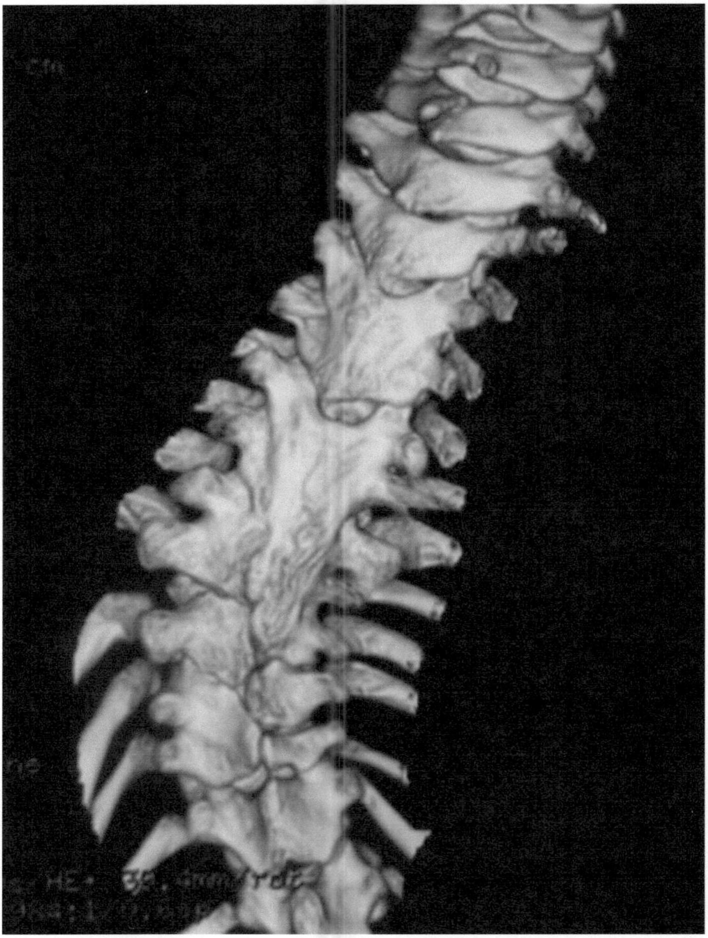

FIGURE 14.2 Computed tomography with 3D reconstruction of the whole spine is essential to understand the pathologic anatomy in detail

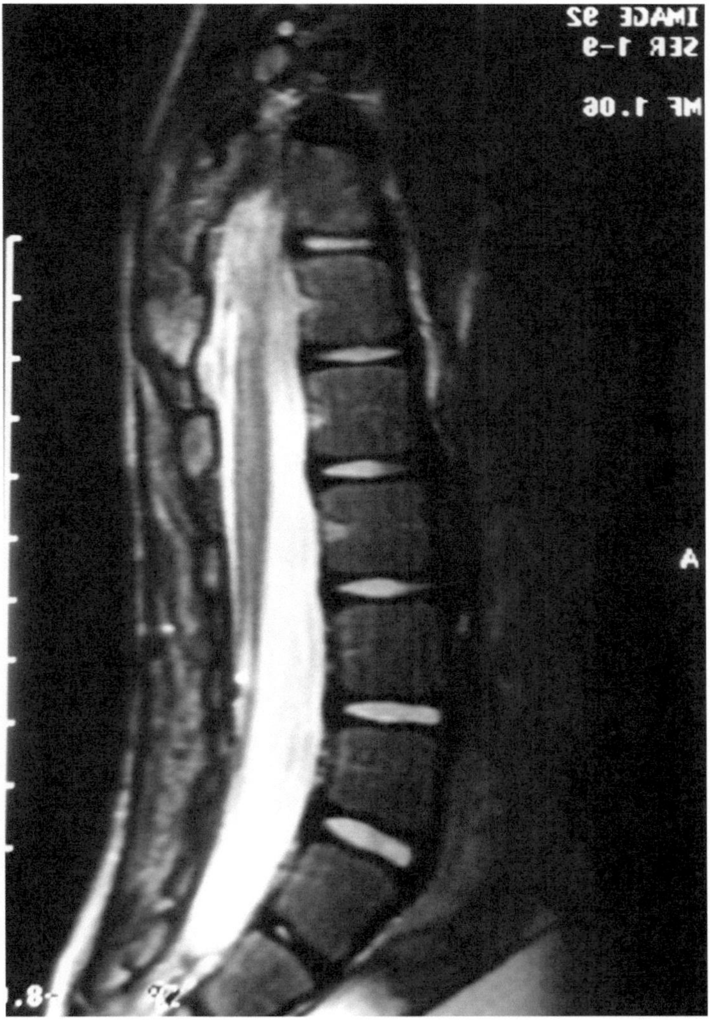

FIGURE 14.3 Magnetic resonance imaging revealed low conus medullaris

In congenital early-onset scoliosis, definitive fusion for such a long sweeping thoracic deformity should be avoided as it may result in the loss of growth potential of the thoracic spine and, consequently, the lungs. Hemivertebrectomy and limited fusion are reasonable alternatives in cases of solitary vertebral formation anomaly. However, in this patient, there were multiple formation and segmentation anomalies involving a long thoracic segment. For this patient, the treatment goal was to achieve deformity correction and maintain spinal alignment while preserving growth. Thus, the preferred method was modulation of spinal growth with posterior instrumented convex hemiepiphysiodesis with distraction of the concave side with a growing rod construct. The specific indications for convex growth arrest (CGA) are (1) early-onset congenital scoliosis in children less than 10 years of age, (2) congenital anomalies involving more than four consecutive thoracic segments, (3) deformity progression of more than 10° per year, and (4) no thoracic insufficiency syndrome.

Surgical Procedure

Intraoperative neuromonitoring was utilized to assess the status of the spinal cord during surgery. Under general anesthesia, the patient was positioned prone, and a straight midline incision was utilized. As a general principle, at the convex side, both cranial and caudal end vertebrae are included in the instrumented fusion. Subperiosteal exposure was performed between T6 and T11 on the convex side, while the concave side was not exposed. After decortication and facetectomy, pedicle screws were inserted into preoperatively determined levels on the convex side and a single rod employed to connect them. Deformity was corrected as much as possible with derotation, compression, and distraction maneuvers. On the concave side, pedicle screws were placed in T2, T3, L2, and L3 in a submuscular fashion. The growing rod construct was completed with two rods and a connector between them (Fig. 14.4).

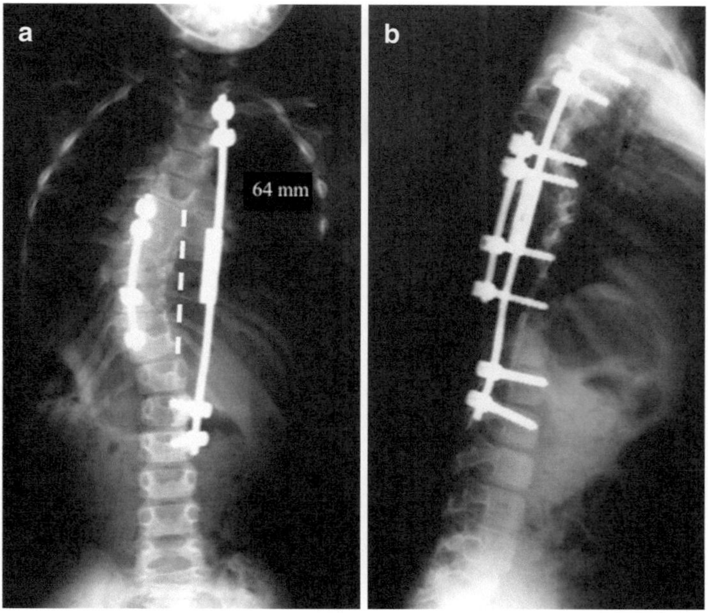

FIGURE 14.4 Early postoperative posteroanterior (**a**) and lateral (**b**) radiographs of the patient after all-posterior instrumented CGA and concave distraction were performed. Please note that the height of unsegmented bar is 64 mm (**a**)

Clinical Course and Outcome

- A custom-made thoracolumbosacral orthosis was used in the postoperative period for 3 months.
- Lengthening of the concave side was routinely performed every 6 months for a total of 10 lengthening procedures during the follow-up of 72 months.
- After index operation, the magnitude of the deformity in the convex instrumented segment was reduced from 57° to 39°.
- After 72-month follow-up, the magnitude of deformity was further decreased to 28° (Fig. 14.5).
- T2–T12 kyphosis was 32° preoperatively, 26° after index operation, and 28° at the last follow-up. The segmental

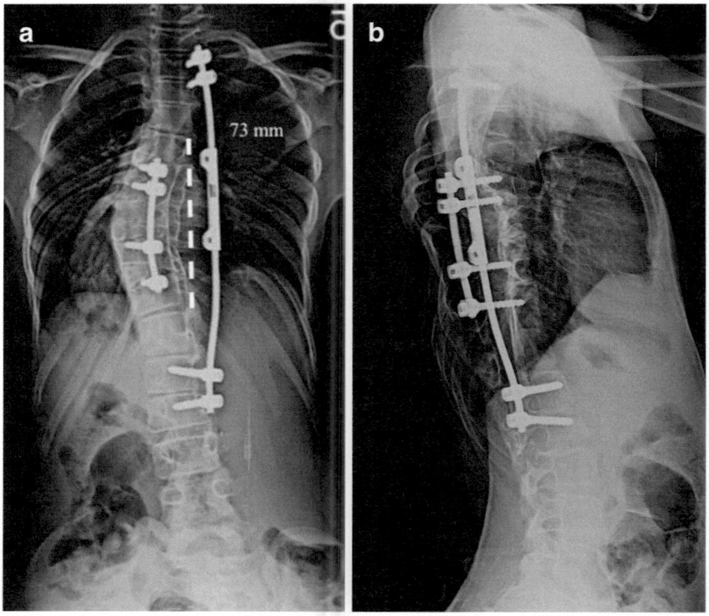

FIGURE 14.5 Posteroanterior (**a**) and lateral (**b**) radiographs of the patient at last follow-up. Please note that deformity was further reduced with growth modulation in the convex side and distraction in the concave side. Please note that the height of unsegmented bar is 73 mm (**a**)

kyphosis between T5 and T10 was 8° preoperatively and 11° at the latest follow-up.

- T1–T12 length of 181 mm after the index operation increased to 213 mm (5.3 mm/year) at the latest follow-up.
- T1–S1 length was 230 mm after the index operation and 290 mm at the latest follow-up (10 mm/year).
- The length of the unsegmented bar in the concave side was 64 mm after the index operation and 73 mm at the latest follow-up (1.5 mm/year).
- No significant complication or unplanned surgery occurred during follow-up.

Clinical Pearls and Pitfalls

- Long sweeping congenital curves including more than four vertebrae are good candidates for CGA and concave distraction treatment.
- Instrumented CGA should include most tilted vertebrae above and below.
- Selection of the distal instrumentation level for the concave growing rod is based upon the stable-to-be vertebra on the supine traction radiograph under general anesthesia.
- Submuscular placement of the growing rod and multilayer closure in both index and lengthening procedures are essential to avoid wound-related complications.
- Regular lengthening procedures of the concave distraction rod are performed at 6–9-month intervals.

Literature Review and Discussion

The rationale behind the CGA procedure is to modulate growth with inhibition on the convex side while allowing growth to continue on the concave side [1]. Its role in the treatment of early-onset congenital scoliosis has been a topic of debate because of previously reported unpredictable results. In the traditional CGA technique, an effective deformity correction is dependent upon the growth potential of the concave side, which is very difficult to assess preoperatively. The traditional technique with the combined anterior and posterior approach has reported failure rates ranging from 8 to 21% [2, 3]. In addition, immediate deformity correction is not possible in non-instrumented procedures (Fig. 14.6).

The instrumented all-posterior CGA technique has been introduced to minimize the unpredictability of the traditional technique (Fig. 14.7). With this modification, pedicle screw instrumentation on the convex side should provide both anterior and posterior growth arrest without the need for

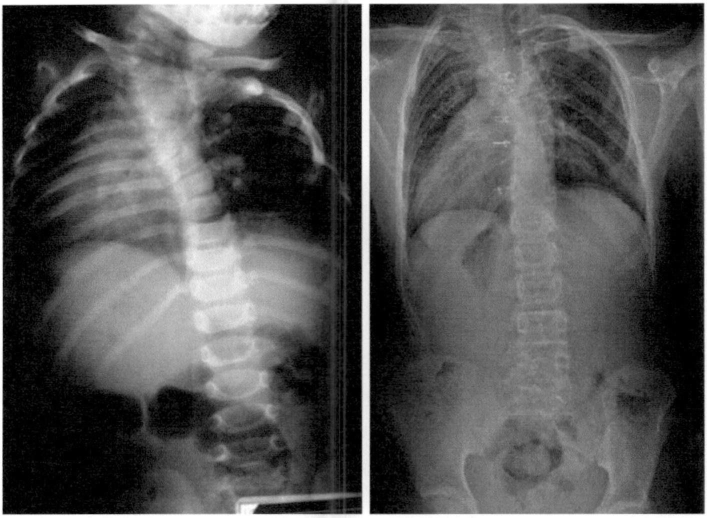

FIGURE 14.6 An example for traditional combined anterior and posterior CGA technique. Please note the gradual correction of the spine deformity after 2 years follow-up. Immediate deformity correction is not possible in the traditional technique

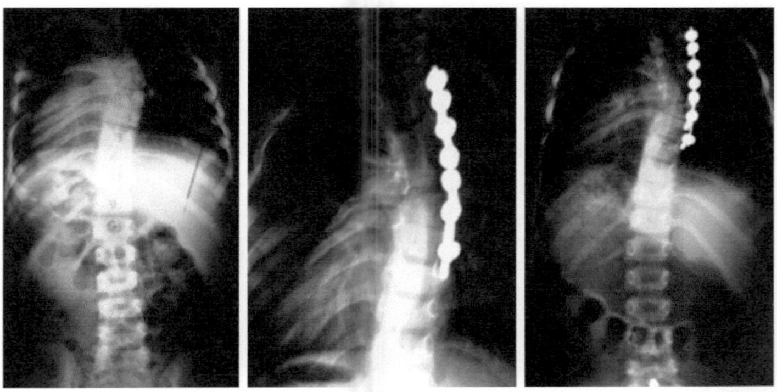

FIGURE 14.7 Another option is the instrumented all-posterior CGA technique. Immediate deformity correction was further improved with growth modulation

anterior surgery. Experimental studies have previously demonstrated that both anterior and posterior vertebral growth can be overpowered with application of posterior instrumented fusion using transpedicular screws and a rod [4, 5]. Another advantage offered by this modification is immediate deformity correction with the effect of instrumentation in addition to gradual correction achieved with the hemiepiphysiodesis effect. Demirkiran et al. [6] reported their experience on instrumented CGA technique in 13 patients with long sweeping congenital scoliosis. According to their results, an average preoperative curve magnitude of 49° was reduced to 38° after the surgical procedure, which was then further reduced to 33.5° after 5 years. They also reported significant improvements in both concave height and T1–T12 height.

The concept of adding concave distraction was initially introduced by Cheung et al. [7], who described using a single Harrington rod and hook construct in addition to a traditional anterior and posterior CGA. Concave distraction produced immediately better coronal balance and decreased the unpredictability of growth modulation achieved by CGA alone.

The instrumented CGA technique has been further modified by adding a concave growing rod construct [8]. In their series of 11 patients with 44.9-month follow-up, Demirkiran et al. [9] reported that segment with CGA was corrected from 60.5 to 40.4° initially and then further improved to 35.5° with growth. The distracted side was corrected from 33.4° to 15.2° initially and then further reduced to 12.7° at the last follow-up. In addition, they noted a 6.4 mm per year increase in T1–T12 height. The authors concluded that the addition of concave growing rods improved curve correction, provided better trunk balance, and stimulated spinal growth without causing any unplanned surgery.

In our case, the average convex instrumented curve magnitude was 57° preoperatively, 42° postoperatively, and 34° at the latest follow-up. The initial correction of the deformity was secondary to intraoperative correction related to the instrumentation, whereas continued improvement can be attributed to the growth modulation effect. The measurements in the sagittal plane remained stable after index surgery and during follow-up.

We noted a 5.3 mm per year increase in thoracic height (T1–T12) that was comparable with a reported 5.2 mm per year increase in congenital scoliosis patients treated with VEPTR [10]. However, this growth rate was still lower than the normative data of healthy children, which was reported as 9.3 mm per year by Dimeglio et al. [11]. In addition, we also noted a 10 mm per year increase in T1–S1 length which was comparable with a reported 11.7 mm per year increase in congenital scoliosis patients treated with dual spine-based growing rods [12].

The height of the unsegmented bar in the concave side increased by 1.5 mm per year during follow-up. Growth of the unsegmented bar in congenital scoliosis patients treated with expansion thoracoplasty has been previously established by Campbell et al. [13]. They reported a 1.1 mm per year increase in length during the follow-up period. The growth that we observed in the unsegmented bar is not consistent with previous reports that unsegmented bars have no growth potential. This phenomenon of growth in the absence of a discernible growth plate may be attributed to appositional bone growth caused by distraction of the concave side. The underlying mechanism for the growth in the unsegmented bar remains unclear and should be further investigated.

A disadvantage of this technique is the necessity for recurrent lengthening procedures on the concave side. To avoid the morbidity caused by recurrent general anesthesia and surgery, magnetically controlled growing rods may be used as a reasonable alternative (Fig. 14.8).

In conclusion, instrumented CGA combined with concave distraction is a reliable treatment option in long sweeping curves of congenital scoliosis. With this technique, it is possible to achieve both an effective immediate and continued gradual deformity correction while allowing for growth of the spine and thorax.

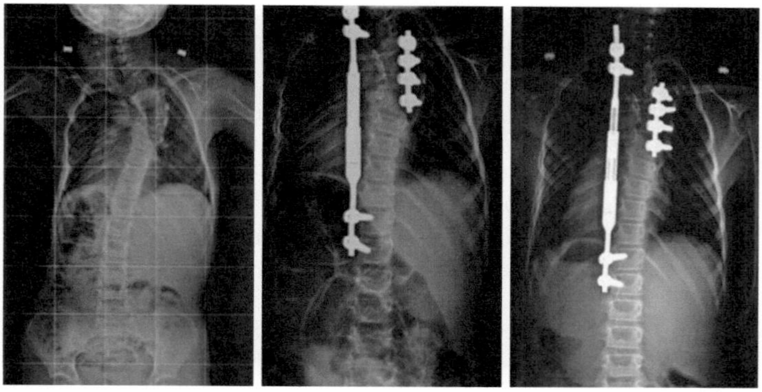

FIGURE 14.8 Using a magnetically controlled device in concave distraction avoids multiple lengthening surgeries throughout growth

References

1. Uzumcugil A, Cil A, Yazici M, et al. Convex growth arrest in the treatment of congenital spinal deformities, revisited. J Pediatr Orthop. 2004;24:658–66.
2. Andrew T, Piggott H. Growth arrest for progressive scoliosis. Combined anterior and posterior fusion of the convexity. J Bone Joint Surg Br. 1985;67:193–7.
3. Kieffer J, Dubousset J. Combined anterior and posterior convex epiphysiodesis for progressive congenital scoliosis in children aged < or=5 years. Eur Spine J. 1994;3:120–5.
4. Kioschos HC, Asher MA, Lark RG, et al. Overpowering the crankshaft mechanism. The effect of posterior spinal fusion with and without stiff transpedicular fixation on anterior spinal column growth in immature canines. Spine (Phila Pa 1976). 1996;21:1168–73.
5. Bekmez S, Demirkiran HG, Yilmaz G, et al. Convex hemiepiphysiodesis: posterior/anterior in-situ versus posterior-only with pedicle screw instrumentation: an experimental simulation in immature pigs. J Pediatr Orthop. 2016;36(8):847–52.
6. Demirkiran G, Yilmaz G, Kaymaz B, et al. Safety and efficacy of instrumented convex growth arrest in treatment of congenital scoliosis. J Pediatr Orthop. 2014;34:275–81.

7. Cheung KM, Zhang JG, Lu DS, et al. Ten-year follow-up study of lower thoracic hemivertebrae treated by convex fusion and concave distraction. Spine. 2002;27:748–53.
8. Alanay A, Dede O, Yazici M. Convex instrumented hemiepiphysiodesis with concave distraction: a preliminary report. Clin Orthop Relat Res. 2012;470(4):1144–50.
9. Demirkiran HG, Dede O, Ayvaz M, et al. Convex instrumented hemiepiphysiodesis with concave distraction: a treatment option for long sweeping congenital curves. J Pediatr Orthop. 2016;36(8):847–52.
10. Murphy RF, Moisan A, Kelly DM, et al. Use of vertical expandable prosthetic titanium rib (VEPTR) in the treatment of congenital scoliosis without fused ribs. J Pediatr Orthop. 2016;36(4):329–35.
11. DiMeglio A, Canavese F, Charles YP. Growth and adolescent idiopathic scoliosis: when and how much. J Pediatr Orthop. 2011;21:28–36.
12. Elsebai HB, Yazici M, Thompson GH, et al. Safety and efficacy of growing rod technique for pediatric congenital spinal deformities. J Pediatr Orthop. 2011;31(1):1–5.
13. Campbell RM, Hell-Vocke AK. Growth of the thoracic spine in congenital scoliosis after expansion thoracoplasty. J Bone Joint Surg Am. 2003;85(3):409–20.

Chapter 15
Congenital Myopathy with Early-Onset Scoliosis

Mark C. Lee and Craig P. Eberson

Case Presentation

History and Physical Examination

The patient initially presented as a 4-year-old girl with nemaline myopathy, a rare, heritable, progressive disorder of skeletal muscles of varying clinical severity. The patient was non-ambulatory and had significant pulmonary impairment, requiring ventilator support via tracheostomy, and used a G-tube for nourishment as a result of dysphagia and intolerance for oral feeds. She demonstrated grossly delayed motor milestones. In follow-up, the patient developed a progressive thoracolumbar scoliosis that interfered with general seating and could not be managed with seating modification or bracing (Fig. 15.1).

M.C. Lee, MD • C.P. Eberson, MD (✉)
Department of orthopedic Surgery, Connecticut Children's, Hartford, CT, USA
Department of Orthopedic Surgery, Brown University/Hasbro Children's Hospital, Providence, RI, USA
e-mail: mlee01@connecticutchildrens.org; Craig_P_Eberson@Brown.edu

R. El-Hawary, C.P. Eberson (eds.), *Early Onset Scoliosis*,
https://doi.org/10.1007/978-3-319-71580-3_15

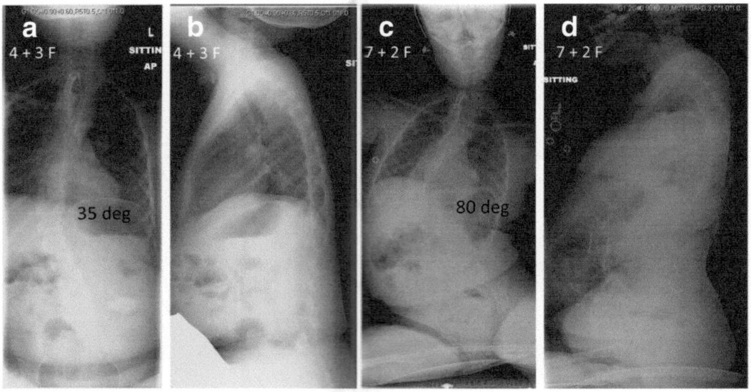

FIGURE 15.1 PA sitting (**a**) and lateral sitting (**b**) radiographs demonstrating an apex right thoracolumbar curve of 35° without significant pelvic obliquity. Over the course of 2 years, repeat PA sitting (**c**) and lateral sitting (**d**) radiographs demonstrate progression of the thoracolumbar curve to 80°. Overall sagittal profile demonstrates mild increase in thoracic kyphosis from 42 to 60°

The patient was dysarthric but communicative via gestures. Note was made of diffuse hypotonia and absent upper and lower extremity reflexes. Bilateral lower extremity equinus contractures were identified. Sensation was intact throughout with limited, but present, volitional movement of the extremities. The patient had a large right thoracolumbar fullness with a marked left-sided waist crease. Significant trunk shift to the right was noted with supported sitting. The skin along the back and the sacrum was intact throughout.

Diagnostic Studies

Radiographic evaluation with the patient in supported sitting demonstrated a right thoracolumbar curve that progressed from 35 to 80° over the course of 3 years. The patient was supported with soft bracing and chair modifications and remained comfortable. Clinical exam confirmed that with gentle support under the arms, the patient's pelvic obliquity was flexible and could be easily corrected. As the curve reached a larger magnitude, traction films were obtained and confirmed that the obliquity was beginning to show signs of losing flexibility (Fig. 15.1). With supine traction, the curve was reduced to 40° (Fig. 15.2). The patient's pelvic obliquity was 40° and reduced to 10° with traction. Because of the curve magnitude and flexibility, surgical management was chosen in order to obtain a level pelvis and support sitting and respiration.

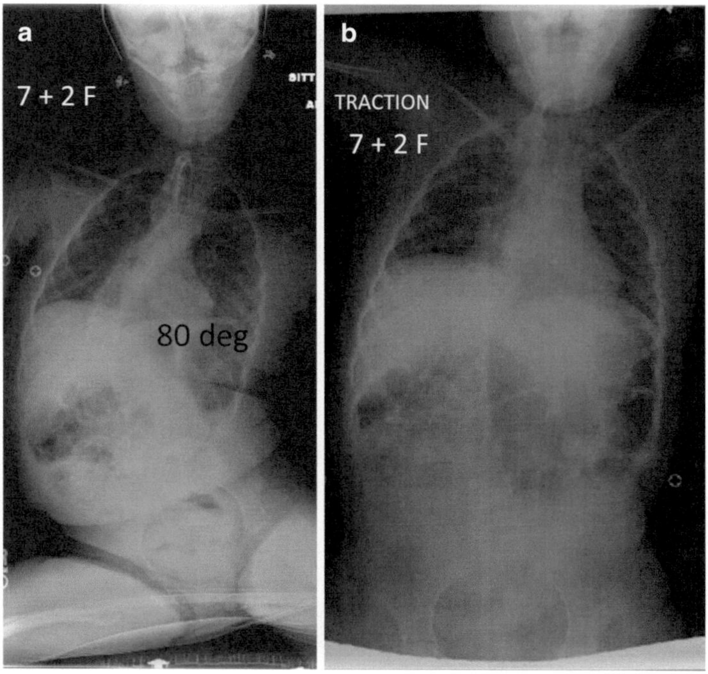

FIGURE 15.2 Supine AP traction radiographs taken in the preoperative period. The traction film demonstrates correction of the scoliosis from 80 to 40°

Management Chosen

The patient underwent growing rod insertion with a pelvis-to-rib construct, with the goal of maintaining pulmonary function while controlling scoliosis progression. Such a construct has the theoretical advantage of avoiding midline dissection over the spine and may impact lung volumes more directly via interaction with the ribs, preventing the so-called collapsing parasol effect seen when using spine-based distraction techniques. Avoiding fusion of the anchor vertebrae may also have the potential benefit of minimizing any effects on the growth of the thoracic cage secondary to upper thoracic fusion. In addition, the relatively anterior placement of the construct may counteract the collapsing kyphosis of muscular disease, when compared to a construct centered on the spine. No preoperative traction was utilized. To minimize anesthetic episodes, the lengthening interval chosen was 9 months, rather than the standard 6 months for idiopathic EOS. As a result, the growing rod construct was subsequently distracted two times over the following 2 years.

Surgical Procedure

First Step: Insertion of Bilateral Pelvis-to-Rib Growing Rod Construct

The patient was placed prone on a radiolucent operating room table. Intraoperative neuromonitoring was established with transcranial motor evoked potentials and somatosensory evoked potentials. An arterial line was placed and a Foley catheter was inserted. No intraoperative traction was utilized, although we have found this helpful for larger or stiffer curves.

A midline incision was made along the upper thoracic spine, and the fascia over the trapezius, just lateral to transverse processes, was split longitudinally, elevating the trapezius and rhomboid muscles in a flap that could be used to cover the hooks. The erector spinae muscles, immediately below the rhomboid muscles, were elevated from lateral to medial to expose the ribs. Ribs on both sides corresponding to the T2, T3, and T4 vertebral bodies were then identified and circumferentially elevated. Rib cradles were then placed along the ribs bilaterally.

A longitudinal incision was then made over the left ilium, and the dissection extended to the fascia. The soft spot just lateral to the longitudinal spinal erectors was developed. The ilium was then partly exposed and an iliac cradle was applied. A short 5.5 mm titanium rod was then contoured into lordosis and attached to the ilium cradle. The same procedure was performed from the right ilium.

A 4.75 mm titanium rod to be placed into the distal end of the sliding sleeve was then measured for appropriate length. The length accounted for the length of the sliding sleeve as well as the distance from the distal end of the sleeve to the iliac cradle. The rod was then contoured to the appropriate lordosis, inserted into the sliding sleeve, and locked in position with a set screw. Another 4.75 mm titanium rod was then cut to a length that spanned the distance from the upper thoracic rib cradles to the proximal 3 cm of the sliding sleeve and contoured to a desired upper thoracic kyphosis. The 4.75 mm rod was then placed into the proximal end of the lengthening sleeve and locked into the lengthening sleeve with a set screw. A distraction ring was fit onto the 4.75 mm rod just distal to the sliding sleeve. The set screws along the proximal portion of the sliding sleeve and sliding ring were tightened to the final torque. The spine was manually corrected in order to estimate the length of the rods to be inserted.

A long Schnidt was then placed from the proximal incision submuscularly to the left ilium incision, and a chest tube was grasped. The chest tube was pulled into the proximal wound, and the rod-sliding sleeve construct was then passed using the chest tube as a guide. We often use this chest tube as a length template, placing it over the anchors to estimate the length of the assembled construct that will be inserted. The proximal 4.75 mm rod was then seated into the left rib anchors, and the distal rod was joined to the 5.5 mm rod associated with the iliac cradle via a rod-to-rod connector. Distraction was then performed distally where the 4.75 mm rod joined the rod-to-rod connector in order to seat the pelvic saddle, beginning on the concavity of the curve. A similar procedure was repeated for the opposite side. The rod-to-rod connectors were finally tightened (Fig. 15.3).

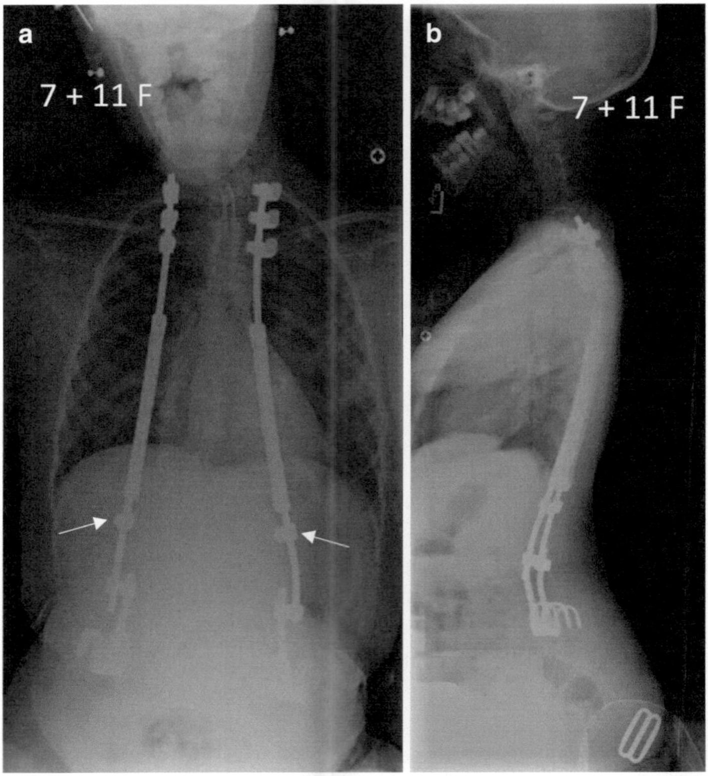

FIGURE 15.3 PA sitting (**a**) and lateral sitting (**b**) radiographs taken 8 months after the index surgery demonstrating a bilateral pelvis-to-rib construct with rib cradles and iliac cradles. Note the rod-to-rod connector distally between the sleeve/rod construct and the iliac cradle. The scoliosis has decreased to [20]. An excellent sagittal profile was achieved

Following copious irrigation, the proximal wound was closed in layers, taking care to re-approximate the trapezius and its associated fascia such that the implants were completely covered. Neuromonitoring remained stable throughout the procedure and no complications occurred.

Subsequent Steps: Growing Rod Distraction

The growing rod construct was distracted serially to allow for patient growth. A small incision was made over the interval between the distraction ring and the lengthening sleeve each time, with loosening and tightening of the sleeve-associated set screw. The first lengthening took place 9 months after the index procedure and the second 11 months after the first lengthening. An attempt was made to space the lengthenings 9 months apart in light of the tenuous medical status of the patient and the inherent risks of repeated anesthesia and repeated surgery. Each lengthening is achieved between 15 mm and 18 mm, with a focus on distracting more along the concavity (Fig. 15.4).

Clinical Course and Outcome

The patient was admitted to the intensive care unit for aggressive pulmonary care and then discharged 4 days after the initial surgical intervention to home without complication. She was evaluated 1 month after the index surgery and subsequently underwent two lengthening procedures, with a follow-up of 2 years. The patient experienced no medical or surgical complications during follow-up. The most recent radiographs obtained 3 years after the index procedure and 6 months after the last lengthening demonstrate well-controlled scoliosis with a stable coronal and sagittal profile (Fig. 15.4). There is no evidence of implant failure. Pelvic obliquity was 10°.

Clinical Pearls and Pitfalls

- Direct rib engagement simplifies proximal fixation and avoids a midline dissection to allow for upper thoracic

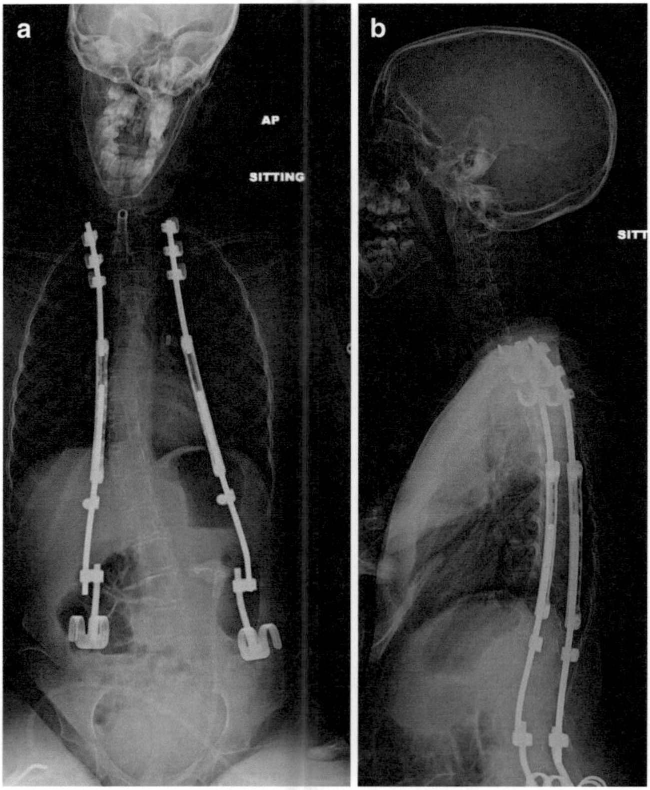

FIGURE 15.4 PA sitting (**a**) and lateral sitting (**b**) radiographs following three distractions. Note the overall maintenance of the thoracolumbar scoliosis with preservation of pelvic obliquity and sagittal profile

spine growth and decrease the complexity of future midline surgeries.

- Using at least five anchors has been shown to decrease the risk of proximal hardware failure (VITALE, SRS 2015).
- Intraoperative neuromonitoring is advised for the rib-to-pelvis construct described, despite performing a procedure that is thought to be generally lateral to the spine.
- The interval between growing rod lengthenings can be increased to potentially minimize perioperative complications over the course of treatment.

- Attention should be directed to preoperative/postoperative cardiac and pulmonary optimization, as these systems are frequently compromised in patients with myopathy. All of our patients are followed closely by a pediatric pulmonologist, so that any precipitous decrease in parameters can be identified and correlated with changes in spine alignment. Pulmonary care tailored to children with muscle disorders is an important step in assuring smooth recovery. Preoperative cardiac exam often reveals subclinical decreases in cardiac function, which are crucial factors in the anesthesia plan. An experienced anesthesia team is mandatory to prevent intraoperative compromise.
- Rib cage support with rib fixation may preserve pulmonary function better than spine-based implants, although respiratory muscle weakness also plays a role, and the ability of the "Eiffel Tower" construct, with or without outriggers, to prevent respiratory decline remains unclear.
- For patients with spinal muscle atrophy, avoiding fusion to permit intrathecal injection of medication is crucial.

Literature Review and Discussion

Nemaline myopathy is a member of the congenital myopathies, a group of rare, heritable muscle-based disorders with an overall incidence of 1:22,480–1:135,000 [1, 2]. The disease group presents in infancy as diffuse hypotonia with symmetrical skeletal muscle weakness. Congenital myopathies are distinguished by static muscle architecture over time, as it is absent in the cycles of progressive muscle necrosis and replacement seen in dystrophies. However, the disease process is often clinically progressive, with insidious onset of pulmonary failure and loss of ambulation [3]. In addition to cardiac and pulmonary involvement seen in most congenital myopathies, nemaline myopathy is notable among myopathies for a 60% prevalence of progressive kyphoscoliosis [4]. The case presented is therefore a useful archetype of the general management of early-onset scoliosis in myopathy. Due to new advances in treatment of other related conditions, such as spinal muscle atrophy, which now has an FDA-approved intrathecal treatment available, the ability to manage these patient's deformities in a fusionless model may even be more important to preserve function while avoiding definitive surgery.

Prior to surgical intervention, attention should be given to the perioperative details of patient management to minimize additional surgical morbidity and mortality. Surgical complication rates for neuromuscular patients are far greater than that for patients with idiopathic deformity. A meta-analysis of 15,218 neuromuscular patients noted a 22.7% rate of pulmonary complications, 12.5% of instrumentation complications, and 3% rate of neurological complications [5]. Growing rod constructs appear to be particularly prone to infection in light of repeated surgeries for lengthening, with a deep wound infection rate of up to 30% [6].

Myopathy patients undergoing surgical management for spinal deformity may experience acute perioperative decompensation of pulmonary and cardiac function [7]. Therefore, thorough preoperative evaluation is required along with the need for collaborative management by multiple medical services in the postoperative period. Avoidance of volatile inhalational anesthetics or depolarizing muscle relaxants is generally recommended for this disease category to guard against the propensity for malignant hyperthermia [8]. An aggressive pain control and respiratory therapy program is required postoperatively to optimize pulmonary function in a patient with acute chest wall discomfort and intrinsically compromised voluntary and involuntary respiratory function. In addition, care should be taken to optimize the patient's nutritional status both before and after surgery in order to minimize wound complications or related skin pressure ulceration [9].

Multiple growth-friendly options are theoretically available for management of early-onset scoliosis in the myopathic neuromuscular population, inclusive of VEPTR (vertical expandable prosthetic titanium rib), growing rods, SHILLA technique, and others [10–14].

The case illustrates the use of an “Eiffel Tower” (EF) construct for management of neuromuscular scoliosis. The design is an extension of the VEPTR instrumentation concept to patients with neuromuscular deformity without primary rib abnormalities [15, 16]. The instrumentation is placed via three or four small incisions and utilizes rib fixation proximally and iliac fixation distally. The reported advantages of this construct include (1) avoidance of a midline dissection of the spine to decrease the likelihood of iatrogenic fusion and to preserve bony architecture for future surgeries, (2) use of a limited dissection to minimize wound complications, (3) direct control of the rib cage for theoretical gains in preserving pulmonary volumes, and (4) relatively anterior placement of instrumentation to counteract the progressive kyphotic tendency of the spine. The EF construct appears to demonstrate an efficacy and complication rate comparable to traditional growing rods, with an average major scoliosis improvement of between 29 and 40% and a complication rate of 10–15% with each intervention [15, 17, 18]. Clear advantages of avoiding a midline spine dissection with this technique are noted in the early-onset myelomeningocele population [19].

The advent of magnetically controlled growing rods (MCGR) may ultimately help to improve the overall complication rates in manual distraction posterior instrumentation constructs by obviating the need for repeated surgical intervention. However, recent studies have suggested that revision rates remain high for patients at 4 years after MCGR implantation and that there may be discordance between lengthening rates reported by the device versus that which is objectively measured on imaging [20, 21]. Additional study is necessary to understand the clinical impact of remotely lengthened growing rods in the neuromuscular population.

Several limitations to the Eiffel Tower construct exist. Smith et al. found that ambulatory neuromuscular patients who received this pelvis-to-rib construct might develop decrements to their baseline ambulation, such as progressive crouch [15]. Therefore, this instrumentation technique should generally be limited to non-ambulatory patients with neuromuscular scoliosis. Additional shortcomings of this approach are common to all growth-friendly, posterior distraction implants, specifically the risks of perioperative or postoperative complications with each surgical distraction procedure, alterations in sagittal balance, and potential for spine auto-fusion despite avoidance of a midline dissection [22, 23].

The surgical management of neuromuscular scoliosis in myopathy has the potential to contribute significantly to the quality of life of a patient. Effective surgical interventions may result in the subjective and objective improvement in pulmonary parameters and can allow for a more stable, upright sitting, which has the benefit of facilitating engagement with the world, caretaker ease, and use of the upper extremity for activities other than trunk support. However, it is helpful to understand that most myopathy patients can be managed conservatively with either observation, wheelchair modifications, or bracing support for early-onset scoliosis. A natural history cohort study of 125 patients with congenital myopathy noted that only 13.6% required surgery for early-onset scoliosis [3]. When considering the high rate of complications from any surgical intervention in this population, it behooves the surgeon to weigh carefully the risks and benefits of the intervention and to undertake a frank discussion with the caretakers regarding surgical goals and known success rates.

References

1. Darin N, Tulinius M. Neuromuscular disorders in childhood: a descriptive epidemiological study from western Sweden. Neuromuscul Disord. 2000;10(1):1–9. http://www.ncbi.nlm.nih.gov/pubmed/10677857.
2. Norwood FLM, Harling C, Chinnery PF, Eagle M, Bushby K, Straub V. Prevalence of genetic muscle disease in Northern England: in-depth analysis of a muscle clinic population. Brain. 2009;132(Pt 11):3175–86. https://doi.org/10.1093/brain/awp236.
3. Colombo I, Scoto M, Manzur AY, et al. Congenital myopathies: natural history of a large pediatric cohort. Neurology. 2015;84(1):28–35. https://doi.org/10.1212/WNL.0000000000001110.

4. Nagai T, Tsuchiya Y, Maruyama A, Takemitsu M, Nonaka I. Scoliosis associated with central core disease. Brain and Development. 1994;16(2):150–2.
5. Sharma S, Wu C, Andersen T, Wang Y, Hansen ES, Bünger CE. Prevalence of complications in neuromuscular scoliosis surgery: a literature meta-analysis from the past 15 years. Eur Spine J. 2013;22(6):1230–49. https://doi.org/10.1007/s00586-012-2542-2.
6. McElroy MJ, Sponseller PD, Dattilo JR, et al. Growing rods for the treatment of scoliosis in children with cerebral palsy: a critical assessment. Spine (Phila Pa 1976). 2012;37(24):E1504–10. https://doi.org/10.1097/BRS.0b013e31826fabd3.
7. North KN, Ryan MM. Nemaline myopathy. In: Pagon RA, Adam MP, Ardinger HH, et al., editors. Seattle, WA; 1993.
8. Zanette G, Robb N, Zadra N, Zanette L, Manani G. Undetected central core disease myopathy in an infant presenting for clubfoot surgery. Paediatr Anaesth. 2007;17(4):380–2. https://doi.org/10.1111/j.1460-9592.2006.02108.x.
9. Pruijs JE, van Tol MJ, van Kesteren RG, van Nieuwenhuizen O. Neuromuscular scoliosis: clinical evaluation pre- and postoperative. J Pediatr Orthop B. 2000;9(4):217–20.
10. McCarthy RE, Sucato D, Turner JL, Zhang H, Henson MAW, McCarthy K. Shilla growing rods in a caprine animal model: a pilot study. Clin Orthop Relat Res. 2010;468(3):705–10. https://doi.org/10.1007/s11999-009-1028-y.
11. Hell AK, Campbell RM, Hefti F. The vertical expandable prosthetic titanium rib implant for the treatment of thoracic insufficiency syndrome associated with congenital and neuromuscular scoliosis in young children. J Pediatr Orthop B. 2005;14(4):287–93.
12. Crawford CH 3rd, Lenke LG. Growth modulation by means of anterior tethering resulting in progressive correction of juvenile idiopathic scoliosis: a case report. J Bone Joint Surg Am. 2010;92(1):202–9. https://doi.org/10.2106/JBJS.H.01728.
13. Betz RR, D'Andrea LP, Mulcahey MJ, Chafetz RS. Vertebral body stapling procedure for the treatment of scoliosis in the growing child. Clin Orthop Relat Res. 2005;(434):55–60.
14. Akbarnia BA. Management themes in early onset scoliosis. J Bone Joint Surg Am. 2007;89(Suppl 1):42–54. https://doi.org/10.2106/JBJS.F.01256.
15. Smith JT. Bilateral rib-to-pelvis technique for managing early-onset scoliosis. Clin Orthop Relat Res. 2011;469(5):1349–55. https://doi.org/10.1007/s11999-010-1700-2.
16. Hasler CC, Mehrkens A, Hefti F. Efficacy and safety of VEPTR instrumentation for progressive spine deformities in young chil-

dren without rib fusions. Eur Spine J. 2010;19(3):400–8. https://doi.org/10.1007/s00586-009-1253-9.
17. Samdani AF, Ranade A, Dolch HJ, et al. Bilateral use of the vertical expandable prosthetic titanium rib attached to the pelvis: a novel treatment for scoliosis in the growing spine. J Neurosurg Spine. 2009;10(4):287–92. https://doi.org/10.3171/2008.12.SPINE08427.
18. Abol Oyoun N, Stuecker R. Bilateral rib-to-pelvis Eiffel Tower VEPTR construct for children with neuromuscular scoliosis: a preliminary report. Spine J. 2014;14(7):1183–91. https://doi.org/10.1016/j.spinee.2013.07.484.
19. Flynn JM, Ramirez N, Emans JB, Smith JT, Mulcahey MJ, Betz RR. Is the vertebral expandable prosthetic titanium rib a surgical alternative in patients with spina bifida? Clin Orthop Relat Res. 2011;469(5):1291–6. https://doi.org/10.1007/s11999-010-1620-1.
20. Teoh KH, Winson DMG, James SH, et al. Magnetic controlled growing rods for early-onset scoliosis: a 4-year follow-up. Spine J. 2016;16(4):S34–9. https://doi.org/10.1016/j.spinee.2015.12.098.
21. Rolton D, Thakar C, Wilson-MacDonald J, Nnadi C. Radiological and clinical assessment of the distraction achieved with remotely expandable growing rods in early onset scoliosis. Eur Spine J. 2016;25(10):3371–6. https://doi.org/10.1007/s00586-015-4223-4.
22. Flynn JM, Tomlinson LA, Pawelek J, Thompson GH, McCarthy R, Akbarnia BA. Growing-rod graduates: lessons learned from ninety-nine patients who completed lengthening. J Bone Joint Surg Am. 2013;95(19):1745–50. https://doi.org/10.2106/JBJS.L.01386.
23. Bekmez S, Dede O, Yazici M. Advances in growing rods treatment for early onset scoliosis. Curr Opin Pediatr. 2017;29(1):87–93. https://doi.org/10.1097/MOP.0000000000000432.

Chapter 16
Cerebral Palsy with Early-Onset Scoliosis

Varun Puvanesarajah and Paul D. Sponseller

Case Presentation

History and Physical Examination

The patient presented as a 10-year-old boy with severe cerebral palsy and a progressive scoliotic thoracolumbar curve. Notably, the patient had a complicated birth history, requiring a Caesarean section after failing forceps delivery. Shortly after birth, he experienced multiple seizures and was intubated, ultimately spending over 2 weeks in the neonatal intensive care unit. At baseline, the patient had a significant developmental delay and spastic quadriplegia—Gross Motor Function Classification System (GMFCS) 5. Prior orthopaedic issues included chronic right hip subluxation.

At initial evaluation, the patient was prepubertal. Posturing of the upper extremities was evident. The patient's trunk was severely rotated with a left thoracolumbar scoliotic curve. Notably, the patient's right ribs were resting on his right iliac

V. Puvanesarajah, MD • P.D. Sponseller, MD (✉)
Department of Orthopedic Surgery, Johns Hopkins Hospital, Baltimore, MD, USA
e-mail: psponse@jhmi.edu

R. El-Hawary, C.P. Eberson (eds.), *Early Onset Scoliosis*,
https://doi.org/10.1007/978-3-319-71580-3_16

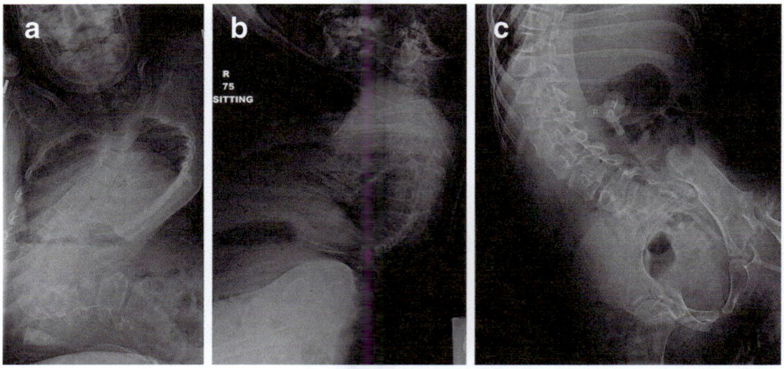

FIGURE. 16.1 Preoperative PA (**a**) and lateral (**b**) radiographs demonstrating a coronal curve of thoracolumbar curve of 135° and pelvic obliquity of 60°. With traction (**c**), this curve reduced to 76°

crest. Significant contracture and stiffness were observed in the right hip. Volitional motor function was completely absent in bilateral lower extremities, though pain sensation was intact.

Diagnostic Studies

Initial radiographic evaluation demonstrated a left thoracolumbar curve measuring 135°. This curve reduced to 76° with traction (Fig. 16.1). His pelvic obliquity was 60°, reducing to 45° with traction.

Management Chosen

The patient underwent halo-gravity traction for 1 week prior to insertion of spine-based growing rods. Growing rods were subsequently distracted five times over the next 5 years, with insertion of new intermediate growing rod segments during the last procedure.

Surgical Procedure

First Step: Halo Traction Application

Given the reduction of approximately 40% of the scoliotic curve with traction, the patient was initially treated with halo traction for 1 week prior to growing rod insertion. This step was chosen to allow the skin, spinal cord and musculature to adapt to a new position. An eight-pin construct, with two pins bilaterally anterolaterally and two pins bilaterally posterolaterally. The pins were tightened to 6 in. pounds, and 10 pounds of traction was applied. This was gradually increased to 40% of body weight over the week between halo and surgery.

Second Step: Growing Rod Insertion

Halo traction was decreased to 10 lbs and continued intraoperatively, after prone positioning in order to achieve deformity correction. No femoral traction was used, but the operating table was placed in 15° reverse Trendelenburg for counter-traction. Intraoperative neuromonitoring was attempted but was not successful and was subsequently abandoned. A long midline incision was made from T2 to S2. Careful dissection of the muscle layer was performed from T2 to T4 and from L5 to S2. Spina bifida occulta was demonstrated at S1 and S2. Pedicle screws were inserted at T2–T4 and L5–S2. Bilateral sacral-alar-iliac (SAI) screws were also inserted. These are placed directly caudal to S1 screws, in the lateral aspect of the first sacral foramen. The trajectory is approximately 40° caudally and 40° laterally. The screws should course above the sciatic notch and aim for the anterior inferior iliac spines. The diameter should be as wide as possible, 7–8 mm if possible. Following screw placement, 5 mm stainless steel growing rods were placed and assembled with a 90 mm tandem connector. The right-sided (concave side of the curve/high side of the pelvis) rod was placed first with distraction. Subsequently, the left-sided rod was placed with

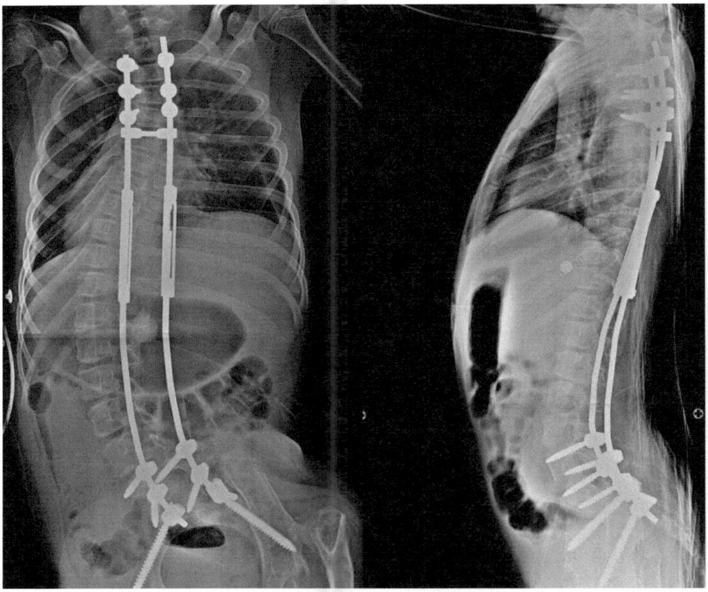

FIGURE. 16.2 Radiographs taken 1 week following the first surgical procedure

little distraction. The linear alignment of the S1 and SAI screws allows longitudinal distraction to level the pelvis. The pelvic obliquity was checked intraoperatively with a T-square, to be sure that the pelvis is perpendicular to the spine. Allograft bone was applied to the instrumented foundations from T2 to T4 and from L5 to S2. No complications occurred. Post-operative images are provided in Fig. 16.2.

Subsequent Steps: Growing Rod Distraction

Nine months after the index procedure, the growing rod construct was distracted to allow for patient growth. In neuromuscular patients, we aim to space out the distraction intervals in order to minimize procedures. Subsequent distraction procedures occurred at intervals between 10 and

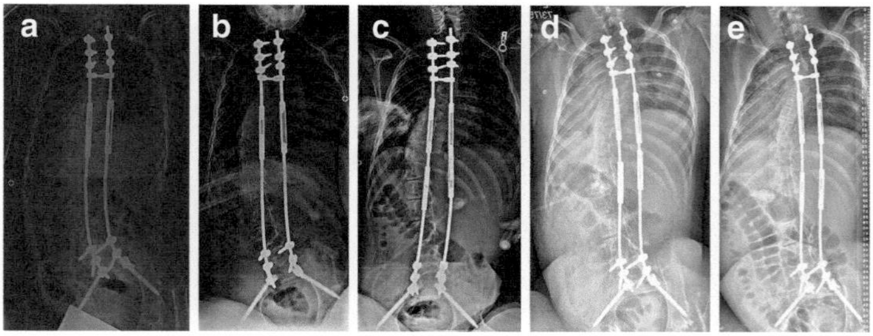

FIGURE. 16.3 Interval PA radiographs taken between subsequent distraction procedures. Radiographs are from after the first distraction (**a**, 9 months following initial surgery, T_i), second distraction (**b**, radiograph taken 28 months following T_i, though second distraction performed 20 months after T_i), third distraction (**c**, radiograph taken 41 months following T_i, though third distraction performed 32 months after T_i), fourth distraction (**d**, 41 months after T_i) and fifth distraction (**e**, 60 months after T_i)

14 months following this initial procedure, with interval placement of additional 70 mm tandem connectors to allow for additional growth potential and later tandem connector replacement. During every distraction procedure, asymmetric right greater than left-sided distraction of 1.0–2.5 cm was accomplished (Fig. 16.3).

Clinical Course and Outcome

Radiographic images demonstrate interval correction over 7 years of follow-up. Of note, the last distraction procedure was performed 2 years prior to the last radiographic study (Fig. 16.4). During the full course of treatment and subsequent follow-up, no complications were noted. At last follow-up, a 50° right-sided curve from T1 to T7 and a 42° left-sided curve from T8 to L3 were present. Pelvic obliquity was 10°. T1–S1 height gained from pre-initial to final was 22 cm, with 7 cm gained from post-initial to final.

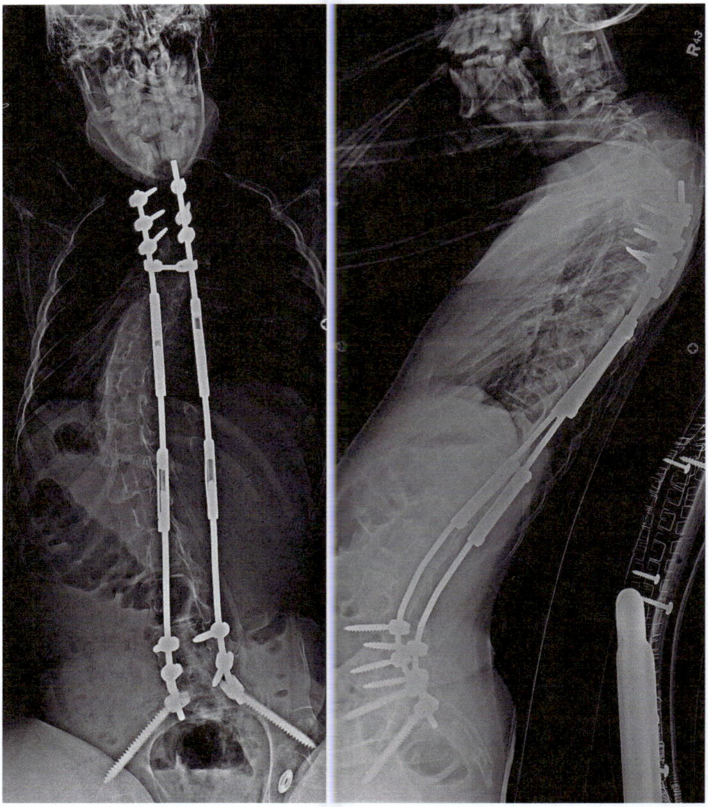

Figure. 16.4 Final PA and lateral radiographs. Images were acquired almost 7 years after the initial surgical procedure. A 50° right-sided curve from T1 to T7 and a 42° left-sided curve from T8 to L3 were present. The patient was 17 years old, and Risser sign was 5. No "final fusion" was planned. A total of 22 cm length was gained from pre-initial surgery to final follow-up, with 7 cm gained from post-initial surgery to final follow-up.

Clinical Pearls and Pitfalls

- Pelvic obliquity correction is the chief aim of surgery in patients with neuromuscular scoliosis. Pelvic screws should be considered as an adjunct to growing rods in this patient population.

- Lengthening procedures are associated with higher complication rates and also may be subject to diminishing returns.
- Though not observed in this patient, infection is a serious risk that must be considered.
- Intraoperative neural monitoring is recommended, though this may be unreliable in patients with neuromuscular scoliosis.

Literature Review and Discussion

Management of neuromuscular scoliosis presents numerous challenges. Patients often have rapidly progressive curves that present early in childhood, requiring preservation of spinal growth while preventing further curve progression. In most neuromuscular patients, bracing does not prevent curve progression. In selected cases, orthopaedic surgeons must rely on surgical intervention. Although definitive fusion is the most efficacious at preventing further curve progression, it is not ideal before age 8–10 [1–5].

To avoid definitive fusion and subsequent growth arrest, there has been a recent trend towards usage of growing rod constructs. Spine-based growing rods were first described by Moe over three decades ago [6] but only came into more popular use recently due to improved construct biomechanics [7], particularly in the development of "dual" growing rods [8]. These require initial implantation followed by several distraction procedures, at regular intervals, to allow for continued vertebral column growth. Often, fusion is undertaken at 2–3 vertebral segments ("foundations") at the cranial and cephalad aspects of instrumentation, with rods connected by tandem connectors to allow for guided growth. Many children with cerebral palsy often have significant pelvic obliquity and require pelvic fixation. Such fixation can be integrated with an existing growing rod construct if appropriate screw trajectories are chosen. For this reason, SAI screws are often used for pelvic fixation with excellent long-term results [9].

Akbarnia et al. demonstrated that on average, the use of dual growing rod constructs resulted in Cobb angle improvement from 82° preoperatively to 38° at last follow-up, with concomitant yearly spine lengthening of 1.2 cm/year [10]. Although a greater number of distraction procedures increases growth potential, each additional procedure has been shown to increase the likelihood of complications by 24% [11]. As such, there has been a recent push to use MAGEC® rods, which can be distracted in an outpatient setting using magnetic technology, without additional surgery.

Though dual growing rods are popular, many surgeons opt to use rib-based techniques (i.e. vertical expandable prosthetic titanium rib prostheses (VEPTR)) or hybrid spine/rib constructs. However, VEPTR may result in more complications per unit growth when compared to dual growing rods [12].

Ultimately, successful management of neuromuscular scoliosis requires critical assessment of a patient's growth potential and risk for developing thoracic insufficiency. As growing rods require more than one procedure, this strategy is indicated only for the largest curves at the youngest ages.

References

1. Campbell RM Jr, Smith MD, Mayes TC, et al. The characteristics of thoracic insufficiency syndrome associated with fused ribs and congenital scoliosis. J Bone Joint Surg Am. 2003;85-A:399–408.
2. Goldberg CJ, Gillic I, Connaughton O, et al. Respiratory function and cosmesis at maturity in infantile-onset scoliosis. Spine. 2003;28:2397–406.
3. Gollogly S, Smith JT, White SK, et al. The volume of lung parenchyma as a function of age: a review of 1050 normal CT scans of the chest with three-dimensional volumetric reconstruction of the pulmonary system. Spine. 2004;29:2061–6.
4. Karol LA, Johnston C, Mladenov K, et al. Pulmonary function following early thoracic fusion in non-neuromuscular scoliosis. J Bone Joint Surg Am. 2008;90:1272–81.
5. Kesling KL, Lonstein JE, Denis F, et al. The crankshaft phenomenon after posterior spinal arthrodesis for congenital scoliosis: a review of 54 patients. Spine. 2003;28:267–71.
6. Moe JH, Kharrat K, Winter RB, et al. Harrington instrumentation without fusion plus external orthotic support for the treat-

ment of difficult curvature problems in young children. Clin Orthop Relat Res. 1984:35–45.
7. Skaggs DL, Akbarnia BA, Flynn JM, et al. A classification of growth friendly spine implants. J Pediatr Orthop. 2014;34:260–74.
8. Thompson GH, Akbarnia BA, Campbell RM Jr. Growing rod techniques in early-onset scoliosis. J Pediatr Orthop. 2007;27:354–61.
9. Sponseller PD, Zimmerman RM, Ko PS, et al. Low profile pelvic fixation with the sacral alar iliac technique in the pediatric population improves results at two-year minimum follow-up. Spine. 2010;35:1887–92.
10. Akbarnia BA, Marks DS, Boachie-Adjei O, et al. Dual growing rod technique for the treatment of progressive early-onset scoliosis: a multicenter study. Spine. 2005;30:S46–57.
11. Bess S, Akbarnia BA, Thompson GH, et al. Complications of growing-rod treatment for early-onset scoliosis: analysis of one hundred and forty patients. J Bone Joint Surg Am. 2010;92:2533–43.
12. Sankar WN, Acevedo DC, Skaggs DL. Comparison of complications among growing spinal implants. Spine. 2010;35:2091–6.

Chapter 17
The Use of the Vertical Expandable Prosthetic Titanium Rib (VEPTR) in Myelomeningocele

Graham Fedorak, John A. Heflin, and John T. Smith

Case Presentation

History and Physical Examination

A 21-month-old female with lumbar myelomeningocele presented with worsening lumbar gibbus deformity. She had undergone neurosurgical closure of the defect after birth, followed by endoscopic third ventriculostomy and choroid plexus coagulation at 1 week of life. Her gibbus subsequently progressed such that it was beginning to interfere with sitting and was at risk for skin breakdown over the apex of the deformity. She was followed in a multidisciplinary spina bifida clinic and had bladder incontinence that was managed with clean intermittent catheterization. Comorbid orthopedic conditions included bilateral dislocated hips, teratologic clubfeet managed with posteromedial releases, and knee flexion contractures treated surgically. She had minimal motor function below the waist but sat well.

G. Fedorak, MD • J.A. Heflin, MD • J.T. Smith, MD (✉)
University of Utah, Salt Lake City, UT, USA
e-mail: John.Smith@hsc.utah.edu

R. El-Hawary, C.P. Eberson (eds.), *Early Onset Scoliosis*,
https://doi.org/10.1007/978-3-319-71580-3_17

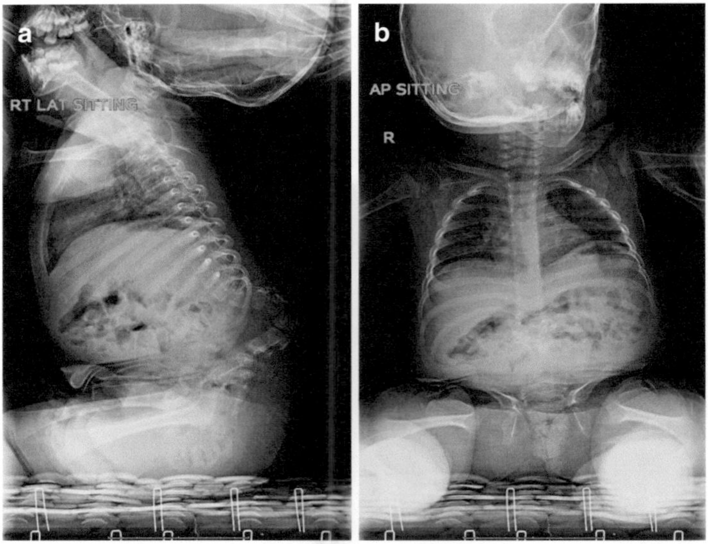

FIGURE. 17.1 (**a**) Sitting lateral view of the spine shows the congenital gibbus deformity of the lumbar spine with the kyphosis measuring 150°. (**b**) Sitting AP view of the spine that shows that the spine is straight in the coronal plane and that there is visible spinal dysraphism in the lumbar spine

- Sat independently without use of hands
- Well-balanced in coronal plane
- Incision well-healed over gibbus, midline soft tissues in good condition
- No useful function in lower extremities

Diagnostic Studies

- Radiographs showed severe lumbar gibbus deformity (Fig. 17.1).
- MRI demonstrates Chiari II anomaly, syringohydromyelia from T3 to the upper lumbar spine (6.3 mm greatest diameter).

Management Chosen

Wheelchair modifications and bracing are ineffective in managing gibbus deformity in spina bifida due to the potential for skin breakdown over the gibbus. Given the large syrinx, there was concern regarding spinal cord tethering and the potential for a de-tethering procedure prior to deformity surgery was considered. However, given minimal lower extremity function, observation of syrinx was chosen with a repeat MRI scheduled in the future. Kyphectomy and fusion at an early age are associated with a high infection risk and potentially result in a shortened trunk from early fusion. We recommend growth-friendly spinal constructs in order to allow further growth of the trunk.

In consultation with the child's parents, a decision was made to proceed with implantation of bilateral rib-to-pelvis VEPTR II devices (VEPTR; Vertical Expandable Prosthetic Titanium Rib, Depuy Synthes Spine, Raynham, MA), with periodic expansion to control the gibbus and allow for continued growth.

Surgical Procedure

- Cephalad midline incision T2–T5 to tip of spinous processes. Bilateral planes are developed between rhomboids and erector spinae to a point lateral to the angle of the rib. Erector spinae are then elevated from lateral to medial, to the tips of transverse processes bilaterally. Superior and inferior aspects of targeted ribs dissected lateral to transverse processes. Two rib hook-cap constructs placed on each side around the ribs.
- Caudally, oblique incisions were made bilaterally, just lateral to the gibbus deformity, lateral to posterior superior iliac spine. After dissection to the lateral margin of the remnants of erector spinae, the inner and outer tables of the ilium were identified. "S" hooks were placed bilaterally over the ilium.

- VEPTR II implant was selected and cut to appropriate length. The implants were then tunneled over a #20 chest tube from proximal to distal and engaged using 5.0–6.0 connectors onto the "S" hooks. The implants were cantilevered to engage the upper rib hooks and secured.
- C-rings were placed, and significant distraction was placed against the pelvic hooks, significantly reducing the gibbus deformity, followed by tightening. This step requires pre-judging the length of the rods prior to insertion to allow maximal correction at the time of initial implantation but also having the correct length when the distal portion of the implant is expanded for maximal length at primary insertion.
- Valsalva maneuvers are always performed with saline over the rib hooks to confirm pleural integrity prior to closure.

Clinical Course and Outcome

- A proximal left prominence was noted 2 weeks postoperatively, and radiographs demonstrated cephalad migration of the left upper rib construct. This was revised at 3 weeks to one VEPTR rib hook and two small USS hooks (USS Universal Spine System, Depuy Synthes Spine, Raynham, MA) connected to the existing VEPTR (Fig. 17.2).
- Three VEPTR expansions have been performed uneventfully at 6-month intervals, with steady improvement in both deformity and T1–S1 height (Fig. 17.3).

Clinical Pearls and Pitfalls

- Preoperative assessment of comorbidities is essential, best done by a multidisciplinary team, and includes hydrocephalus requiring shunting, tethered cord, Arnold-Chiari

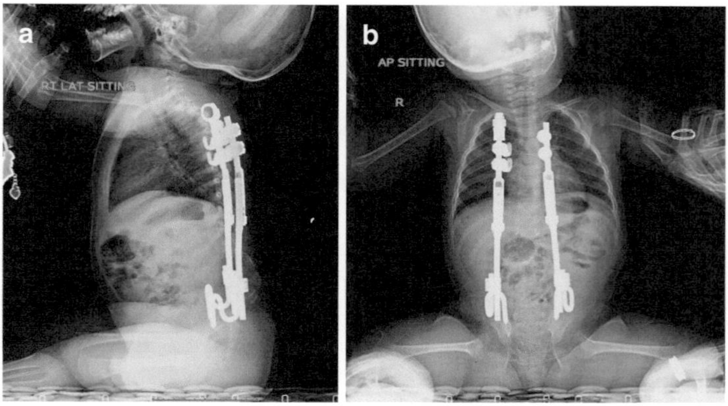

FIGURE. 17.2 (**a**) Sitting lateral view of the spine shows the rib-to-pelvis VEPTR construct with significant improvement in the severity of the gibbus deformity. (**b**) Sitting AP view of the spine demonstrated a significant improvement in spinal height and improved positioning of the pelvis for sitting

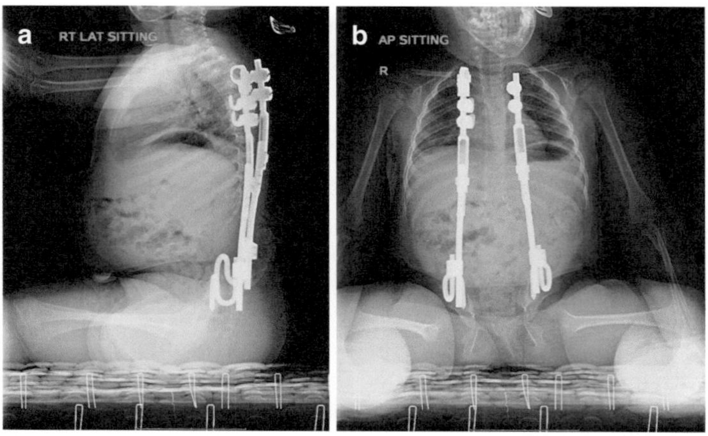

FIGURE. 17.3 (**a**) Sitting lateral view of the spine after three operative expansions of the VEPTR implants. (**b**) Sitting AP view of the spine after three operative expansions

malformation, insensate skin, latex allergy, renal anomalies, bacterial colonization of the urinary tract, bowel and bladder incontinence, and lower extremity and foot deformities.

- If a shunt is in place, its function should be confirmed as there is always a risk of shunt malfunction after correction.
- When the soft tissue envelope is attenuated, consider plastic surgery consultation for placement and expansion of soft tissue expanders prior to spine surgery.
- Fixation points away from the gibbus avoid the typically poor-quality midline skin.
- The use of pelvic S-hooks at the PSIS places the distraction vector for gibbus correction anterior to the spine, and thus, distraction of the construct produces lordosis and further correction of the kyphotic deformity.

Literature Review and Discussion

Spinal deformities in patients with myelomeningocele are common and are often complicated by several factors: (1) deficient posterior elements and lack of muscular support contribute to multi-planar instability; (2) poor midline skin susceptible to breakdown; (3) secondary thoracic insufficiency syndrome [1]; (4) concomitant congenital defects cephalad or caudad to the level of the defect; and (5) the presence of central nervous system anomalies including hydrocephalus, Arnold-Chiari malformation, and intrathecal anomalies [2].

The reported incidence of kyphotic deformity in patients with myelomeningocele ranges between 8 and 21% and most commonly occurs in the thoracolumbar or upper lumbar spine [3–5]. When the kyphosis is rigid (gibbus), these deformities will progress rapidly in early childhood, at rates from 6.4 to 12.1° per year [3, 6, 7].

Nonsurgical interventions such as wheelchair modifications and bracing have proven minimally effective at preventing deformity progression [8–10]. Furthermore, bracing creates potential for skin ulceration, impaired respiration, and may interfere with G-tubes. Serial casting has the same difficulties, with less opportunity to attend to skin issues. While kyphectomy and limited spinal fusion are an established technique to address gibbus deformity, complication rates are high [9, 11–16] Furthermore, early fusion may result in crankshaft deformity, a foreshortened trunk height, and inhibition of lung growth [2, 11].

Nonambulatory patients with myelomeningocele often develop secondary thoracic insufficiency syndrome due to collapsing spinal deformity and a shortened trunk [1, 2, 17, 18]. Growth-friendly procedures are necessary in early-onset spinal deformity to allow continued growth of the trunk and thorax. Limited reports of the use of VEPTR to address early-onset spinal deformity in myelodysplasia exist [2, 19, 20]. First described by Smith and Novais [20], and subsequently dubbed the "Eiffel Tower" construct [19], bilateral rib-to-pelvis fixation is the preferred growth-friendly approach to manage gibbus deformity in myelomeningocele. This is typically limited to non-ambulators or, as a last resort in ambulators, due to the high incidence of crouch gait postoperatively [21].

VEPTR allows relatively low-profile fixation away from the gibbus and the typically attenuated midline tissues. Furthermore, the use of pelvic S-hooks places the moment arm anterior to the apex of the deformity, promoting efficient improvement of the kyphosis. In small children, the placement of these hooks just lateral to the gibbus on the ileum is critical to prevent migration over time. S-hooks are relatively low profile and can be used in small children. Once children become larger, pelvic saddles are an alternative. We feel that it is important to correct this deformity as early as possible prior to the child developing skin breakdown over the gibbus. Subsequent distraction procedures allow continued growth of the spine as well as further correction of deformity. Gibbus deformity in myelomeningocele is a challenging problem in a complex patient population, which the VEPTR device is particularly well-suited to manage.

References

1. Campbell RM, Smith MD, Mayes TC, Mangos JA, Willey-Courand DB, Kose N, Pinero RF, Alder ME, Duong HL, Surber JL. The characteristics of thoracic insufficiency syndrome associated with fused ribs and congenital scoliosis. J Bone Joint Surg Am. 2003;85:399–408.
2. Flynn JM, Ramirez N, Emans JB, Smith JT, Mulcahey MJ, Betz RR. Is the vertebral expandable prosthetic titanium rib a surgical alternative in patients with Spina bifida? Clin Orthop Relat Res. 2011;469:1291–6.
3. Carstens C, Koch H, Brocai DR, Niethard FU. Development of pathological lumbar kyphosis in myelomeningocele. J Bone Joint Surg Br. 1996;78:945–50.
4. Hoppenfeld S. Congenital kyphosis in myelomeningocele. J Bone Joint Surg Br. 1967;49:276–80.
5. Lindseth RE, Stelzer L Jr. Vertebral excision for kyphosis in children with myelomeningocele. J Bone Joint Surg Am. 1979;61:699–704.
6. Doers T, Walker JL, van den Brink K, Stevens DB, Heavilon J. The progression of untreated lumbar kyphosis and the compensatory thoracic lordosis in myelomeningocele. Dev Med Child Neurol. 1997;39:326–30.
7. Mintz LJ, Sarwark JF, Dias LS, Schafer MF. The natural history of congenital kyphosis in myelomeningocele. A review of 51 children. Spine. 1991;16(8 Suppl):S348–50.
8. Hall JE, Poitras B. The management of kyphosis in patients with myelomeningocele. Clin Orthop Relat Res. 1977;(128):33–40.
9. Leatherman KD, Dickson RA. Congenital kyphosis in myelomeningocele. Vertebral body resection and posterior spine fusion. Spine. 1978;3:222–6.
10. Lintner SA, Lindseth RE. Kyphotic deformity in patients who have a myelomeningocele. Operative treatment and long-term follow-up. J Bone Joint Surg Am. 1994;76:1301–7.
11. Akbar M, Bremer R, Thomsen M, Carstens C, Abel R. Kyphectomy in children with myelodysplasia: results 1994–2004. Spine. 2006;31:1007–113.
12. Banta JV, Hamada JS. Natural history of the kyphotic deformity in myelomeningocele [abstract]. J Bone Joint Surg Am. 1976;58:279.

13. Heydemann JS, Gillespie R. Management of myelomeningocele kyphosis in the older child by kyphectomy and segmental spinal instrumentation. Spine. 1987;12:37–41.
14. Karline LI. Kyphectomy for myelodysplasia. Neurosurg Clin N Am. 2007;18:357–64.
15. Ko AL, Song K, Ellenbogen RG, Avellino AM. Retrospective review of multilevel spinal fusion combined with spinal cord transection for treatment of kyphoscoliosis in pediatric myelomeningocele patients. Spine. 2007;32:2493–501.
16. Sharrad WJ. Spinal osteotomy for congenital kyphosis and myelomeningocele. J Bone Joint Surg Br. 1968;50:466–71.
17. Campbell RM, Smith MD, Mayes TC, Mangos JA, Willey-Courand DB, Kose N, Pinero RF, Alder ME, Duong HL, Surber JL. The effect of opening wedge thoracostomy on thoracic insufficiency syndrome associated with fused ribs and congenital scoliosis. J Bone Joint Surg Am. 2004;86:1659–74.
18. Campbell RM, Smith M. Thoracic insufficiency syndrome and exotic scoliosis. J Bone Joint Surg Am. 2007;89:108–22.
19. Oyoun NA, Stuecker R. Bilateral rib-to-pelvis Eiffel Tower VEPTR construct for children with neuromuscular scoliosis: a preliminary report. Spine J. 2014;14:1183–91.
20. Smith JT, Novais E. Treatment of gibbus deformity associated with myelomeningocele in the young child with use of the vertical expandable prosthetic titanium rib (VEPTR)—a case report. J Bone Joint Surg Am. 2010;92:2211–5.
21. Smith JT. Bilateral rib-to-pelvis technique for managing early-onset scoliosis. Clin Orthop Relat Res. 2011;469:1349–55.

Chapter 18
Early-Onset Scoliosis in Skeletal Dysplasia

David Tager, Suken Shah, and William G. Mackenzie

Case Presentation

History and Physical Examination

The patient is a female with spondylometaphyseal dysplasia Kozlowski type (SMDK) who initially presented at 5 years old with a history of progressive kyphoscoliosis. She was diagnosed with skeletal dysplasia at 9 months of age. Her kyphoscoliosis had been managed at an outside institution with nighttime bracing for the previous 2 years, and due to the family's relocation in our region, further management was

D. Tager, MD
West Virginia University Hospital,
Morgantown, WV, USA
e-mail: david.tager@hsc.wvu.edu

S. Shah, MD
The Spine and Scoliosis Center, Nemours/Alfred I. duPont Hospital for Children, Wilmington, DE, USA
e-mail: Suken.Shah@nemours.org

W.G. Mackenzie, MD (✉)
Department of Orthopedic Surgery, Nemours/Alfred I. duPont Hospital for Children, Wilmington, DE, USA
e-mail: wmackenz@nemours.org

R. El-Hawary, C.P. Eberson (eds.), *Early Onset Scoliosis*,
https://doi.org/10.1007/978-3-319-71580-3_18

sought at our institution. She denied back pain, radicular pain, or myelopathic symptoms. She denied any additional musculoskeletal complaints. She remained an active participant in age-appropriate sports.

Vital signs were obtained on presentation: weight 17.5 kg (16 percentile) and height 106 cm (5 percentile). The patient's neck demonstrated full, nonpainful range of motion. Spine examination revealed level shoulders with a prominent kyphosis in the thoracolumbar region. The back was observed to have both flank asymmetry and a right-sided thoracolumbar prominence consistent with concurrent coronal plane deformity. The kyphoscoliosis exhibited moderate flexibility. The patient had a mild pelvic obliquity with the left leg approximately 1 cm shorter than the right. Hip range of motion was symmetric, with 100° of flexion, 30° of abduction, and 50° of internal and external rotation. Motor strength in the lower extremities was grade 5/5 and symmetric. Reflexes at the knees and ankles were 1+ and symmetric, and abdominal reflexes were intact and symmetric. A downgoing plantar reflex was elicited, and no clonus was appreciated in the lower extremities. Examination of the skin revealed no lesions.

Diagnostic Studies

Full-length standing X-rays were obtained with ultra-low dose slot scanning imaging in the PA and lateral positions to assess overall balance in the coronal and sagittal planes and regional deformities and to check the hips and pelvis for LLD, dysplasia, and sagittal mismatch. The major coronal curve measured 69°, and the kyphosis in the thoracolumbar junction measured 94° (Fig. 18.1). Supine bending and pull films were obtained to characterize the flexibility of the major and minor curves and plan anchor sites (Fig. 18.2). A full spinal MRI scan was obtained to evaluate the neural axis and screen for stenosis (Fig. 18.3).

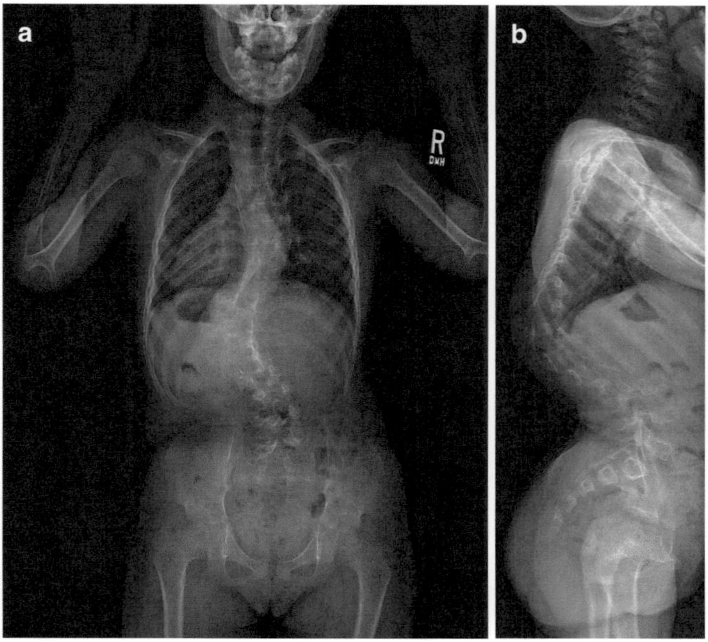

FIGURE. 18.1 Erect PA and lateral X-rays of the spine demonstrating the major coronal thoracolumbar curve and the sagittal thoracolumbar kyphosis

Management Chosen

Since the patient presented at 5 years old with a moderately flexible curve confirmed on pull and bending films, initial management consisted of application of spinal elongation, derotation, and flexion (EDF) casting (Fig. 18.4). Our goal was to temporarily halt progression of the kyphoscoliosis and allow the patient to grow prior to surgical management. Two spine EDF casts were applied for 4-month intervals which delayed surgical management for approximately 1 year (Fig. 18.5). At 1 year, her kyphoscoliosis had progressed and

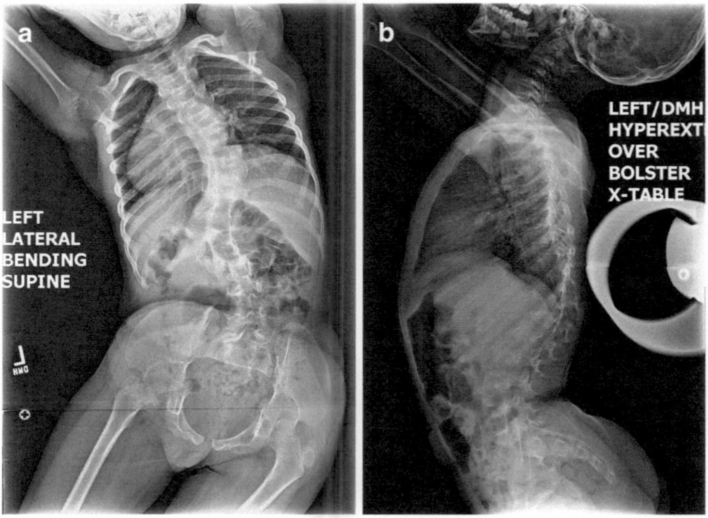

FIGURE. 18.2 Supine bending and pull X-rays demonstrating the flexibility of the major and minor curves

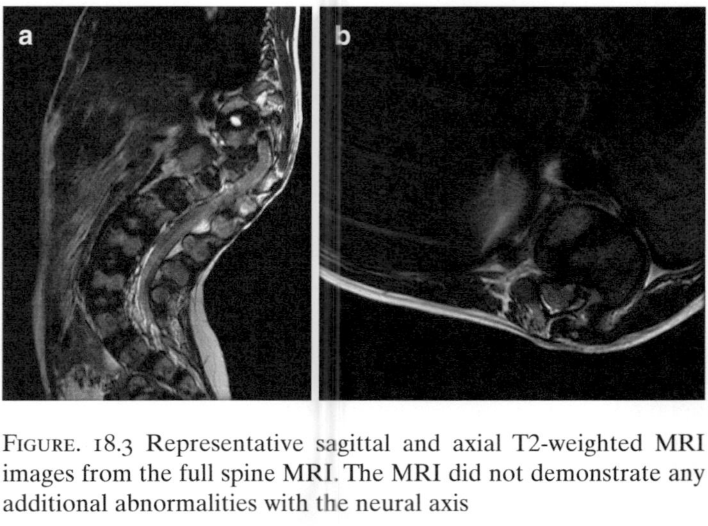

FIGURE. 18.3 Representative sagittal and axial T2-weighted MRI images from the full spine MRI. The MRI did not demonstrate any additional abnormalities with the neural axis

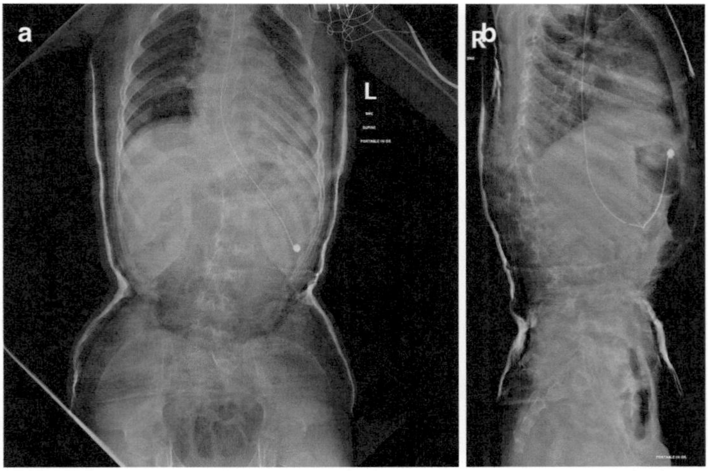

FIGURE. 18.4 Supine AP and lateral X-ray following application of the elongation, derotation, and flexion (EDF) casting

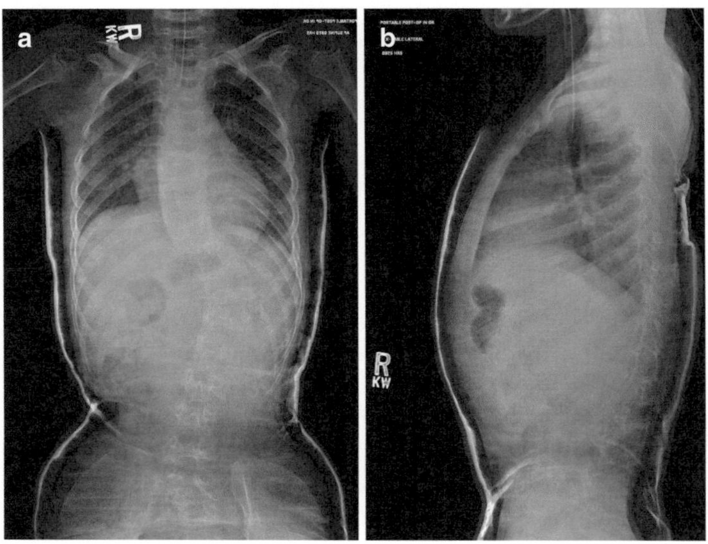

FIGURE. 18.5 Supine AP and lateral X-ray following application of the second EDF casting

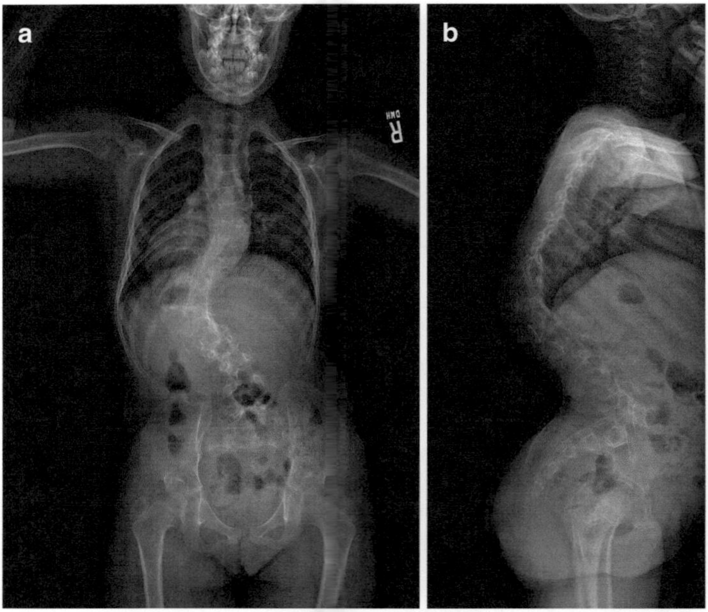

FIGURE. 18.6 Erect PA and lateral spine XR demonstrating progression of the kyphoscoliosis

become more rigid, and the family elected to discontinue casting and move to surgical treatment at our recommendation (Fig. 18.6).

Surgical Procedure

At 7 years +7 months old, the patient underwent placement of magnetically controlled growing rods (MCGR) to allow for concurrent control of the progressive kyphoscoliosis and growth of the spine (Fig. 18.7). Central to management of this complex, early-onset deformity was the presence of severe kyphosis at the thoracolumbar junction, severe scoliosis just distal to the apex of the kyphosis, and increasing rigidity of the curves in a spine with poor bone density. Intraoperative cranial tongs were used for positioning, and

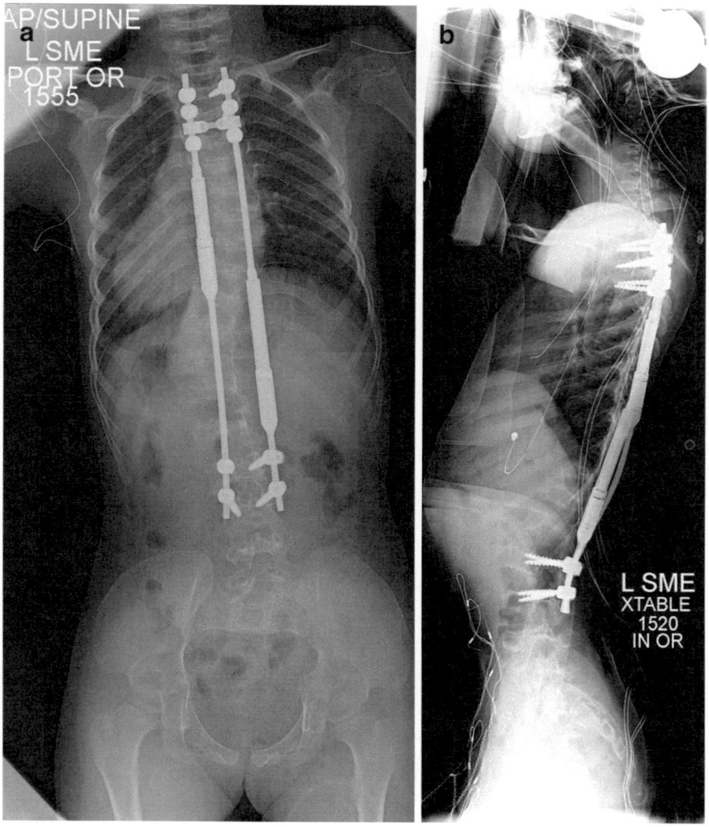

FIGURE. 18.7 Supine intraoperative AP and lateral X-ray following placement of magnetically controlled growing rods. Proximal and distal anchor sites were placed at T2–T4 and L2–L3, respectively

traction of 25% body weight was applied with noninvasive skin traction to obtain initial correction. The procedure was performed through two posterior incisions just at the levels of the planned proximal and distal spinal anchor sites. Pedicle screws were placed at T2–T4 and at L2–L3. Care was taken to preserve cephalad and caudal facets of the two fusion areas. A MCGR with a 90 mm actuator was placed in the standard configuration on the concavity of the thoracolumbar curve. A magnetically controlled growing rod with an offset configuration 70 mm actuator was placed on the convexity of the curve, reversed so that substantially more rod was available for contour over the kyphosis and convexity. Both rods were tunneled subfascially to connect the proximal and distal pedicle screw constructs. Translation and cantilever correction were employed over the apex of the kyphoscoliotic curve. No brace was utilized postoperatively.

Clinical Course and Outcome

At 4 months postoperative, the patient had returned to swimming, running, and biking. The patient was brought back to the clinic at 3–4-month intervals for lengthening of her magnetically controlled growing rods. Approximately 2–3 mm of length was achieved at each session in a noninvasive fashion, in the clinic, without sedation. To date, she has undergone eight sessions of lengthening in the clinic. Measurements pre- and post-lengthening were confirmed by ultrasound and annual X-rays to confirm integrity of the implants and to assess overall balance (Fig. 18.8). During the MCGR treatment period, she has gained 54 mm of total height, 11 mm of spinal height from T1 to T12, and 20 mm in spinal height from T1 to S1. The patient has experienced no complications in her postoperative course. She is currently 9 years old. When her spine has achieved sufficient growth, her posterior instrumentation will likely be revised to a segmental posterior spinal fusion with pedicle screw instrumentation.

Clinical Pearls and Pitfalls

- Care must be taken during the procedure to preserve soft tissue attachments and facets cephalad and caudal to the fusion points to prevent premature fusion of unintended levels and development of junctional deformity, which primarily occurs proximally.

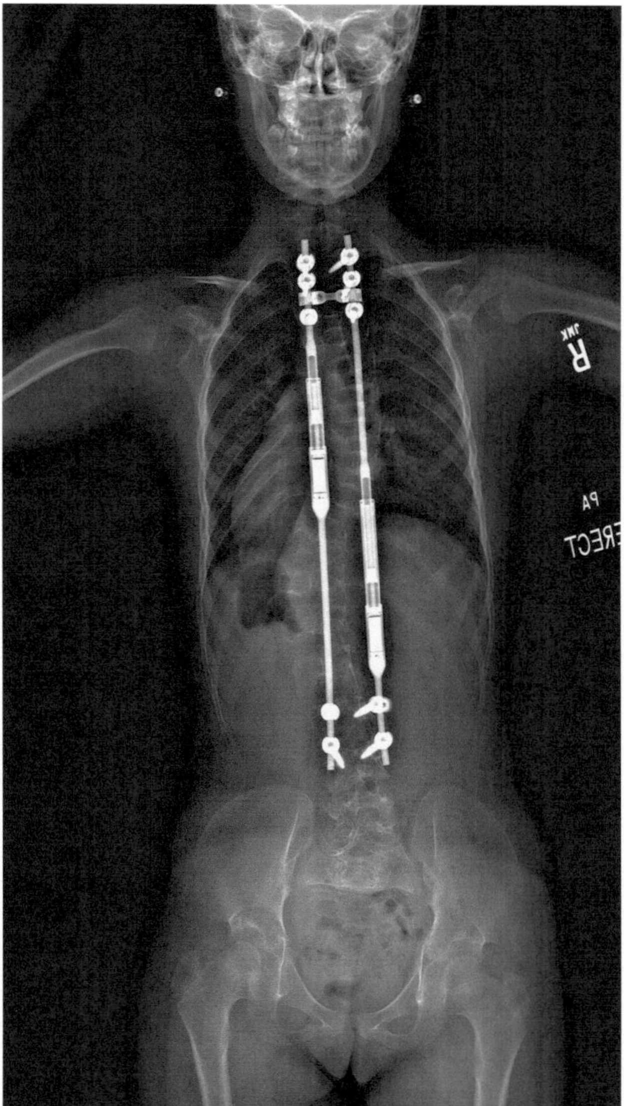

FIGURE. 18.8 Standing PA X-ray after eight sessions of MCGR lengthenings in the clinic. During this treatment period, she has gained 54 mm of total height, 11 mm of spinal height from T1 to T12, and 20 mm in spinal height from T1 to S1

- For the current magnetically controlled rods for spine implantation, the patient must be able to accommodate, at a minimum, a 70 mm actuator that must rest over a relatively neutral area of the patient's spine (preferably the TL junction). Magnetically controlled rods with 70 mm actuators need 90 mm of flat spine, while 90 mm actuators require 110 mm. The actuator region of the rod cannot be contoured. If the size of the patient's spine cannot accommodate this size actuator, then a traditional growing rod can be utilized. Both options should be discussed at length with the family preoperatively, and proper planning is necessary to be prepared intraoperatively.
- Rods must be carefully tunneled from proximal to distal to avoid iatrogenic injury to the thoracic cavity. A chest tube can be utilized to aid in rod passage.
- If bone quality is a significant concern, the procedure can be staged with anchor placement to first achieve fusion regions at the cephalad and caudal screw constructs. The patient can be brought back in 3–4 months later for correction and placement of traditional or magnetically controlled growing rods. Halo gravity traction can be used in between stages.
- Patients with skeletal dysplasia create significant challenges for the spinal deformity surgeon. Except in a specialty referral practice, they are rarely encountered and have considerable comorbidities for the anesthesiologist (airway and chest compliance), orthopedic surgeon (cervical spine instability, stenosis, hip, and lower extremity deformities),and pulmonologist (decreased pulmonary function). Multidisciplinary care with the aid of a geneticist is essential for successful outcomes.

Literature Review and Discussion

The chronological parameters of early-onset scoliosis (EOS) have been debated, but the consequences of progressive curves in the young child have been established. Children who develop large curves before 5 years of age can develop life-threatening respiratory and cardiovascular sequelae [1, 2]. Currently EOS is widely considered to include children who develop spinal deformity prior to 10 years. Genetic skeletal disorders represent a large heterogenous group with multiple underlying etiologies. The 2015 revision from the *Nosology and Classification of Genetic Skeletal Disorders* identified 436 conditions placed into 42 groups [3]. Because of this variability, patients with skeletal dysplasia have varying degrees of spinal involvement which can affect the entire spine, from the cranio-vertebral junction to the sacrum.

Spondylometaphyseal dysplasia (SMD) is a rare skeletal dysplasia affecting both vertebral bodies and metaphyseal regions of long bones. It was first described by Kozlowski in 1967 [4], and up to ten subtypes have been described. The Kozlowski type of SMD (SMDK), or SMD type I, is the most common form, and the transmission is largely autosomal dominant [5]. Clinical manifestations of SMD include rhizomelic shortening of the limbs, shortening of the trunk, respiratory problems, cervical spinal instability, kyphoscoliosis, and extremity malalignment [6].

The kyphoscoliosis present in our patient can closely resemble the spinal deformity seen in other skeletal dysplasias. Complicating the presentation of our patient was the early onset of her disease. Therefore, the preservation of thoracic growth in an individual already susceptible to respiratory compromise from a shortened trunk is essential. The priority with our patient was to control kyphoscoliosis progression and delay spinal fusion. While a case report demonstrated the potential efficacy of brace treatment for thoracolumbar kyphosis in SMDK [7], our patient had failed this course of treatment. Therefore, we pursued spinal casting as a temporary measure prior to operative treatment. Our utilization of a spinal cast in this instance allowed for approximately 1 year of continued spinal growth prior to surgical management.

Once our patient's kyphoscoliosis progressed and became more rigid, surgical management was indicated. The use of growth-friendly implants in patients with skeletal dysplasia is not well described. As our patient had pronounced thoracolumbar kyphosis and scoliosis, we sought to utilize an intervention that allowed for fewer procedures and decreased chance of wound breakdown over the kyphosis. Therefore, we chose to implant magnetically controlled growing rods to reduce the number of procedures during lengthening and reduce the risk of wound breakdown over the kyphoscoliosis.

Cranial tongs were used for intraoperative traction, and cantilever correction was employed over the kyphosis of the spinal deformity. The pedicle screw fixation was sufficient to use the cantilever strategy. This resulted in good correction of the kyphoscoliosis. If poor bone quality does not allow for this method and degree of correction, the procedure can be staged. The pedicle screws are inserted into the cephalad and caudal anchor regions for the spinal instrumentation. These are allowed to fuse, and 3 months later, the growth-friendly implants are inserted in a second procedure. This two-stage growing rod strategy can be utilized for both traditional growing rods and magnetically controlled growing rods [8].

Our patient's kyphoscoliosis has been well controlled for 1.3 years and eight noninvasive lengthenings. Each lengthening has achieved approximately 2–3 mm of construct length confirmed by ultrasound. She will continue to be managed by a form of growth-friendly spinal instrumentation until her skeletal maturity and thoracic height are conducive to a definitive fusion, but since no norms are available for children with rare disorders, the later treatment phases must be customized to preserve growth, avoid thoracic insufficiency syndrome, and preserve health-related quality of life.

References

1. Pehrsson K, et al. Long-term follow-up of patients with untreated scoliosis a study of mortality, causes of death, and symptoms. Spine. 1992;17(9):1091–6.
2. Swank SM, Winter RB, Moe JH. Scoliosis and cor pulmonale. Spine. 1982;7(4):343–54.
3. Bonafe L, et al. Nosology and classification of genetic skeletal disorders: 2015 revision. Am J Med Genet A. 2015;167(12):2869–92.
4. Kozlowski K. La dysostose spondylometaphysaire. Presse Méd. 1967;75:2769–74.
5. Nural MS, et al. Kozlowski type spondylometaphyseal dysplasia: a case report with literature review. Diagn Interv Radiol. 2006;12(2):70–3.
6. Duarte ML, et al. Spondylometaphyseal dysplasia: an uncommon disease. Radiol Bras. 2017;50(1):63.
7. Ibrahim S, Labelle H, Mac-Thiong J-M. Brace treatment of thoracolumbar kyphosis in spondylometaphyseal dysplasia with restoration of vertebral morphology and sagittal profile: a case report. Spine J. 2015;15(6):e29–34.
8. Gomez JA, et al. Staged growing rods with preimplantation of spinal anchors for complex early onset scoliosis. J Pediatr Orthop. 2017;37(8):e606–11.

Chapter 19
Complications with Early Onset Scoliosis

Brandon A. Ramo and Charles E. Johnston

Case Presentation

History and Physical Examination

A 16-month-old boy presented with a left trunk shift and left thoracic prominence to an outside institution. Previous medical history was noncontributory. A left thoracic scoliosis was noted with a Cobb angle of 45°. A CT scan of the entire spine was obtained to rule out a congenital anomaly (none found), and TLSO bracing was initiated. Of note, no spine MRI was obtained to evaluate for intrathecal anomaly. By age 26 months, despite family-reported good brace compliance, the curve had progressed to 69° (Fig. 19.1).

Implantation of a single concave VEPTR device was performed by the initial treating surgeon at age 2 years + 2 months. The upper rib cradle was inserted under the fifth rib, and a down-going L2 laminar hook was inserted

B.A. Ramo, MD • C.E. Johnston, MD (✉)
Texas Scottish Rite Hospital for Children, Dallas, TX, USA

Department of Orthoapedic Surgery,
University of Texas Southwestern, Dallas, TX, USA
e-mail: brandon.ramo@tsrh.org; charles.johnston@tsrh.org

R. El-Hawary, C.P. Eberson (eds.), *Early Onset Scoliosis*,
https://doi.org/10.1007/978-3-319-71580-3_19

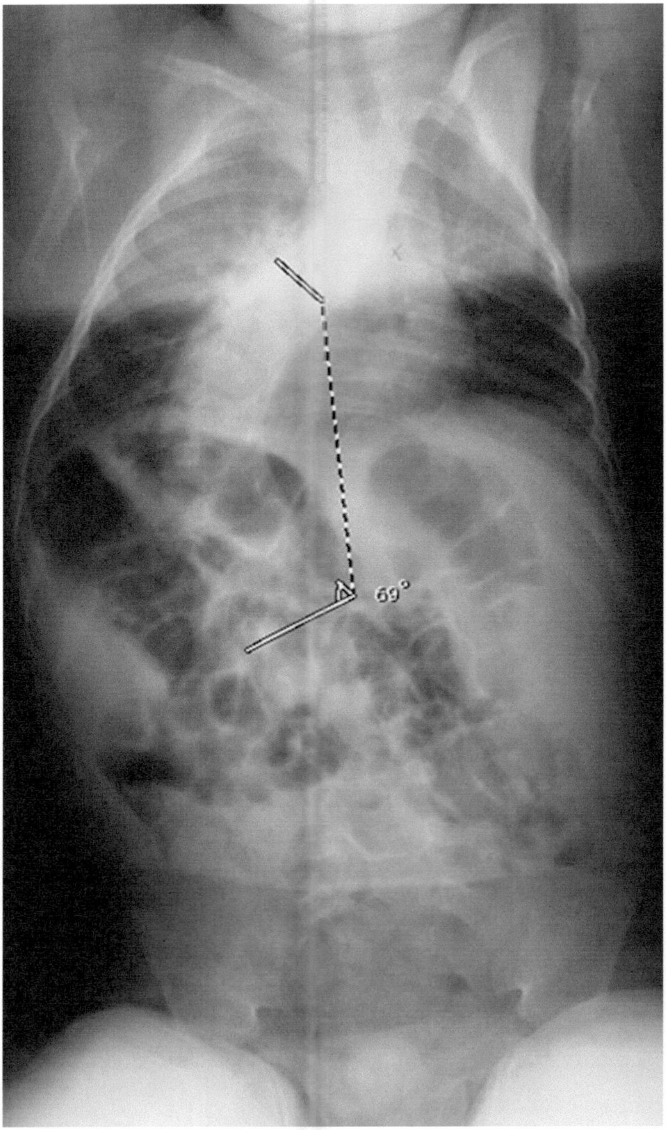

FIGURE 19.1 Supine AP radiograph at age 2 + 2 demonstrating 69° left thoracic scoliosis

at the LIV, as was commonly performed at that time. A superficial wound dehiscence resolved with local wound care and antibiotics. Seven months later, upper cradle revision from rib 5 to 7 was performed due to progression of the main thoracic curve. He then underwent uneventful VETPR lengthening at age 3 years + 4 months and age 3 years + 11 months (Fig. 19.2).

He underwent his fifth procedure at age 4 years + 11 months, a lengthening which was noted to obtain minimal distraction intraoperatively with minimal correction radiographically, followed by another distraction at age 5 years + 5 months.

At age 5 years + 10 months, he was noted to have rib fracture and loss of correction and was returned to the operating room for his seventh procedure and second upper cradle revision where the upper cradle was moved to rib 4–5. Postoperative radiographs (Fig. 19.3) demonstrate further loss of deformity correction, sagittal imbalance, but increasing T1–T12 height.

He then underwent uneventful lengthening of the VEPTR at 6 years + 2 months but was noted to have upper cradle plow postoperatively and underwent another revision of the upper cradle back to the fourth rib, his nineth total procedure, and third upper cradle revision.

At the time of presentation to our institution, the child had severe clinical deformity (Fig. 19.4a–d). He had a shortened trunk with positive forward balance and stiff chest wall. He had a left trunk shift and left rib razorback prominence. He also had prominent implants on the right rib cage and healed multiply operated scars.

Diagnostic Studies

His radiographs demonstrated uncontrolled deformity with a major Cobb angle exceeding 110° and substantial loss of the previously obtained T1–T12 height of only 14 cm. Additionally, his kyphosis has not been well controlled (80°) which has contributed to the loss of upper cradle fixation (Fig. 19.5).

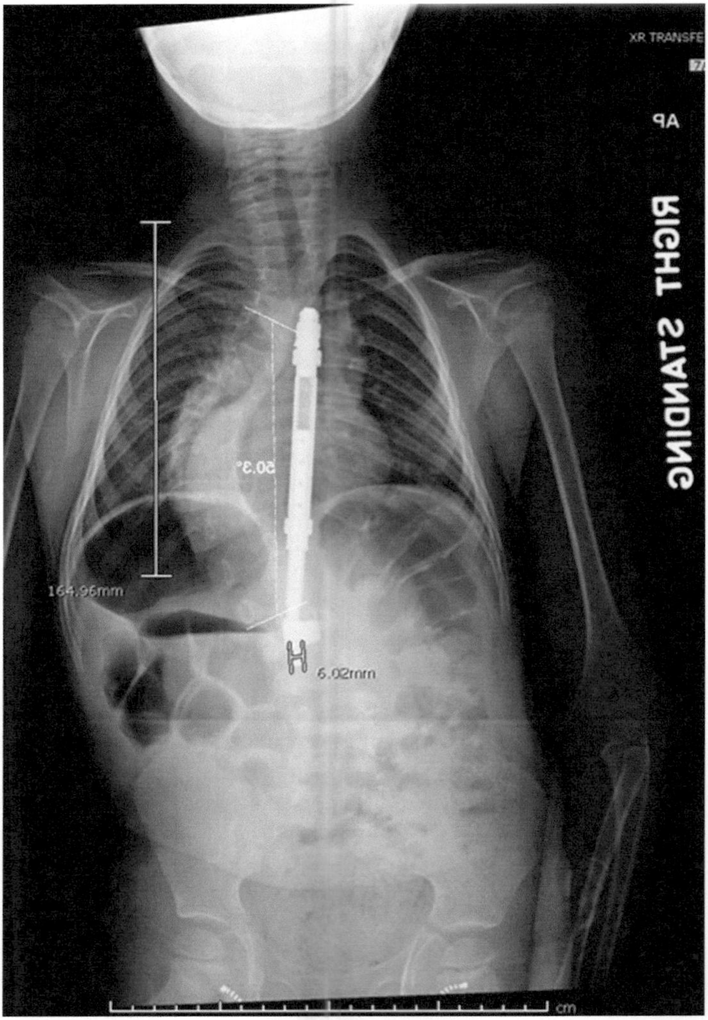

FIGURE 19.2 Age 4 + 3 after VEPTR insertion at age 2 + 2, upper cradle revision at age 2 + 10, and two subsequent uneventful lengthenings at age 3 + 4 and 3 + 11. After 21 months and four procedures, the major Cobb has improved from 69° to 50°, and the T1–T12 height is now 16.5 cm

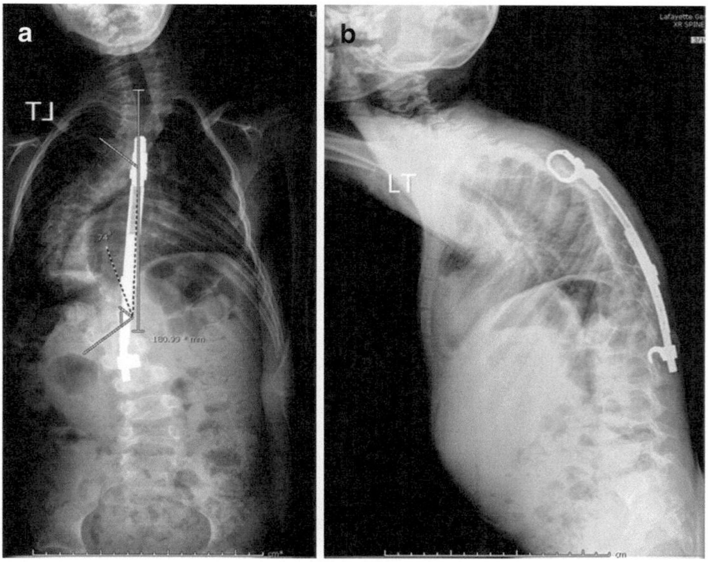

FIGURE 19.3 (**a**, **b**) Age 5 + 10 after revision of upper cradle. After sixth procedure and second upper cradle revision, the child has loss of deformity correction with major Cobb angle now 74°, but T1–T12 height has improved to 18.1 cm. Notice that the sagittal plane is not well accommodated or matched by the device chosen

Pulmonary function tests demonstrated an FVC = 53% predicted and FEV1 = 55% predicted for age. An MRI was obtained due to the lack of CNS evaluation during his previous course of treatment. A pineal tumor and Chiari malformation were identified and eventually underwent surgical treatment by a neurosurgeon with excision of the tumor and Chiari decompression at age 8 years + 5 months.

Management Chosen

Because of the severity and stiffness of the deformity as well as kyphotic sagittal plane, the decision was made to remove

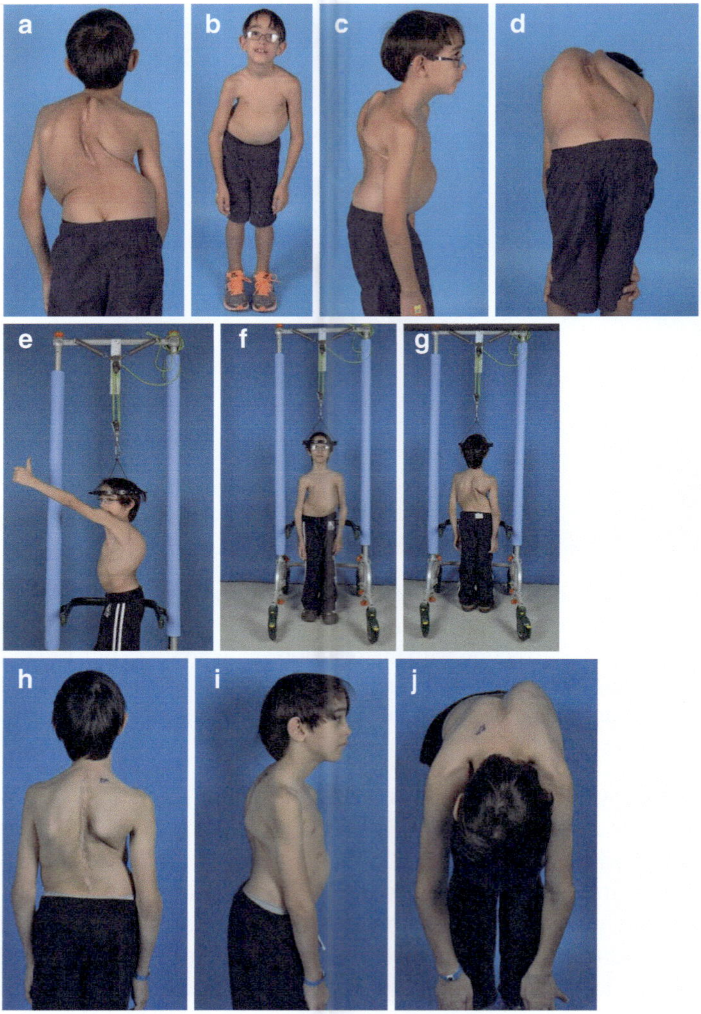

FIGURE 19.4 (**a–d**) Age 7 + 5 at presentation to our institution. (**e–g**) 7 + 10 in HGT. (**h–j**) Age 8 + 10 after implant of growing rods. (**k–m**) Age 9 + 10 after lengthenings. (**n–q**) Age 10 + 10. (**r–u**) Age 11 + 10 before "final" fusion

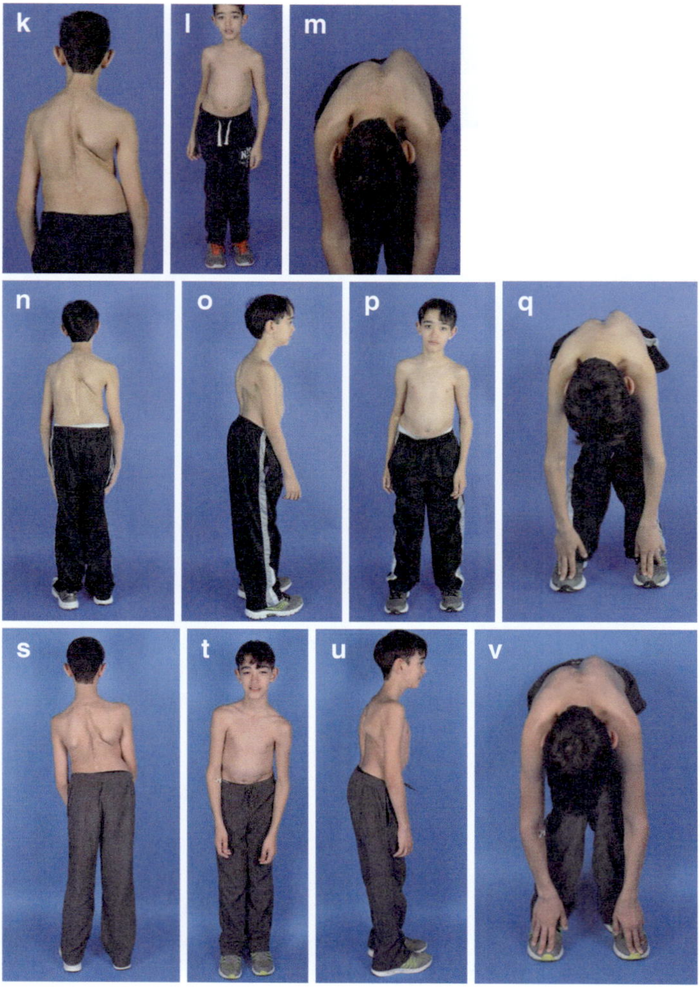

FIGURE 19.4 (continued)

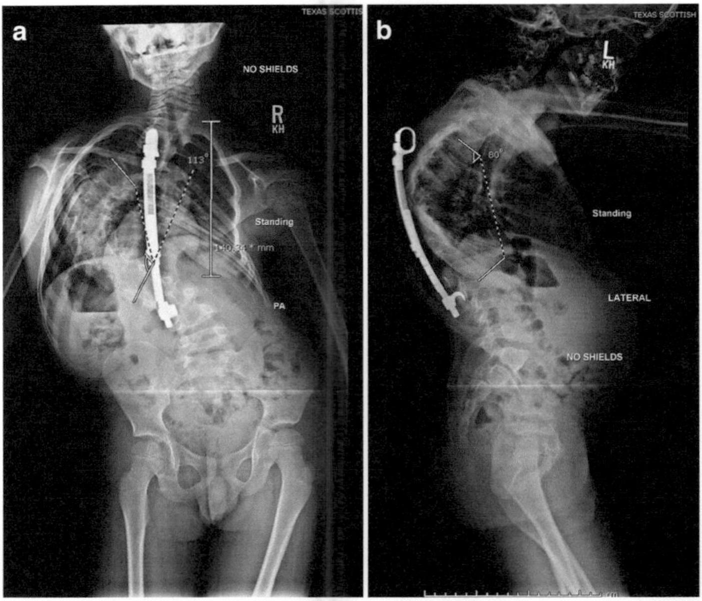

FIGURE 19.5 (**a**, **b**) Age 7 + 0 at presentation to our institution. Following nine procedures including three revisions over 4.8 years, the patient now has a fourth proximal implant failure, uncontrolled deformity with a major Cobb angle exceeding 110°, and substantial loss of previously obtained T1–T12 height of only 14 cm. Additionally, his kyphosis has not been well controlled with kyphosis of 80°

implants and proceed with halo-gravity traction for adjunctive preoperative deformity correction to gain length of the spine and to improve the kyphosis. This allowed the skin, spinal cord, and musculature to adapt to a new position gradually over time employing the viscoelasticity of the tissues while stretching the deformity while the patient is awake and their neurological status can be easily monitored with serial physical exams (Fig. 19.4f–g). This is typically employed at our institution for an 8–12-week period. The next step is then the implantation of dual, tandem growing rods. Our preference is to use spine-based fixation for deformities that do not involve the chest wall and in order to control any major or structural curve within the levels of instrumentation.

Surgical Procedure

First Step: Halo-Gravity Traction Application

The VEPTR was removed and a halo applied with a typical 8-pin construct, with two pins bilaterally anterolaterally and two pins bilaterally posterolaterally. For an older child such as this 7-year-old, we utilize 2 anterior pins and 4–6 posterior pins tightened to 6-inch pounds. Traction is introduced via both walker and wheelchair setup on post-halo application day #1 and then gradually increased over approximately 1–3 weeks to a goal weight that is typically 50–60% of the child's body weight. Cranial nerves and lower extremity strength and reflexes are assessed daily, and weight can be titrated taking in consideration the child's comfort level as some will develop mild neck pain. The use of a double windlass mechanism spring traction system (Fig. 19.4e–g) improves patient comfort compared to weight and pulley or fish-scale systems, as well as improves safety, as the patient can self-discontinue traction by standing or pushing up on wheelchair/walker armrests. We aim for 12 h of traction per day with a goal of 4 h in the walker for ambulatory patients. This is typically performed as an in-patient, although can be done at home with reliable families and weekly checks in clinic.

Second Step: Anterior Release and Growing Rod Insertion with Apical Control

This child spent approximately 5 months in halo-gravity traction, with one complication occurring during traction which was pin loosening necessitating a return to the OR for pin revision approximately 3 months into traction(Fig. 19.6). At age 7 years + 10 months, an anterior release from T7 to T11 was

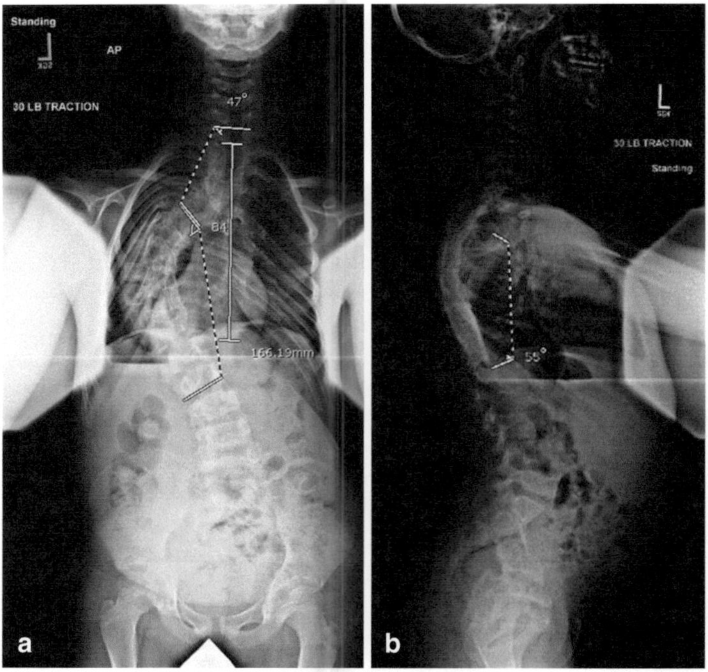

FIGURE 19.6 (**a**, **b**) Appearance of the spine after 4 months of halo-gravity traction. The coronal plane deformity now measures 84° (27.5% improvement), and the sagittal major Cobb has improved to 55° (37% improvement)

performed to address the stiffness of the rib cage and the apical penetration of the spine into the thorax (Fig. 19.7). The seventh rib was selected as the entry point for the thoracotomy. With retractors in place, it was noted clinically that the spine essentially touched the lateral chest wall at the apex of the deformity. This made dissection of the upper and lower ends of the curve difficult due to the marked obliquity of the disc spaces falling away from the apex. Following discectomy, no attempt to fuse the anterior interbody spaces was made. The sole purpose of the anterior procedure was to provide some flexibility to this patient's exceedingly stiff and rotated apex.

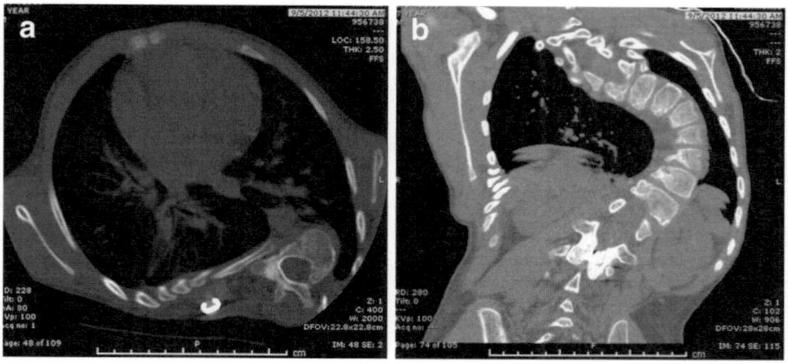

FIGURE 19.7 (**a**, **b**) CT scan demonstrating significant apical penetration of the spine into the left thorax with the spine nearly abutting the left ribs due to its rotation

The thoracotomy was closed, and the patient was repositioned prone and halo traction installed at 30 pounds on the head and 10 lbs on each leg via skin tape. Use of intraoperative traction assists with deformity correction prior to implant placement and improves access to upper implant points, particularly in proximal kyphotic deformities where placing pedicle screws in the upper thoracic spine can require steep angles. Intraoperative neuromonitoring using TcMEPs and SSEPs is standard.

The previous midline incision was utilized taking care to expose spinal elements subperiosteally only at levels intended for anchor placement. In this case, T3–5 and L2–4 were exposed. The L2 segment (the site of the previous VEPTR sublaminar hook) was noted to have spontaneously fused. Pedicle screws were placed on the left side of L2, L3, and L4 and on the right side at L3 and L4 using standard technique.

An extensive rib fusion was found from the transverse processes at T4–5, probably due to the previous VEPTR cradle. The ribs were dissected laterally and then cut using osteotome and Kerrison Rongeur to free the upper thoracic spine from these rib fusions. Because of a significant rib fusion on the concavity of the right side, an up-going laminar hook site was created in the rib mass underneath the expanded transverse process. A claw construct was created using the transverse process of T4 medially above it. On the left side, a T4 pedicle screw was placed with a down-going hook placed over the T3 transverse process to create a claw construct.

The convex apex (left side) was then approached lateral to the paraspinous musculature (direct approach to pedicles due to rotation) to place T9 and T10 pedicle screws, to provide control of the apex of the deformity and be able to translate it medially toward the concavity. Facet joints were excised from these two levels and screws placed.

A rod of the appropriate length was contoured and tunneled under the musculature of the convex side to connect the proximal thoracic anchors on the left side to the apical screws which had just been placed at T9 and T10. A second rod requiring complex contouring to accommodate lordosis and apical rotation was then "dominoed" to the proximal rod. During the assembly of this construct, a significant amount of lateral translation was achieved using the apical screws. Once the cantilever connecting maneuvers had been completed, the right rod construct (two rods connected by domino) was then distracted directly, with concave length and opening of the hemithorax being achieved.

Locally harvested rib and spine autograft was applied to the instrumented foundations from T3 to T4 and from L2 to L4. No complications occurred. Postoperative images are provided in Fig. 19.8.

Subsequent Steps: Growing Rod Distractions and Rod Revisions

At age 8 years + 9 months, approximately 1 year following implantation, during the planned growing rod distraction, a rod fracture on the left was noted intraoperatively necessitating rod revision. Both left and right rods were then distracted at the level of the domino. During every distraction procedure, asymmetric concave greater than convex distraction of 1.0–2.5 cm was attempted.

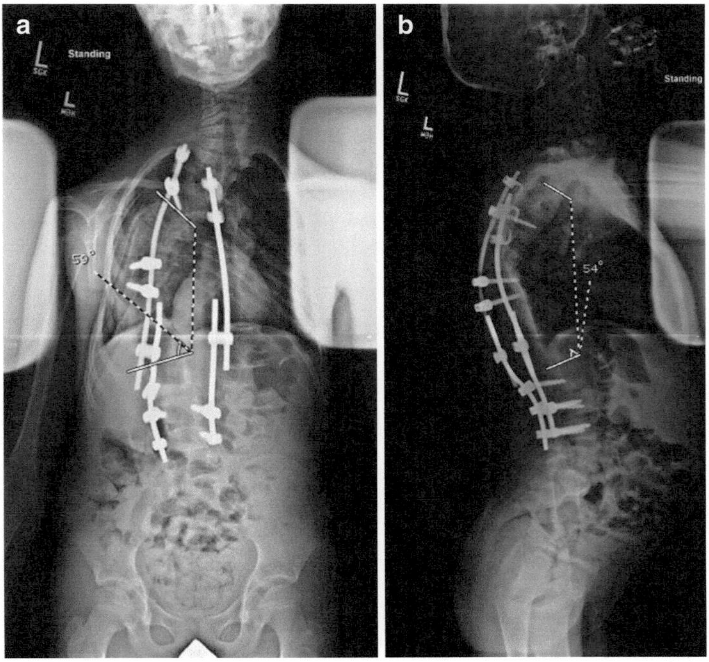

FIGURE 19.8 (**a**, **b**) Postoperative images at age 8 + 0. There has been further correction of the coronal plane deformity after traction, and the sagittal kyphosis remains stable at 54° from correction achieved while in traction. The apical screws seen on the left at T9 and T10 represent an option to try and decreased apical penetration of the spine into the left chest wall and to allow in situ contouring during future lengthenings to translate the apex further to the midline

The child underwent uneventful distraction at age 9 years + 10 months, 1 year later (Fig. 19.9).

At age 10 years + 8 months, a second rod fracture on the right was noted after the child felt a "pop" near his right scapula. The right rod was replaced at the time of a planned lengthening at age 10 years + 10 months, exchanging a titanium rod for cobalt chrome (Fig. 19.10). Utilizing the concept of apical control: during the lengthening procedure, the apical set screws are loosened to allow the rod to slide, and then the rods

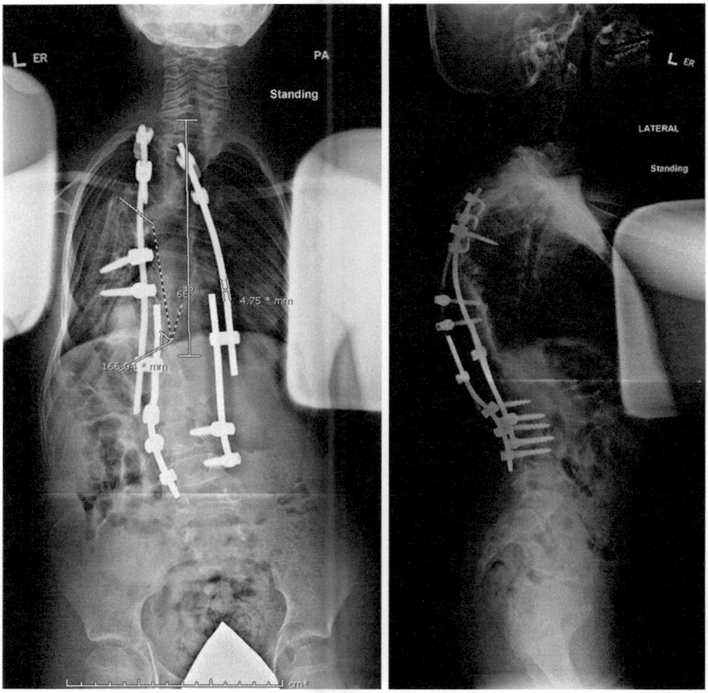

FIGURE 19.9 Age 9 + 10 after first lengthening of the new growing rod system. Major Cobb has improved to 68° coronally, and T1–T12 height is now 16.7 cm

are bent in situ to translate the apex toward the concavity while the screws can be rotated. The changing contour of the distal left rod is noted from Figs. 19.8, 19.9, 19.10, 19.11 with resulting improvement in the apical penetration.

Final Fusion

At age 11 years + 5 months, the child was evaluated and found to have stable spinal deformity and radiographs, and consideration was given to observation without final fusion. However, at age 11 years + 10 months, the child fractured his right rod again while playing baseball (Fig. 19.11). The decision was

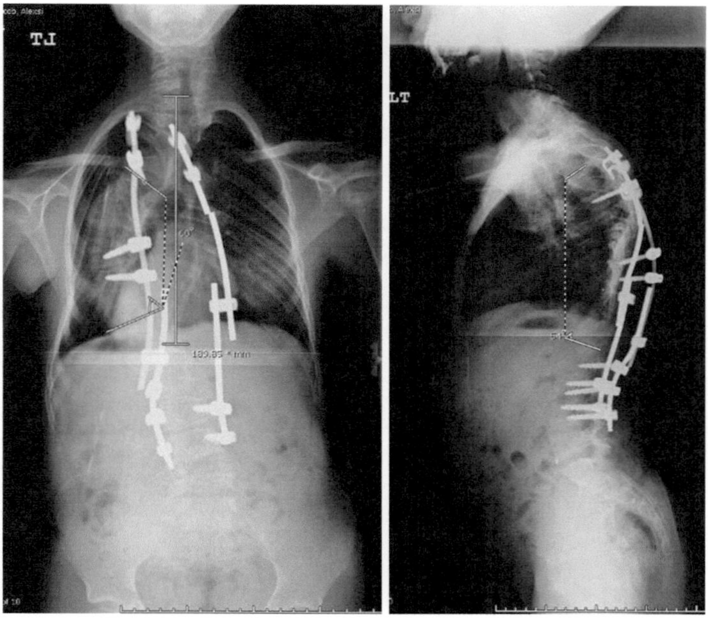

FIGURE 19.10 Age 10 + 10 immediately prior to revision incorporated into planned lengthening for fractured rod. Coronal Cobb angle is stable at 60°, and coronal T1–T12 height is now 19.0 cm. Sagittal Cobb has stabilized at 54°

therefore made to proceed with final fusion. This was performed by accepting the spinal deformity as is, replacing all growth constructs with new 5.5 mm cobalt chrome rods, decorticating previously unexposed areas of the spine, and laying in the newly contoured rods with additional new intercalary anchors to improve stability (Fig. 19.12). This procedure was performed and healed without complication.

Clinical Course and Outcome

Radiographic images demonstrate interval correction over 4 years of follow-up. During the full course of treatment and subsequent follow-up, two complications of rod fracture were

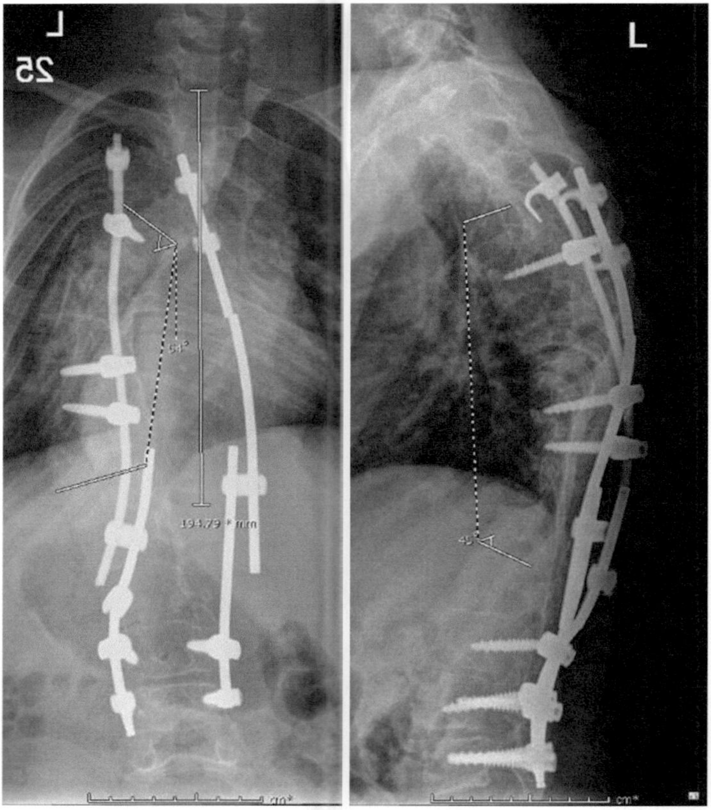

FIGURE 19.11 Age 11 + 10 second rod fracture at same location. Coronal major Cobb is now 54°, and coronal T1–T12 height is 19.5 cm. Sagittal Cobb has improved at 45°

noted. These both occurred immediately prior to planned interval lengthening at the 1 year mark and therefore resulted in no additional anesthetic or procedures. *At last follow-up, a 50° right-sided curve from T1 to T7 and a 42° left-sided curve from T8 to L3 were present.* Coronally measured T1–T12 height improved from 14 cm at presentation at age 7 years to 19.4 cm at final fusion at age 11 years + 10 months. Coronal Cobb angle improved from 113° to 50°, while sagittal major Cobb kyphosis improved from 80° to 44°. Additionally, coronal

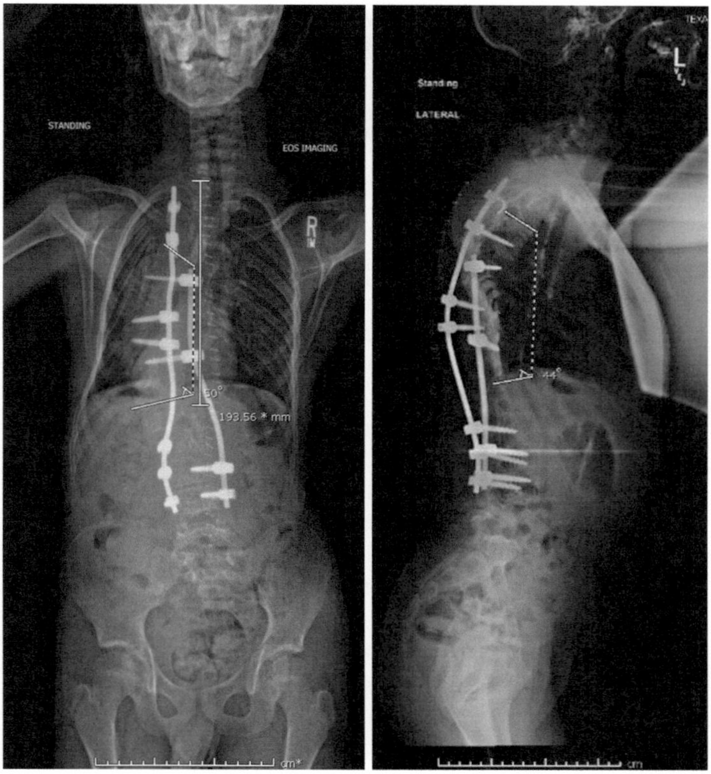

FIGURE 19.12 Age 11 + 10 after "final" fusion. Coronal Cobb is 50°, and coronal T1–T12 height is 19.4 cm. Sagittal Cobb (T4–T12) is now 44°

plane balance was clearly improved as was the patient's cosmetic deformity (Fig. 19.4a–k). At age 11 years + 5 months, PFTs obtained demonstrated slight improvement of FVC to 63% predicted for age and FEV1 of 61% predicted for age.

Clinical Pearls and Pitfalls

- Our preference is for delay tactics, such as casting with or without early application of halo-gravity traction, to be attempted instead of surgical implantation at age

2 years + 2 months. Delay would have allowed more robust anchors and more growing instrument options. Premature implantation of unilateral constructs provides poor deformity control and has unacceptable complication rates.

- Halo-gravity traction is a useful pre-growing rod implantation adjunct to improve deformity correction and to nutritionally optimize patients.
- Stable proximal fixation is critical and becomes more so in the setting of excessive kyphosis.
- Idiopathic infantile scoliosis is a diagnosis of exclusion requiring formal assessment of the spinal canal and brainstem with the use of magnetic resonance imaging. One may speculate that the early severe progression was related to the pineal tumor and Chiari malformation diagnosed only after initial and repetitive treatments at age 7.
- Rod fracture is a known complication of growing rod treatment, but when occurring in dual-growing rod constructs, it often results in no increase in reoperation rate as rod revision can be incorporated into planned interval lengthening.
- It is unknown at this time whether all patients require "final" fusion, but it is clear that many patients require future procedures even after the treating surgeon feels treatment is final.

Literature Review and Discussion

Complications related to the surgical management of early onset scoliosis are myriad and ubiquitous. At our institution, parents are informed of a nearly 100% likelihood of any individual patient having a complication during what is, by definition, a prolonged treatment course. Several key studies have supported the incredibly high rate of complications associated with EOS [1–3], and a new disease-specific complication system has been devised [2] (Table 19.1).

It is important to apply certain principles which have been elucidated and supported in the literature. First, Bess et al. [1]

TABLE 19.1 Complications classification system

Grading	Device related	Disease related
I	Does not require unplanned surgery	Outpatient medical management only
II		Impatient medical management
IIA	Requires 1 unplanned surgery	
Ii B	Requires multiple unplanned surgeries	
III	Requires abandoning growth-friendly strategy	Requires abandoning growth-friendly strategy
IV	Death	Death

reported that the risk of complication, particularly surgical site infection, increases by 20% with each subsequent surgical procedure. Therefore, any non-operative method which can control the deformity while delaying surgical intervention is a useful one. Fletcher et al. [4] demonstrated that casting offers an opportunity, in patients who can tolerate serial anesthesia and a compressive force on the chest, to delay surgical intervention on average 39 months, in a cohort of patients who were specifically identified as expected to eventually require management (not those infantile idiopathic curves attempting a cure) [4]. Other studies have found similar results using casting to delay timing to surgery [5]. While a legitimate criticism of casting is the concern over effects on the immature cerebrum from repetitive anesthesia in children under 3, it clearly avoids the complications inherent to surgical management such as infection, scarring, creation of chest wall stiffness, and others [6–8].

In the case of our patient, had casting been employed, while unlikely to be curative, it may have allowed a curve to be controlled for at least a year and with transition to a TLSO after improvement of the major Cobb with casting, an additional several years of delay may have been achieved [9]. The psychological effects of repetitive surgical treatment of EOS on children are now more well understood, and it cannot be overstated that the child in the case above had 15 separate spinal surgeries during his treatment course over a decade [10, 11]. Especially in light of the data presented by Bess et al. [1] and noted above, any opportunity to reduce the number of total surgeries has value. The authors feel that halo-gravity traction offers an opportunity to delay surgery while controlling and even improving spinal deformity and have employed it at our institution in difficult circumstances as a repetitive instrument combined with aggressive casting and bracing to delay surgical treatment for years. HGT is in general safe when patients are monitored routinely. Known complications including cervical distraction and cranial nerve deficit, particularly in the setting of cervical spine fusions, are rare. Common complications are pin track infection and pin loosening necessitating halo pin revision [12–15].

This patient suffered proximal anchor failure on three separate occasions during the first 4 years of treatment. While the contour of the implant may be partially to blame, this is a known complication of growth-friendly implants, and increased kyphosis has clearly been linked with the risk of proximal implant/anchor failure [3, 16]. Recent evidence has suggested that the number of proximal anchors, specifically more than five, may help diminish the odds of implant failure, regardless of whether rib or spine anchors are used [17].

We note that an MRI was not obtained during the initial 4 years of treatment at the first facility, therefore delaying the knowledge that this might not be an idiopathic scoliosis but rather a curve associated with an underlying CNS abnormality. One study has suggested a 16% incidence of positive CNS MRI findings in presumed idiopathic infantile scoliosis [18]; thus, it is the authors' belief that any child with a presumed diagnosis of IIS should receive an MRI at least before the onset of surgical management. The diagnosis of a Chiari-associated scoliosis may have alerted the treating physician to a potentially more challenging treatment course.

It is well established that EOS patients can receive elevated amounts of ionizing radiation during multiple diagnostic studies during their childhood, and thus unnecessary or injudicious use of radiation should be considered as a complication [19]. CT tomography represents the largest contributor to ionizing radiation doses these children receive, and therefore the use of a CT scan to evaluate an idiopathic-like deformity in a 1-year-old such as in this case is not indicated and clearly inferior to MRI. MRI offers not only considerably more information toward a diagnosis but also no unnecessary radiation exposure. We often incorporate the timing of the MRI with initial treatment such as a cast or halo to minimize the number of anesthetics.

The recently developed Classification for Early Onset Scoliosis (C-EOS) system may eventually be validated as a useful prognostic tool, and in this case, by establishing an accurate diagnosis may have aided in expectations for complications [20]. This will be a valuable tool to compare various growth-friendly treatment options (guided growth technique vs distraction-based techniques, or rib anchors vs. spine anchors) [2]. The senior author of this chapter campaigned for a separate category of complication to identify when there is a complication related to inappropriate use of an expandable device which due to its subjective nature was not incorporated into the classification system [2] (Table 19.1). It is our opinion that the device employed in this child which utilizes a rib anchor system without the ability to contour for the pre-existing kyphosis represents an inappropriate use of that device which was initially designed for chest wall deformities. Attempting to use rib anchors in a 2-year-old, and the three proximal anchor revisions required over the first 4 years of treatment, speaks to the issue of inappropriate use. When the system was converted to a dual spine-based growing rod system which could be contoured to accommodate for kyphosis, there were no further proximal anchorage failures. The authors' opinion is that rib-based constructs should be used primarily for chest wall deformities and that spine-based constructs should be employed for purely spinal deformities. Further, dual-rod treatment regardless of implant utilized now has multiple citations in the literature demonstrating superiority over single-rod instrumentation [1, 21]. Bess et al. [1] demonstrated the lowest complication rates in patients treated with dual submuscular growing rods. This makes inherent sense as it allows dispersement of forces over 100% more implant, and the case presentation above may have been improved by the use of a dual-rod implant from initial treatment. Significant control of axial plane deformity ("crankshaft") has also been described in dual-rod constructs [22]—a significant component of this patient's uncontrolled deformity prior to transfer of care was the associated crankshaft and rib hump deformity (Fig. 19.4a–d).

Rod breakage is an expected consequence of any growth-friendly rod of early onset scoliosis, which is an inherent risk of trying to maintain motion of a spine with implants that are not currently designed to accommodate motion and therefore are subject to metal fatigue stresses. That two rod fractures occurred in this case simply illustrates that once the end anchors of a growth-friendly construct are stabilized, fatigue failure is inherent and is proof of the concept that the intercalary vertebral segments are still moving and thus can be lengthened or manipulated. Rod fracture occurs in 15% of patients with fusionless constructs, occurring more often in ambulatory patients (21%) [23]. An important point is that rod fractures are usually addressed at the time of anticipated lengthening surgery, and therefore, while they often represent a grade 1 complication as an unintended event, additional unplanned surgery is unnecessary, avoiding converting the rod fracture to a grade IIA complication [2]. However, should the rod fracture be so symptomatic or be associated with such an excessive loss of correction that an unplanned revision is performed, the opportunity for an additional lengthening should in most cases be utilized at the time of rod revision. The decision to replace an intact rod at the time of fractured rod revision must be made on an individual case basis, taking into consideration, among other things, the amount of time the intact rod has been implanted and the amount of remaining rod overlap available for future lengthenings.

Infection, although it did not occur in this case, is one of the most common complications of growing rod surgery because of repetitive soft tissue intrusion and micromotion of the implants, resulting in implant debris in the soft tissue envelope which can incite an inflammatory response. Careful attention to management of the soft tissues and layered, staggered wound closure may obviate some infection risk [24]. *Any* infection around growing rod implants should be treated with aggressive irrigation and debridement and i.v. antibiotics followed by suppressive oral antibiotics. In cases where gross infection cannot be cleared, we have employed a period of halo-gravity traction to allow complete implant removal while still controlling the deformity until inflammatory markers return to normal and reimplantation can occur.

Finally, it has been proposed, particularly in light of complications which can occur with final treatment, that observation may be appropriate in some patients rather than attempting a final fusion if the surgeon feels growth has been maximized [25, 26]. In our patient, we attempted this observation strategy, but he fractured a rod through an area of persistent motion near the apex of his deformity. He recently underwent "final" fusion, but, as reported by Poe-Kochert [27], there is significant potential for further surgical treatment due to a number of possible complications, and thus "final" fusion may not yet have been realized.

The complications illustrated by this case include:

1. Failure to accurately diagnose the etiology of the scoliosis. At a minimum, an MRI should have been performed prior to surgical treatment.
2. Failure to use delay tactics to avoid or reduce complications inherent in early surgical treatment. Early surgery by definition means more operations, with the incidence of complications increasing with each subsequent operation.
3. Inappropriate use of CT radiation to "evaluate" a non-congenital deformity, rather than appropriate use of MRI.

4. Inappropriate implant which is ineffective in controlling coronal and axial plane deformity and does not accommodate sagittal plane consideration.
5. Halo pin loosening necessitating repeat anesthetic.
6. Growing rod fractures × 2 which in this case did not require additional unplanned surgery but are an expected consequence of growth-friendly constructs.
7. Additional potential for procedure necessary after presumed final treatment (observation)—to be determined.

References

1. Bess S, Akbarnia BA, Thompson GH, et al. Complications of growing-rod treatment for early-onset scoliosis: analysis of one hundred and forty patients. J Bone Joint Surg Am. 2010;92:2533–43.
2. Smith JT, et al. A new classifcation system to report complications in growing spine surgery: a multicenter consensus study. J Pediatr Orthop. 2015;35:798–803.
3. Watanabe K, et al. Risk factors for complications associated with growing-rod surgery for early-onset scoliosis. Spine (Phila Pa 1976). 2013;38(8):E464–8.
4. Fletcher ND, et al. Serial casting as a delay tactic in the treatment of moderate-to-severe early-onset scoliosis. J Pediatr Orthop. 2012;32:664–71.
5. Baulesh DM, et al. The role of serial casting in early-onset scoliosis. J Pediatr Orthop. 2012;32:658–63.
6. Backeljauw B, Holland SK, Altaye M, Loepke AW. Cognition and brain structure following early childhood surgery with anesthesia. Pediatrics. 2015;136(1):e1–e12.
7. Ing C, DiMaggio C, Whitehouse A, et al. Long-term differences in language and cognitive function after childhood exposure to anesthesia. Pediatrics. 2012;130(3):e476–85.
8. Sun LS, et al. Association between a single general anesthesia exposure before age 36 months and neurocognitive outcomes in later childhood. JAMA. 2016;315(21):2312–20.
9. Johnston CE, et al. Comparison of growing rod instrumentation versus serial cast treatment for early-onset scoliosis. Spine Deform. 2013;1(5):339–42.

10. Matsumoto H, et al. Psychosocial effects of repetitive surgeries in children with early-onset scoliosis: are we putting them at risk? J Pediatr Orthop. 2014;34(2):172–8.
11. Flynn JM, et al. Psychological dysfunction in children who require repetitive surgery for early onset scoliosis. J Pediatr Orthop. 2012;32(6):594–9.
12. Sink EL, et al. Efficacy of perioperative halo-gravity traction in the treatment of severe scoliosis in children. J Pediatr Orthop. 2001;21(4):519–24.
13. Nemani VM, et al. Preoperative halo-gravity traction for severe spinal deformities at an SRS-GOP site in West Africa: protocols, complications, and results. Spine. 2015;40(3):153–61.
14. Grabekyan T, et al. The results of preoperative halo-gravity traction in children with severe spinal deformity. J Pediatr Orthop B. 2014;23(1):1–5.
15. Bogunovic. Preoperative halo-gravity traction for severe pediatric spinal deformity: complications, radiographic correction and changes in pulmonary function. Spine Deform. 2013;1(1):33–9.
16. Schroerlucke SR, et al. How does thoracic kyphosis affect patient outcomes in growing rod surgery? Spine. 2012;37(15):1303–9.
17. Vitale et al. Proximal Rib vs Proximal Spine Anchors in Growing Rods: A Multicenter Prospective Study. Spine Deformity. 2015;3(6): 626–627
18. Martin BD, et al. Intrathecal anomalies in presumed infantile idiopathic scoliosis: when is MRI necessary? Spine Deform. 2014;2(6):444–7.
19. Khorsand D, et al. Iatrogenic radiation exposure to patients with early onset spine and chest wall deformities. Spine. 2013;38(17):E1108–14.
20. Williams BA, et al. Development and initial validation of the classification of early-onset scoliosis. J Bone Joint Surg Am. 2014;96:1359–67.
21. Akbarnia BA, Marks DS, Boachie-Adjei O, et al. Dual growing rod technique for the treatment of progressive early-onset scoliosis: a multicenter study. Spine. 2005;30:S46–57.
22. Kamaci S, et al. The effect of dual growing rod instrumentation on the apical vertebral rotation in early-onset idiopathic scoliosis. J Pediatr Orthop. 2014;34(6):607–12.
23. Yang JS, Sponseller PD, et al. Growing rod fractures: risk factors and opportunities for prevention. Spine. 2011;36(20):1639–44.

24. Grzywna AM, et al. Offset layered closure reduces deep wound infection in early-onset scoliosis surgery. J Pediatr Orthop B. 2016;25(4):361–8.
25. Jain A, et al. Avoidance of "final" surgical fusion after growing-rod treatment for early-onset scoliosis. J Bone Joint Surg Am. 2016;98(13):1073–8.
26. Sawyer JR, et al. Complications and radiographic outcomes of posterior spinal fusion and observation in patients who have undergone distraction-based treatment for early onset scoliosis. Spine Deform. 2016;4(6):407–12.
27. Poe-Kochert C, et al. Final fusion after growing-rod treatment for early onset scoliosis: is it really final? J Bone Joint Surg Am. 2016;98(22):1913–7.

Chapter 20
Spine Growth Assessment of Growth-Friendly Surgery

Ron El-Hawary and Félix Brassard

Case Presentation

A 6-year-old boy presented with early onset scoliosis secondary to neurofibromatosis. His parents first noticed an asymmetric appearance of his scapulae 1 year prior to his presentation. They also observed a significant and worsening deformity of his posterior chest wall, especially when the patient was bending forward.

History and Physical Examination

There is no known family history of spinal deformity; however, his father has neurofibromatosis, type 1 with multiple cutaneous neurofibromas and café-au-lait spots. There were no complications during pregnancy or delivery, which was a vaginal cephalic delivery. His APGAR score at birth was 9-10-10. The patient presents with otherwise normal global development. He walked at the age of 13 months. He has no

R. El-Hawary, MD, MSc, FRCS(C) (✉) • F. Brassard, MD, FRCS(C)
IWK Health Centre, Halifax, NS, Canada
e-mail: ron.el-hawary@iwk.nshealth.ca; felix.brassard@hotmail.com

R. El-Hawary, C.P. Eberson (eds.), *Early Onset Scoliosis*,
https://doi.org/10.1007/978-3-319-71580-3_20

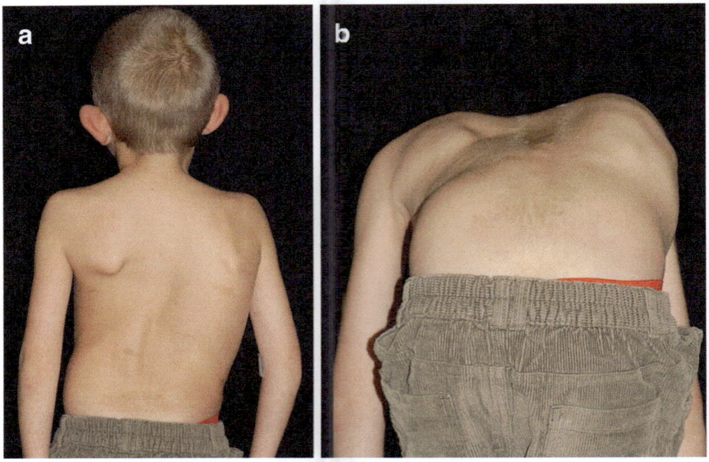

FIGURE 20.1 Healthy-appearing 5-year-old male. (**a**) Standing clinical photograph demonstrating multiple café-au-lait spots, axillary and inguinal freckling, shoulder asymmetry with right scapula lateralized and elevated, right trunk shift, asymmetry of waistline, and no pelvic tilt. (**b**) Adam's forward bending test demonstrates right rib prominence (14° scoliometer)

allergies and is not taking any medication. There are no motor or sensory symptoms. He has normal sphincter function. The patient never complained of backache or headache. There is no history of recurrent pulmonary infection, weight loss, or constitutional symptoms.

Spine examination is presented in Fig. 20.1. Neurological examination:

- Normal motor, sensory, and reflex function in upper and lower extremities
- Normal superficial abdominal reflexes
- Normal tone, no clonus, and normal cutaneous plantar reflexes (Babinski test)
- Normal gait with no evidence of hip, knee, or foot anomaly

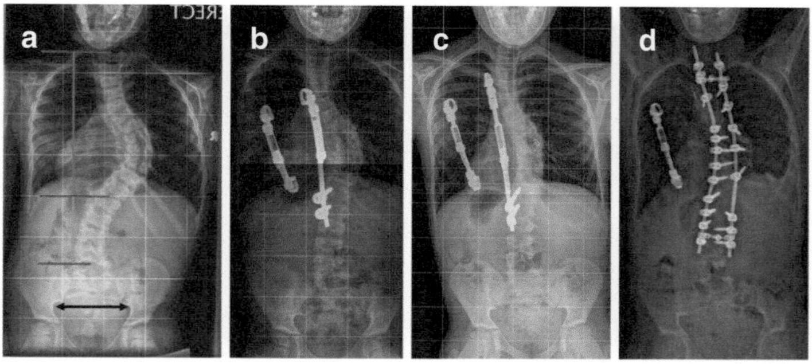

FIGURE 20.2 Serial standing PA radiographs. (**a**) Preoperative at age 7.3 years. Thoracic spine height is measured by drawing a horizontal line from the middle of the superior end plate of T1 (*red*) and drawing a second horizontal line from the middle of the superior end plate of L1 (*red*). Connecting these two parallel lines with a vertical line (*blue*) is the thoracic spine height. Lumbar spine height is measured by a horizontal line from the midpoint of the superior end plate of L1 (*red*) and drawing a perpendicular line (*green*) connecting this horizontal line to the S1 horizontal line. The vertical distance between these lines is the lumbar spine height. Total spine height is the summation of thoracic and lumbar spine heights. The *black* line represents the maximum pelvic inlet width (PW). (**b**) Post-implantation. (**c**) 5 years post-implantation. (**d**) Post-graduate surgery

Diagnostic Studies

At the age of 7 years, standing postero-anterior (PA) and lateral X-rays of the spine revealed no congenital anomalies and close proximity (but no fusion) of the sixth to the tenth ribs on the left side. The patient was skeletally immature with open triradiate cartilage (Figs. 20.2a and 20.3a). There was a 63° right thoracic scoliosis from T6 to T11, the thoracic height was 17 cm, and the total spine height was 26.4 cm (Fig. 20.2a). There was a thoracic kyphosis of 21° with thoracic sagittal spine length (SSL) of 17.6 cm and the total sagittal spine length (SSL) of 31.7 cm (Fig. 20.3a).

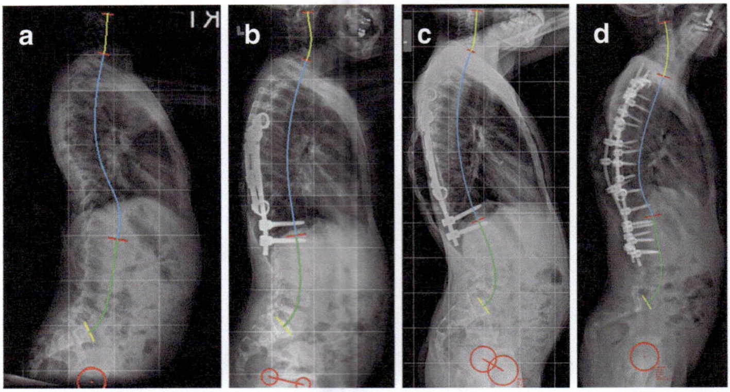

FIGURE 20.3 Serial standing lateral radiographs. (**a**) Preoperative at age 7.3 years. Thoracic sagittal spine length is measured by a curved arc along the length of the thoracic spine in the sagittal plane from upper end plate of T1 to upper end plate of L1 (*blue*). Lumbar spine length is measure by a curved arc along the length of the lumbar spine in the sagittal plane from upper end plate of L1 to upper end plate of S1 (*green*). Total sagittal spine length is the summation of thoracic and lumbar sagittal spine lengths. (**b**) Post-implantation. (**c**) 5 years post-implantation. (**d**) Post-graduate surgery

A complete spine MRI was performed showing no sign of spinal cord anomaly or dural ectasia. Using the Classification for Early Onset Scoliosis (C-EOS), this patient was classified as S3 N [1].

Management Chosen

The Scoliosis Research Society Growing Spine Committee defined the goals of treatment for patients presenting with early onset scoliosis: minimize spinal deformity over the life of the patient; maximize thoracic volume and function over the life of the patient; minimize the extent of any final spinal fusion; maximize motion of the chest and spine; minimize complications, procedures, hospitalizations, and burden for the family; and consider overall development of the child [2].

Achieving these goals should allow better alveolar lung development, potentially avoiding thoracic insufficiency syndrome and associated respiratory and heart failure [3]. Improving global spinal balance and alignment will also have a positive impact on energy expenditure of upright standing, neurologic function, pain, and clinical appearance.

Depending on skeletal maturity, nature of deformity, magnitude of curvature, and the progression of spinal deformity over time, a specific avenue of treatment must be methodically chosen for each individual patient [4]. The various management options available are:

(a) Observation
(b) Casting/bracing
(c) Growth-friendly spine implants

Distraction-based systems (rib or spine-based)
Compression-based systems (vertebral body stapling, vertebral body tethering)
Guided growth systems (Luque Trolley, Shilla technique)

In rare scenarios, spinal fusion and instrumentation may be chosen; however, this treatment violates several principles of growth-friendly treatment for early onset scoliosis [5].

After detailed evaluation and explanation of the different treatment options, a distraction-based growth-friendly implant (VEPTR; DePuy Synthes Spine, Raynham, Ma) was chosen.

Surgical Procedure

After detailed preoperative planning for implant insertion and anchor levels, two VEPTR rods were inserted from a posterior approach with minimal dissection. A medial rod was anchored on the fifth rib proximally and distally on T12 and L1. A lateral rod was also inserted from the sixth to the 11th ribs. Initial distraction was performed. Multimodal neurophysiologic monitoring did not show any significant changes during the procedure (Fig. 20.2b).

Clinical Course and Outcome

Surgical Course

After the initial implantation surgery, serial surgical procedures were performed every 6–9 months [6, 7]. Between implantation surgery at age 7 years and his last lengthening surgery at age 12 years, the patient had nine uncomplicated lengthening surgeries and one planned rod exchange. Just prior to "graduation" surgery, at age 14 years, the patient had an implant failure with disengagement of the superior medial rib hook from the medial rod. The patient proceeded to his "graduation" surgery which involved prone right thoracoscopic anterior fusion from thoracic vertebrae 7 to thoracic vertebrae 11, removal of medial VEPTR device, posterior spinal fusion, and instrumentation from thoracic vertebrae 2 to lumbar vertebrae 3 with allograft. The anterior procedure was performed to decrease the risk of pseudarthrosis in this patient with neurofibromatosis (Figs. 20.2 and 20.3) [8].

Assessment of Growth

Table 20.1 outlines the growth of this patient's spine throughout his growth-friendly surgical treatment. These measurements of spine growth include the standard of care coronal plane vertical height measurements of thoracic spine height and total spine height (Fig. 20.2a). As these coronal plane measurements do not take into account any out-of-plane sagittal length changes, the table also includes thoracic and total sagittal spine length measurements (Fig. 20.3a).

Coronal plane growth can be assessed during the following phases of treatment:

- Implantation Phase: During insertion of the growth-friendly device, "growth" is mainly the result of deformity correction (biomechanical distraction) plus any growth from implantation to just before the first lengthening surgery.

TABLE 20.1 Summary of spinal parameters from the preoperative, post-implant, 5 years post-implant, and at the time of the graduation surgery for the presented patient

Time	Age (year)	Kyphosis (°)	Thoracic height (cm)	SSL-Thoracic (cm)	Total spine height (cm)	SSL-Total (cm)
Preoperative	7.3	21	17.0	17.6	26.4	31.7
Post-implant	7.3	22	20.5	23.0	32.2	35.4
5 years post-implant	12.6	34	24.7	27.3	37.0	41.7
Graduation	14.9	23	25.4	26.0	37.4	42.4

Ht height, *SSL* sagittal spine length

– Growth from Implantation Phase	= (Post-Implant–Pre-Operative) Ht
– Thoracic Growth Implantation Phase	= 20.5 cm–17.0 cm
	= 3.5 cm
– Total Spine Growth Implantation Phase	= 32.2 cm–26.4 cm
	= 5.8 cm

- Distraction Phase: During periodic serial lengthening procedures, "growth" is related to a combination of the height gained from each lengthening surgery (biomechanical distraction) plus any growth from the time of each lengthening surgery to just before the subsequent lengthening surgery. These measurements may also include the potential growth stimulation from the effects of mechanical distraction.

– Growth from Distraction Phase	= (Final Post–Immediate Post) Ht
– Thoracic Growth Distraction Phase	= 24.7 cm–20.5 cm
	= 4.2 cm
– Total Spine Growth Distraction Phase	= 37.0 cm–32.2 cm
	= 4.8 cm

- Graduation Phase: During graduation, there may be further height gained from deformity correction (biomechanical distraction).

– Growth from Graduation Phase	= (Graduation–Final Post) Ht
– Thoracic Growth Graduation Phase	= 25.4 cm–24.7 cm
	= 0.7 cm
– Total Spine Growth Graduation Phase	= 37.4 cm–37.0 cm
	= 0.4 cm

TABLE 20.2 Summary of values for spine growth parameters according to Dimeglio [10]

T1/S1 expected growth rate in relationship to patient's age (years)	Under 5	>2 cm/year
	Between 5 and 10	0.9 cm/year
	>10 to skeletal maturity	1.8 cm/year
Proportion of sitting height in relationship to standing height	At birth	66%
	At 5 years	56%
	At the end of growth	52%
Average absolute T1/S1 height according to age (years)	Newborn	19.5 cm
	5 years	29.0 cm
	Adult	44.5 cm

During this patient's treatment course, he had actual coronal plane thoracic spine growth of 8.4 cm of which 3.5 cm was from the initial implantation, 4.2 cm from serial lengthening procedures, and 0.7 cm from the graduation surgery. He had *actual coronal plane total spine growth of 11.0 cm* of which 5.8 cm was from the initial implantation, 4.8 cm from serial lengthening procedures, and 0.4 from the graduation surgery.

Dimeglio described an average growth per vertebrae of 0.07 cm/year [9]. One can easily estimate the expected final spinal height loss at skeletal maturity according to the age at the time of fusion and the number of fused levels. He also described the expected growth rate of the spine from birth to skeletal maturity (Table 20.2) [10]. Using Dimeglio's data for expected total spine growth, we can determine the percentage of expected total spine growth that this patient obtained.

Expected growth age 5–10 years = 0.9 cm/year

This patient's implantation age was 7.3 year	= 2.7 years of growth <10 years of age
	= 2.7 years of growth × 0.9 cm/year
	= 2.4 cm

Expected growth age >10 years = 1.8 cm/year

This patient's graduation age was 14.9 year	= 4.9 years of growth >10 years of age
	= 4.9 years of growth × 1.8 cm/year
	= 8.8 cm

Total expected growth for this patient	= 2.4 cm + 8.8 cm
	= 11.2 cm

Percentage of growth achieved for this patient	= (Actual growth)/(Expected growth).
	= 11.0 cm/11.2 cm
	= 98% of normal

Considering only the growth achieved during the *distraction phase* of treatment:

Percentage of growth achieved for this patient	= (Actual growth distraction)/(expected)
	= 4.8 cm/11.2 cm
	= 43% of normal

Although 98% of normal age-matched spine growth was achieved for this patient, the majority of this growth was gained through the implantation phase, and approximately 43% of age-matched normal spine growth was achieved during the 7 years in the distraction phase.

It has been published that coronal plane total spine height of an adult is 44.5 cm [10]. According to this value, the percentage of normal adult spine height that our patient achieved was 84% (37.4 cm/44.5 cm).

Gold et al. proposed a method to estimate the expected total spine growth and the thoracic dimension according to the maximal pelvic inlet width [11]. Using these data, we can determine the percentage of expected total spine growth that this patient obtained during distraction phase.

Expected spine height based upon maximal pelvic width (PW):

Thoracolumbar Height (Male) = 3.0 × (PW + 44.8)–99.3 mm [11]

Post-operative PW = 95 mm

Post-operative Spine Height (Expected) = 3.0 × (PW + 44.8) –99.3 mm = 320 mm

Graduation PW = 121 mm

Graduation Spine Height (Expected) = 3.0 × (PW + 44.8) –99.3 mm = 398 mm

Expected Spine Growth = (Expected Graduation–Expected Post-Op) Spine Height

= 398 mm–320 mm

= 78 mm

Actual Spine Growth = (Actual Graduation–Actual Post-Op) Spine Height

= 374 mm–322 mm

= 52 mm

Percentage of growth achieved for this patient during distraction phase

= (Actual growth)/(Expected growth)

= 52 mm/78 mm

= 67% of normal

As current published reference data is only for the coronal plane, we can only estimate expected spine growth in one dimension. As posterior distraction-based growth-friendly treatments are known to be kyphogenic, it is important to also recognize potential out-of-plane growth. By evaluating the sagittal spine length (SSL), the effects of thoracic kyphosis (and to a lesser extent the effects of lumbar lordosis) can be considered (Fig. 20.3). By taking into account sagittal plane curvature, it should be noted that SSL is consistently greater than coronal plane spine heights (Table 20.1).

Clinical Pearls and Pitfalls

- Efforts should be made to critically evaluate growth achieved during treatment of early onset scoliosis. This should include evaluation of the implantation, distraction, and graduation phases of treatment.
- During the implantation phase, significant apparent "growth" is achieved though deformity correction (biomechanical distraction). This apparent "growth" can be considered to be analogous to the final height achieved if the patient simply underwent spinal fusion surgery.
- To evaluate the true benefit of growth-friendly surgery, the distraction phase should be critically evaluated.
- Reference data has been published for normal coronal plane spine growth for children and can be used to estimate percentage of age-matched normal growth achieved with growth-friendly surgeries (Table 20.2).
- In patients with significant kyphosis, sagittal spine length (SSL) is an important tool to measure continued out-of-plane growth that may not be apparent with standard of care coronal plane measurements of spine height.

Literature Review and Discussion

Orthopedic surgeons should understand the different characteristics and the various changes of spine growth to adequately treat any patient in the skeletally immature population with a spinal pathology. Many complex variables have to be taken in account for any specific individual prior to the initiation of a treatment. A myriad of constantly evolving anatomical, biological, and mechanical factors need to be evaluated during each phase of growth in a child before reaching full skeletal maturity.

Spinal growth initially occurs around the third week of gestation, time at which the cardiac and genitourinary systems are also beginning their development. In early spine development, 42 to 44 pairs of somites are derived from the paraxial mesoderm. After cranio-caudal differentiation, each somite will grow and coalesce around the notochord, giving rise to their respective sclerotomes, eventually forming a complete vertebrae. Abnormalities in sclerotomal signaling and posterior arc closure could further produce a spinal dysraphism [12, 13].

Dimeglio published an anatomic description of spine growth in 1993. In his original article, he evaluated the rate of growth of the thoracic and the lumbar spine from early infancy until skeletal maturity. According to Dimeglio, the T1-S1 rate of growth is >2 cm/year during the first 5 years of life. This rate will then decrease to 0.9 cm/year between 5 and 10 years and increase again to1.8 cm/year until full skeletal maturity (Table 20.2). He also established the average absolute height for the thoracic and lumbar segments of the spine [10]. Dede et al. more recently published a radiologic evaluation of the T1–T12 spine growth based on 194 thoracic CT scans. According to his works, the thoracic spine growth rate between 0 and 4 years was 1.37 cm/year; 4–10 years, 0.68 cm/year; 10–12 years, 1.33 cm/year; and 13–17 years, 0.75 cm/year [14]. With these values, one can easily estimate the predicted final spine length or height deficiency after a paravertebral fusion procedure in the skeletally immature population.

As there are several potential confounders that may result in variable growth rates for given individuals, it has been described to use the patient's own anatomy to predict their expected thoracic dimensions (Fig. 20.2). The maximum pelvic inlet width (PW) can be measured on radiographs or CT scan and can be used to predict maximum chest width, thoracic height, lumbar height, and thoracolumbar height [11].

In 2008, Karol et al. published an evaluation of pulmonary function following early thoracic fusion in non-neuromuscular scoliosis in 28 patients. They found that increasing the number of thoracic levels included in the fusion as associated with a worsening of the forced vital capacity (FVC) especially when more than four levels were fused. Also, they concluded that a minimal T1–T12 height of 18 cm and if possible 22 cm was required for minimal adequate thoracic function [15].

With the popularization of growth-friendly treatment for early onset scoliosis, efforts have been made to quantify the effects that these treatments have on spine growth. Sankar et al. published that a "law of diminishing returns" exists in the increase in vertical spine height achieved with serial posterior spine-based distraction surgeries [16]. They theorized that the diminishing returns were related to auto fusion of the spine that occurs after the initial lengthening procedures. Their results have helped popularize the trend of serial casting prior to the start of surgical intervention as a "delay tactic" for the treatment of EOS [17]. Sankar et al. did not specifically evaluate the effects of serial lengthening surgeries on thoracic kyphosis. As it has previously been published that spine-based distraction surgeries are kyphogenic, there may be sagittal plane increases in length that may not be identified by coronal plane measurements which may have led to an underrepresentation of the growth achieved through spine-based distraction surgery. The Children's Spine Study Group has evaluated the effects of rib-based distraction surgeries on spine growth and demonstrated that rib-based distraction maintains 75% of the expected T1-S1 growth up to the age of 10 years [18]. In that same cohort of subjects, there was a significant increase in their mean kyphosis from 44° at first lengthening to 65° by the 15th lengthening surgery. The group hypothesized that these traditional coronal plane measurements of spine length may not account for any out-of-plane length increases that may lead to an underestimation of the growth effects of the surgical interventions.

To take into account these potential increases in out-of-plane spine length, the sagittal spine length (SSL) concept was created and studied [19]. SSL is a measure of the curved arc length of the spine in the sagittal plane and takes into account the effects of thoracic kyphosis and lumbar lordosis

(Fig. 20.3a). With excellent reliability, this measurement demonstrated a progressive difference between traditional coronal plane spine height measurements and sagittal spine length as kyphosis increased. In an effort to provide more comprehensive data on the effects of growth-friendly treatment on spine growth, we encourage the use of the SSL measurement in order to complement the current coronal plane measurements of spine growth.

As there are likely growth changes in all three dimensions, the three-dimensional true spine length (3D–TSL) has recently been designed and evaluated. 3D–TSL is a biplanar, three-dimensional measurement technique that follows the true path of the spine (Figs. 20.4 and 20.5). It has been found to be accurate (0.4% error), precise (0.944 ICC), and reliable (0.952 ICC) and may be useful for more complex spinal pathology [20].

Dimeglio's group has also published on three-dimensional and volumetric thoracic growth using trunk surface topography. For young patients, they quantified the transverse thoracic dimension as 30%, anteroposterior thoracic dimension as 20%, and thoracic perimeter as 100% as compared to sitting height. This was the same for subjects without spinal pathology and for patients with mild to moderate idiopathic scoliosis [21].

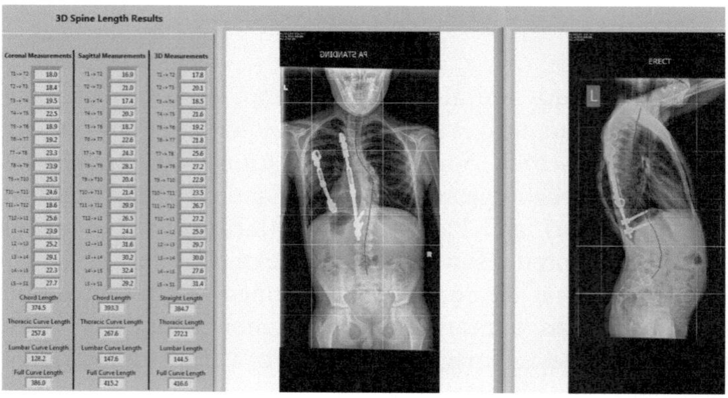

Figure 20.4 Three-dimensional true spine length (3D–TSL) is a biplanar, three-dimensional technique that follows the true path of the spine

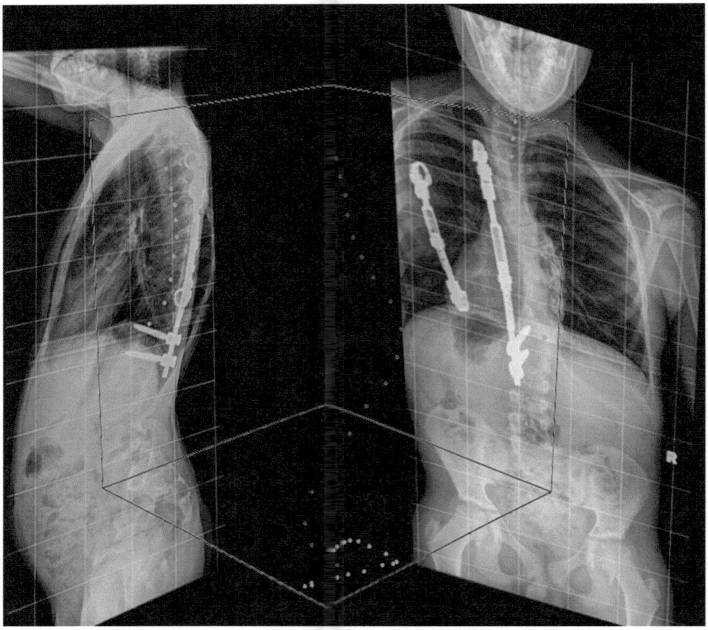

FIGURE 20.5 A graphical representation of the 3D–TSL created from the results of this patient's 5-year postoperative PA and lateral radiographs

Other groups are also evaluating spine growth utilizing modern techniques. At the 2015 Annual Meeting of the Scoliosis Research Society presentations were made by Balasubramanian's group (CT scan), Sanders' group (anthropometric data), and Parent's group (biplanar radiographs) who all presented results utilizing novel modalities [22–24]. It is our hope that the results of these ongoing studies will be integrated, and a more complete understanding of spine growth will be achieved. In the future, a three-dimensional reference for normal spine growth can be used to more completely assess the results of growth-friendly surgery and may also be used to predict the timing of interventions such as growth modulation surgeries (i.e., vertebral body tethering).

References

1. Williams BA, Matsumoto H, McCalla DJ, Akbarnia BA, Blakemore LC, Betz RR, et al. Development and initial validation of the Classification of Early-Onset Scoliosis (C-EOS). J Bone Joint Surg. 2014;96(16):1359–67.
2. Skaggs DL, Guillaume T, El-Hawary R. Early onset scoliosis consensus statement, SRS Growing Spine Committee. Spine Deform. 2015;3(2):107.
3. Campbell RM Jr, Smith MD, Mayes TC, Mangos JA, Willey-Courand DB, Kose N, et al. The characteristics of thoracic insufficiency syndrome associated with fused ribs and congenital scoliosis. J Bone Joint Surg Am. 2003;85(3):399–408.
4. Gomez JA, Lee JK, Kim PD, Roye DP, Vitale MG. “Growth friendly” spine surgery: management options for the young child with scoliosis. J Am Acad Orthop Surg. 2011;19:722–7.
5. Skaggs DL, Akbarnia BA, Flynn JM, Myung KS, Sponseller PD, Vitale MG, Chest Wall and Spine Deformity Study Group, Growing Spine Study Group, Pediatric Orthopaedic Society of North America, Scoliosis Research Society Growing Spine Study Committee. A classification of growth friendly spine implants. J Pediatr Orthop. 2014;34(3):260–7.
6. Campbell RM. Operative strategies for thoracic insufficiency syndrome by vertical expandable prosthetic titanium rib expansion thoracoplasty. Oper Tech Orthop. 2005;15:315–25.
7. Campbell RM, Smith MD, Hell-Vocke AK. Expansion thoracoplasty: the surgical technique of opening wedge thoracotomy, surgical technique. J Bone Joint Surg Am. 2004;86(Suppl. 1): 51–64.
8. Crawford AH. Pitfalls of spinal deformities associated with neurofibromatosis in children. Clin Orthop Relat Res. 1989;245:29–42.
9. Dimeglio A, Bonnel F. Le rachis en croissance. Paris: Springer; 1990. p. 392–4.
10. Dimeglio A. Growth of the spine before age 5 years. J Pediatr Orthop B. 1993;1:102–7.
11. Gold M, Dombek M, Miller PE, Emans JB, Glotzbecker MP. Prediction of thoracic dimensions and spine length on the basis of individual pelvic dimensions. Spine. 2013;1:74–80.
12. Larsen W. Human embryology. New York: Churchill Livingstone; 1993.
13. Gammill LS, Bronner-Fraser M. Neural crest specification: migration into genomics. Nat Rev Neurosci. 2003;4:795–805.

14. Dede O, Demirkiran G, Buyukdogan K, Olgun ZD, Akpinar E, Yazici M. Growth of the thoracic spine re-visited: is the Dimeglio data accurate? Spine Deform. 2015;3(6):613.
15. Karol LA, Johnston C, Mladenov K, Schochet P, Walters P, Browne RH. Pulmonary function following early thoracic fusion in non-neuromuscular scoliosis. J Bone Joint Surg. 2008;90(6):1272–81.
16. Sankar WN, Skaggs DL, Yazici M, Johnston CE, Shah S, Javidan P, et al. Lengthening of dual growing rods and the law of diminishing returns. Spine. 2011;35(10):806–9.
17. Fletcher ND, McClung A, Rathjen KE, Denning JR, Browne R, Johnston CE. Serial casting as a delay tactic in the treatment of moderate-to-severe early-onsetscoliosis. J Pediatr Orthop. 2012;32(7):664–71.
18. El-Hawary R, Samdani A, Wade J, Smith M, Heflin JA, Klatt JW, et al. Children's spine study group, rib-based distraction surgery maintains total spine growth. J Pediatr Orthop. 2016;36(8):841–6.
19. Spurway AJ, Chukwunyerenwa CK, Kishta WE, Hurry JK, El-Hawary R. Sagittal spine length measurement: a novel technique to assess growth of the spine. Spine Deform. 2016;4(5):331–7.
20. Spurway AJ, Hurry JK, Gauthier L, Orlik B, Chukwunyerenwa CK, Kishta WE, et al. Three dimensional true Spine length: a novel technique for assessing the outcomes of scoliosis surgery. J Paediatr Orthop. 2017;37(8):e631–7.
21. Charles YP, Marcoul A, Schaeffer M, Canavese F, Diméglio A. Three-dimensional and volumetric thoracic growth in children with moderate idiopathic scoliosis compared with normal. J Paediatr Orthop B. 2017;26:227–32.
22. Peters J, Bisirri E, Campbell RM, Balasubramanian S. Age-related shape characterization of the pediatric thoracic Spine using generalized procrustes analysis. Presented at the 50th Annual Meeting of Scoliosis Research Society, Minneapolis, MN, Sept 2015.
23. Sanders JO, Karbach L, Osinski T, Liu R, Qiu X, Cooperman D. Normal human Spine growth and prediction of final spine height developed from a longitudinal cohort of children followed through their growth until completion. Presented at the 50th Annual Meeting of Scoliosis Research Society, Minneapolis, MN, Sept 2015.
24. Tremblay L, Tohmé P, Roy-Beaudry M, Beauséjour M, Labelle H, Parent S. Spinal growth in normal children between 3 and 11 years old using 3D reconstruction: a longitudinal study. Presented at the 50th Annual Meeting of Scoliosis Research Society, Minneapolis, MN, Sept 2015.

Chapter 21
The Role of Traction in Early-Onset Scoliosis

Benjamin Orlik and Craig P. Eberson

Case Presentation

History and Physical Examination

The patient, a 5-year-old female with neuromuscular scoliosis, was born preterm and was diagnosed, in infancy, with spastic, quadriplegic cerebral palsy. Her gross motor functional classification scale (GMFCS) level was V. She had a VP shunt, was G-tube fed, and had a seizure disorder treated with valproic acid. She had multiple emergency visits and admissions for respiratory complications.

On exam she was nonverbal but responded with smiles, to sound and touch. She sat comfortably in her wheelchair and had a mild apex right, C-shaped curve, without significant pelvic obliquity. Her curve was flexible to stretch and side bending, and she did not have any areas of skin breakdown or deep creases.

B. Orlik, MD • C.P. Eberson, MD (✉)
Division of Pediatric Orthopedic Surgery, IWK Heath Centre and Dalhousie University, Halifax, NS, Canada

Division of Pediatric orthopedic Surgery, Hasbro Children's Hospital and Alpert Medical School of Brown University, Providence, RI, USA
e-mail: benjamin.orlik@iwk.nshealth.ca; Craig_P_Eberson@Brown.edu

R. El-Hawary, C.P. Eberson (eds.), *Early Onset Scoliosis*,
https://doi.org/10.1007/978-3-319-71580-3_21

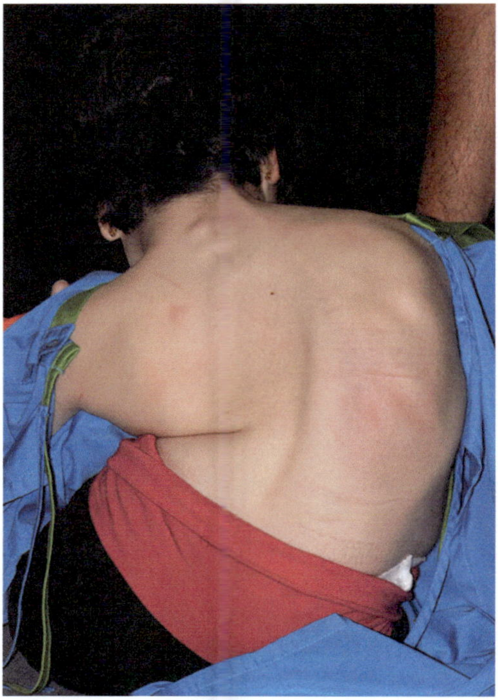

FIGURE 21.1 Preoperative clinical photos

She was observed and managed conservatively over the next 5 years with modifications to her custom-molded insert, in her powered wheelchair, as her curve progressed. By age 9, she developed clinically apparent, pelvic obliquity, and her curve became more rigid. As she was still prepurbertal, she was managed conservatively with clinical exam and radiographs every 6 months. By age 10, she developed deep skin creases and rib impingement on the pelvis and had difficulty sitting for prolonged periods of time. She weighed 30 kg.

Her clinical photos are seen in Fig. 21.1.

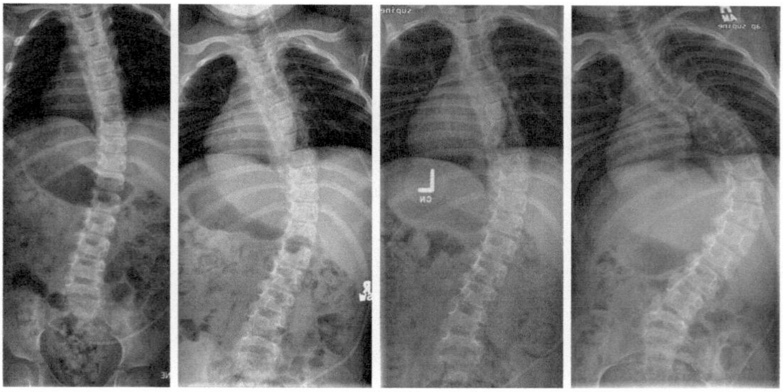

FIGURE 21.2 Supine AP radiographs at age 5, 7, 8, and 9 years old

Diagnostic Studies

Supine, AP radiographs at age 5, 7, 8, and 9 are seen in Fig. 21.2. She remained Risser 0, with an open triradiate cartilage, during this time period. Upright AP, lateral, and supine stretch radiographs at age 10 are seen in Fig. 21.3. By age 10, her triradiate cartilage had closed, and her Risser classification was still zero. Her major curve Cobb angle measured 110° from T7 to L2 and stretched to 75° (flexibility index of 32%). Her pelvic obliquity measured 25°. Her femoral heads were spherical, congruent, and reduced in the acetabulum, with a migration percentage of less than 20°.

Management Options

Management options for early-onset scoliosis of a neuromuscular etiology are numerous. Surgical options include growth-friendly surgery, definitive posterior spinal instrumentation and fusion (PSIF), and anterior release and posterior spinal instrumentation and fusion (APSIF) [1, 2].

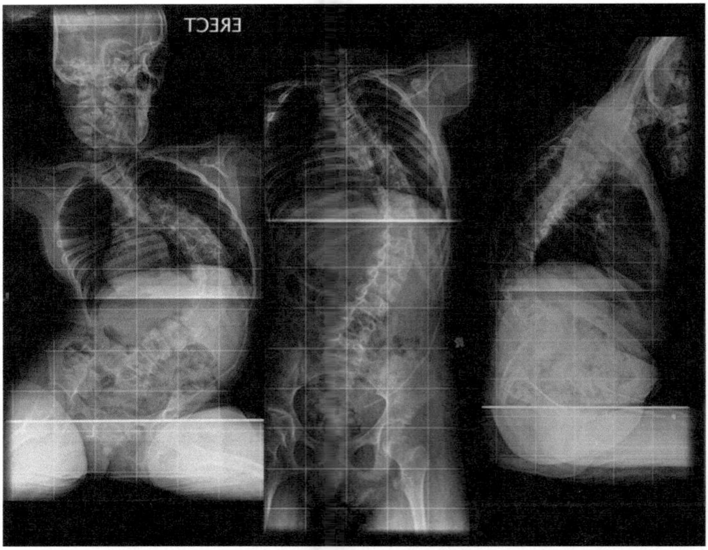

FIGURE 21.3 Preoperative: upright AP, supine stretch and upright, lateral radiographs

Growth-friendly options would typically be a distraction-based implant, which could either be rib-based (e.g., VEPTR), spine-based (e.g., dual growing rods), hybrid, or a remotely expandable device (e.g., MAGEC) [3].

All of these procedures could be augmented with traction. Traction options include:

1. Preoperative halo-gravity traction
2. Halo-gravity traction between staged, anterior release and PSIF
3. Intraoperative skull-femoral traction

Typical skull traction options include Halter, Halo, Gardner-Wells, and Mayfield. Femoral traction includes skeletal traction and skin traction.

Management Chosen

The author chose to wait until the triradiate cartilage closed, acknowledging and allowing the Cobb angle to progress (>100°) and become stiffer (stretch/bend >70°). A single-stage PSIF with intraoperative skull-femoral traction was performed.

The author felt that this would avoid the higher complication rate and morbidity seen with distraction-based systems or anterior surgery and anticipated that intraoperative traction and modern posterior instrumentation would allow for a powerful correction to achieve a level pelvis and a well-balanced spine. Closure of the triradiate cartilage was the trigger for surgery, to avoid crankshaft deformity [4–8] or the loss of correction over time.

Surgical Procedure

Gardner-Wells tongs were used for the skull, and 5/64th, smooth, stainless steel, Kirschner wires with traction bows were used for the femoral traction (see Figs. 21.4 and 21.5). 10 lbs (15% body weight) of traction were placed on the head; 7 lbs (10% BW) and 21 lbs (30% BW) were placed on the right and left legs, respectively. The weight was applied every 5 min, in three increments, ensuring stable neuromonitoring signals (somatosensory- and motor-evoked potentials). The weights were applied pre-incision and removed prior to closure.

A standard posterior approach was used. Facetectomies were performed at each level, but no further osteotomies were done. Bilateral pedicle screws were placed at L4, L5, and S1, with bilateral S2-alar-iliac screws to achieve a stable base, and alternating screws were then placed up to T3 with placement of down-going, transverse process hooks at T2 for a "soft landing" [9, 10]. A 6.0 mm cobalt-chrome rod was

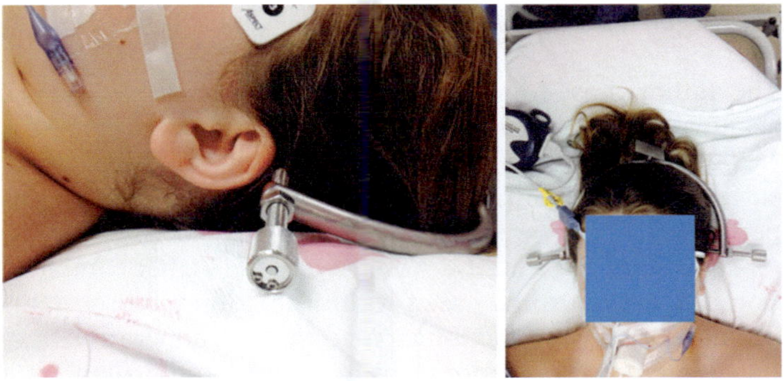

FIGURE 21.4 Placement of Gardner-Wells tongs

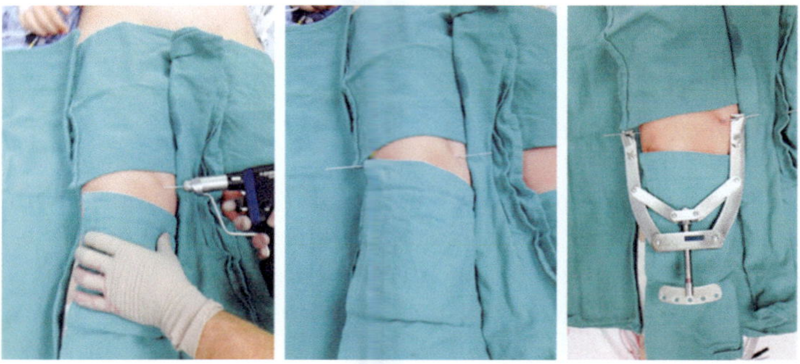

FIGURE 21.5 Placement of femoral traction pin and bow

placed on the left side followed by a 5.5 titanium alloy rod on the right. The spine was reduced to the left-sided rod (with reduction tubes) while simultaneously performing rod rotation and vertebral body manipulation.

Clinical Course and Outcome

The patient tolerated the procedure well; stayed in the pediatric intensive care unit overnight, prior to transfer to the surgical inpatient unit; had an uneventful recovery; and was discharged home post-op day 5. Wheelchair modifications

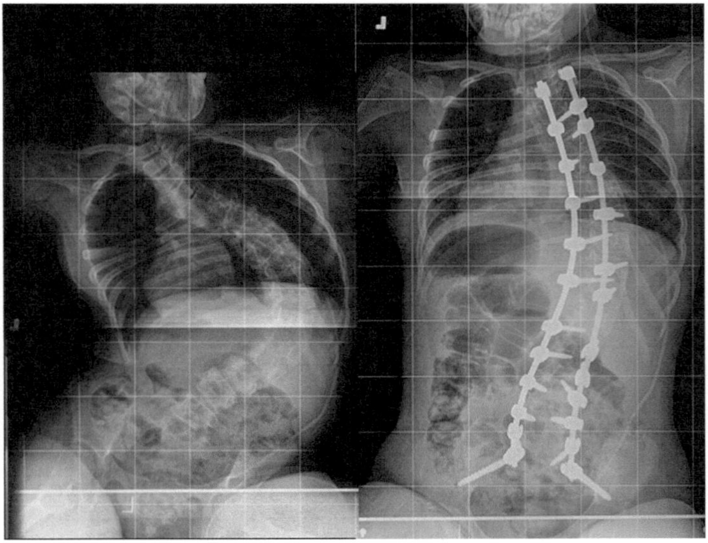

FIGURE 21.6 Pre- and postoperative upright AP radiographs

were made in the hospital. Skin creases, sitting balance, and sitting duration were significantly improved and maintained at 1-year follow-up. There were no complications. Pre- and postoperative X-rays are seen in Fig. 21.6.

The major coronal Cobb angle corrected from 110° to 35° (correction index of 68%), which was two times better than the flexibility index (32%). The pelvic obliquity corrected from 25° to 4° (correction index of 84%).

Clinical Pearls and Pitfalls

- Traction can provide a significant corrective force to the spine, facilitating correction of large curves.
- Small patients with thin skull osteology are at risk for pin penetration and dural injury/infection. A halo ring with multiple anchor points allows distribution of forces to decrease this risk, while standard Gardner-Wells tongs can be used for adult-sized patients.

- If traction is used intraoperatively, reliable neuromonitoring is mandatory to prevent iatrogenic neurologic injury.
- Countertraction can be provided via femoral traction pin, traction tape, or fracture table traction boot. Care to avoid excessive lordosis from hip extension should be taken. Asymmetric application of femoral countertraction is useful to correct pelvic obliquity.

Literature Review and Discussion

Spinal traction was first described by Hippocrates [11, 12]. The two types of traction that will be discussed in this chapter are halo-gravity traction (HGT) and intraoperative skull-femoral traction (IOT) as these are the types most commonly reported in the literature. Traction for spinal deformity is almost exclusively used in conjunction with surgery.

Potential benefits of traction are [13–19]:

1. To improve final correction of spinal deformity
2. To allow for gradual rather than acute correction to reduce neurologic injury
3. To reduce the magnitude of acute correction of deformity
4. To reduce forces on implants when less acute correction is applied
5. To aid in surgical exposure with improved patient positioning
6. To aid in pedicle screw placement when three-dimensional deformity, on table, is improved
7. To improve rod contouring and seating into pedicle screws or hooks
8. To improve pulmonary function
9. To improve nutritional status

Perioperative Halo-Gravity Traction

Halo-gravity traction (HGT) was introduced by Stagnara in 1969 [20]. Perioperative refers to the use of HGT in three ways [18]:

1. **TF**: **T**raction—**F**usion
2. **RTF**: surgical **R**elease—**T**raction—**F**usion
3. **TRTF**: **T**raction—surgical **R**elease—**T**raction—**F**usion

There is no consensus for the specific indications for using traction nor to guide which type of traction to use. As halo-gravity traction requires a separate anesthetic for application and there is a duration traction, it tends to be used for severe, stiff, kyphoscoliotic curves.

Halo-Gravity Traction Technique and Protocols

The patient undergoes a general anesthetic for application of the halo fixator. Application is described by Mubarak [21] and involves using the appropriate number of pins (usually six to eight), at the appropriate torque (usually 6–8 lbs per in.^{2}), for the patient's age, size, and bone quality [14, 21, 22]. The patient is then awoken prior to application of weight, so neurologic status and tolerance can be monitored. The halo is typically attached to a spring and then a scale followed by the rope, pulley, and weights. It can be configured to a bed, wheelchair, or walker, to accommodate lying down (sleeping), sitting, and walking. It is typically used 24 h per day. The "dose" (starting weight, incremental weight increase, total weight, and duration) is variable in the literature. In a review, Neal and Siegall (2017) tabulated the dose of traction used in 17 articles, of which 12 used preoperative HGT. Typical initial weight was 3–5 lbs (range 3–10 lbs), with daily increases of 2–3 lbs (range 1–6 lbs), up to a final weight of 30–50% of body weight, for a duration range of 2–28 weeks. Anterior surgical release was also used all of the time in two (17%) studies, some of the time in seven (58%) studies, and none of the time in two (17%) studies. The remaining studies did not specify [17]. The authors have used as much as 75% of body weight in some patients.

The effect of duration was studied by Park et al. (2013), who found that 66% of the coronal correction obtained by traction was achieved in the first 2 weeks, 21.7% more in the 3rd week, and 7.5% in the 4th week. Sagittal correction was

Table 21.1 Recommended dose, using average reports in literature

Initial weight	3–5 lbs
Frequency of increases in weight	Daily
Magnitude of weight increase	2–3 lbs
Total weight	30–50% of lean body weight
Duration	2–6 weeks

similar at 62.7, 24.3, and 15.9%, at 2, 3, and 4 weeks, respectively [15] (Table 21.1).

Efficacy of Halo-Gravity Traction

In a 2016, systematic review of 16 studies and 351 patients, Yang et al. [18] found coronal plane correction was 24% (194 pts., in nine studies) and sagittal plane correction was 19% (92 pts., in four studies), in patients that had an initial, average, coronal Cobb angle of 101° and a sagittal Cobb angle of 80°.

However, only four studies reported on preoperative flexibility index, which had a mean of 12.9%, while the preoperative curve, after halo-gravity traction, improved by 19%, which was only 6.1% better than the flexibility. The average initial curve was 107.7 in this pooled sub-analysis [18].

Only three studies had a control group, but they were too heterogeneous to pool the data. One study showed no significant differences pre- or post-op, in terms of coronal Cobb angle, sagittal Cobb angle, flexibility, or correction, though the patients in the traction group were less likely to undergo vertebral column resection [23]. The second study did show a significant improvement in postoperative correction, in the traction group (59%), versus the non-traction group (47%), and the traction group had less OR time and less blood loss [24].

The third study compared preoperative halo-gravity traction ($n = 12$), with surgical release ($n = 13$), prior to implantation of a VEPTR or growing rod construct. A control ($n = 72$)

and disc excision (n = 9) group was also studied. The halo-gravity traction (HGT) group had a higher, pre-op, scoliosis of 92.0° and kyphosis of 99.5°, compared to the surgical group (SR) of 73.3 and 67.6, respectively. Postoperatively, they found better scoliosis correction in the surgical release group (46°, 63%) than the HGT group (37°, 40%); however they did not report on preoperative curve flexibility. The kyphosis correction was better in the HGT group (48°, 48%) than in the SR (27°, 41%). The increase in thoracic spine height and thoracic spine length significantly was larger in the HGT group [25].

Intraoperative Skull-Femoral Traction

A MEDLINE search failed to find any studies of intraoperative skull-femoral traction, in a population with, specifically, early-onset scoliosis or in cases of growth-friendly surgery.

A recent systematic review found nine studies that met their inclusion criteria, and six studies had a control group; however, all studies were retrospective. Three studies looked at adolescent idiopathic scoliosis (AIS), four studies looked at neuromuscular (NM) patients, and the rest were combined. The traction protocols were variable, with one, out of the nine studies, using halter and skin traction, as opposed to skeletal pin fixation. Halo or Gardner-Wells tongs were used for skull traction, and weights varied between 15 lbs and 25% body weight. Four studies used unilateral femoral pins, three used bilateral, and one study used both (bilateral for AIS and unilateral for NM). Femoral weight varied between 25 lbs and 50% body weight [26] (Table 21.2).

The studies' outcomes were heterogeneous and, therefore, were not pooled, for analysis. Seven, of the nine, studies showed positive outcomes, for the intervention. These included:

1. Improved pelvic obliquity
2. Improved sitting balance
3. Improved major curve correction
4. Improved apical vertebral rotation

TABLE 21.2 Dose of intraoperative traction

Initial skull weight	5% (max 5 lb)
Initial femoral weight	5% each leg (max 5 lb)
Time interval between increases	Minimum 5 min with stable MEPs and SSEPs
Final skull weight	15–20% to max of 15 lbs
Final femoral weight	15–25% per leg, if bilateral
	30–50% between both legs
	Consider unilateral or asymmetrical in neuromuscular cases with pelvic obliquity

5. Less blood loss
6. Less transfusions
7. Shorter OR time

Interestingly, none of the studies with a comparative group showed a significant improvement in the major curve correction between groups. The study by Keeler et al., however, compared traction (in posterior-only fusion) to no traction (in combined anterior and posterior surgery), and concluded that anterior release may not be necessary, with the use of intraoperative traction [27].

The study by Takeshita et al. had a significantly better correction of pelvic obliquity in the traction group (26°–5.5°, 78%) vs. the no traction group (17°–5.2°, 52%). The increased improvement in coronal Cobb angle from 87.3° to 35.3° (59%) in the traction group compared to the no traction group of 66.9° to 32.3° (51%) did not reach statistical significance. Although in a sub-analysis, of only cases with posterior fusion, their correction rate of 64% (76°–27°), in the traction group, was significantly better than the 46% correction rate (67°–36°) in the no traction group [28].

TABLE 21.3 Complications in spinal traction

Complication	Rate (%)	Study
Pin related (loosening/irritation/infection, etc.)	9–16	[14, 18, 29]
Transient nystagmus	9	[14]
Upper extremity numbness	3	[14]
Acute brachial plexus neuropathy	Single case report	[30]
Decreased bone mineral density	45	[31]
Other neurologic	1	[18]
Hypoglossal nerve injury	Single case report	[32]
Transient motor-evoked potential changes	47	[33]

Complications

Spinal traction is not without complications. A compilation of reported complications is seen in Table 21.3. From most studies, the rate of minor complications is relatively high, but the rate of severe complications is quite low. Many studies also report the surgical complications, and as they do not have a control group, it is difficult to ascertain whether the traction component of the procedure increased the risk.

In the meta-analysis by Yang et al., they found a pooled prevalence of 22%, for non-neurologic traction-related complications. Three neurologic complications were seen in 13 studies and 293 patients [18].

An example of how these techniques can be combined can be found when preparing patients with stiff, kyphotic EOS curves for growing rods. Particularly if MAGEC rods are being contemplated, it is imperative to correct the kyphosis enough to allow insertion of the straight actuator portion of the rod. By obtaining maximal correction prior to rod insertion, excessive stress on anchor points can be

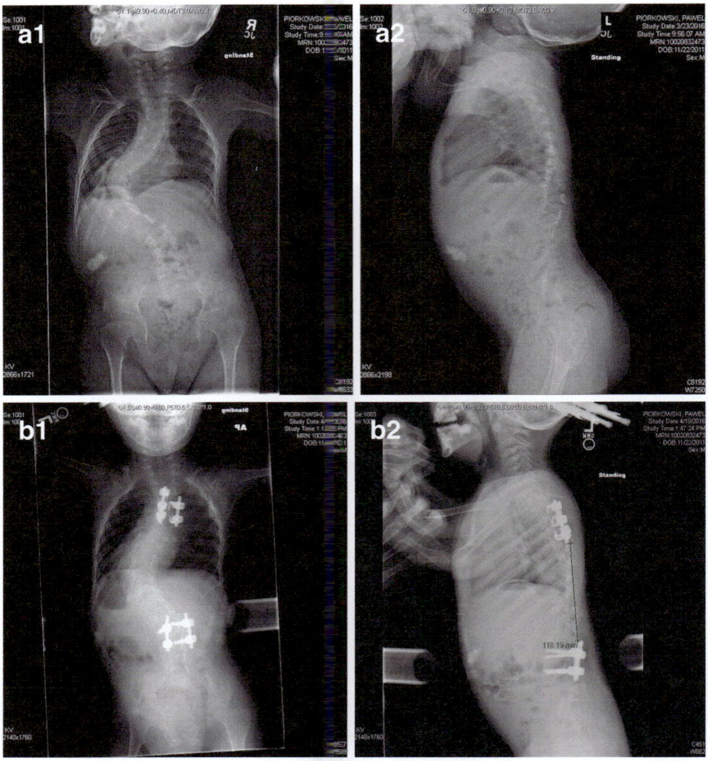

FIGURE 21.7 Five-year-old patient with diastrophic dysplasia with progressive kyphoscoliosis initially treated with cast application. While there was improvement in the kyphosis with casting, the scoliosis was rigid, and some thoracolumbar kyphosis persisted (**a**). A multipin halo was applied in the OR, using ten pins, finger-tightened. Proximal and distal anchors were inserted under the same anesthesia. After 2 months of daily traction (wheelchair and walker), the patient retuned to the OR for rod insertion (**b**). Halo-skin traction was used to facilitate intraoperative correction, seen here in another patient (**c**). Final films with MAGEC rod inserted at 1 year postoperatively (**d**)

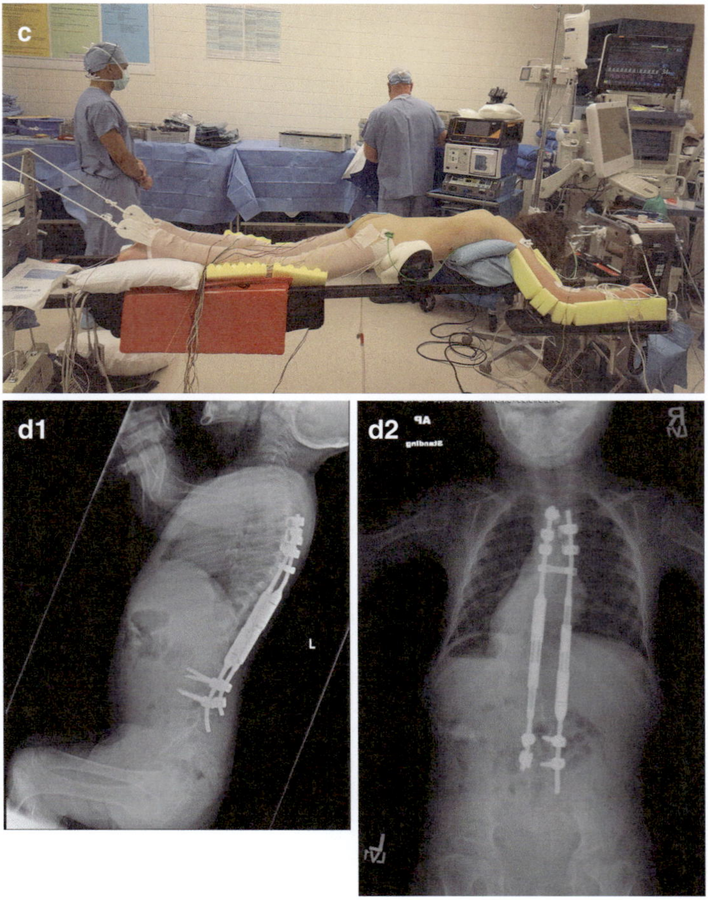

FIGURE 21.7 (continued)

avoided. Anchors can be inserted, if fusion at the sites is desired, at the time of initial halo application, to allow fusion to begin prior to rod insertion. At the time of rod insertion, halo-skin traction can obtain additional correction (Fig. 21.7).

References

1. El-Hawary R, Chukwunyerenwa C. Update on evaluation and treatment of scoliosis. Pediatr Clin North Am. 2014;61:1223–41.
2. Cunin V. Early-onset scoliosis—current treatment. Orthop Traumatol Surg Res. 2015;101:S109–18.
3. El-Hawary R, Akbarnia BA. Early onset scoliosis—time for consensus. Spine Deform. 2015;3:105–6.
4. Yaszay B, Sponseller PD, Shah SA, Asghar J, Miyanji F, Samdani AF, Bartley C, Newton PO. Performing a definitive fusion in juvenile CP patients is a good surgical option. J Pediatr Orthop. 2016;37(8):e488–91. https://doi.org/10.1097/BPO.0000000000000793.
5. Roberto RF, Lonstein JE, Winter RB, Denis F. Curve progression in Risser stage 0 or 1 patients after posterior spinal fusion for idiopathic scoliosis. J Pediatr Orthop. 1997;17:718–25.
6. Sponseller PD, Jain A, Newton PO, Lonner BS, Shah SA, Shufflebarger H, Bastrom TP, Marks MC, Betz RR. Posterior spinal fusion with pedicle screws in patients with idiopathic scoliosis and open Triradiate cartilage: does deformity progression occur? J Pediatr Orthop. 2016;36:695–700.
7. Hamill CL, Bridwell KH, Lenke LG, Chapman MP, Baldus C, Blanke K. Posterior arthrodesis in the skeletally immature patient. Assessing the risk for crankshaft: is an open triradiate cartilage the answer? Spine. 1997;22:1343–51.
8. Sponseller PD, Betz R, Newton PO, et al. Differences in curve behavior after fusion in adolescent idiopathic scoliosis patients with open triradiate cartilages. Spine. 2009;34:827–31.
9. Hassanzadeh H, Gupta S, Jain A, El Dafrawy MH, Skolasky RL, Kebaish KM. Type of anchor at the proximal fusion level has a significant effect on the incidence of proximal junctional kyphosis and outcome in adults after long posterior spinal fusion. Spine Deform. 2013;1:299–305.

10. Helgeson MD, Shah SA, Newton PO, Clements DH, Betz RR, Marks MC, Bastrom T, Harms Study Group. Evaluation of proximal junctional kyphosis in adolescent idiopathic scoliosis following pedicle screw, hook, or hybrid instrumentation. Spine. 2010;35:177–81.
11. Wang JH, Daniels AH, Palumbo MA, Eberson CP. Cervical traction for the treatment of spinal injury and deformity. JBJS Rev. 2014;2:1.
12. D'Astous JL, Sanders JO. Casting and traction treatment methods for scoliosis. Orthop Clin N Am. 2007;38:477–84.
13. Garabekyan T, Hosseinzadeh P, Iwinski HJ, Muchow RD, Talwalkar VR, Walker J, Milbrandt TA. The results of preoperative halo-gravity traction in children with severe spinal deformity. J Pediatr Orthop B. 2014;23:1–5.
14. Bogunovic L, Lenke LG, Bridwell KH, Luhmann SJ. Preoperative halo-gravity traction for severe pediatric spinal deformity: complications, radiographic correction and changes in pulmonary function. Spine Deform. 2012;1:33–9.
15. Park DK, Braaksma B, Hammerberg KW, Sturm P. The efficacy of preoperative halo-gravity traction in pediatric spinal deformity the effect of traction duration. J Spinal Disord Tech. 2013;26:146–54.
16. Sink EL, Karol LA, Sanders J, Birch JG, Johnston CE, Herring JA. Efficacy of perioperative halo-gravity traction in the treatment of severe scoliosis in children. J Pediatr Orthop. 2001;21:519–24.
17. Neal KM, Siegall E. Strategies for surgical management of large, stiff spinal deformities in children. J Am Acad Orthop Surg. 2017;25:e70–8.
18. Yang C, Wang H, Zheng Z, Zhang Z, Wang J, Liu H, Kim YJ, Cho S. Halo-gravity traction in the treatment of severe spinal deformity: a systematic review and meta-analysis. Eur Spine J. 2016;9:486.
19. Pourtaheri S, Shah SA, Ditro CP, Holmes L, Mackenzie WG. Preoperative halo-gravity traction with and without thoracoscopic anterior release for skeletal dysplasia patients with severe kyphoscoliosis. J Child Orthop. 2017;10:135–42.
20. D'Astous JL, Sanders JO. Casting and traction treatment methods for scoliosis. Orthop Clin North Am. 2007;38:477–84.
21. Mubarak SJ, Camp JF, Vuletich W, Wenger DR, Garfin SR. Halo application in the infant. J Pediatr Orthop. 1989;9:612–4.

22. Bono CM. The halo fixator. J Am Acad Orthop Surg. 2007;15:728–37.
23. Sponseller PD, Takenaga RK, Newton P, et al. The use of traction in the treatment of severe spinal deformity. Spine. 2008;33:2305–9.
24. Koptan W, ElMiligui Y. Three-staged correction of severe rigid idiopathic scoliosis using limited halo-gravity traction. Eur Spine J. 2011;21:1091–8.
25. Caubet JF, Emans JB. Halo-gravity traction versus surgical release before implantation of expandable spinal devices: a comparison of results and complications in early-onset spinal deformity. J Spinal Disord Tech. 2011;24:99–104.
26. LaMothe JM, Sayeg Al S, Parsons DL, Ferri-de-Barros F. The use of intraoperative traction in pediatric scoliosis surgery: a systematic review. Spine Deform. 2015;3:45–51.
27. Keeler KA, Lenke LG, Good CR, Bridwell KH, Sides B, Luhmann SJ. Spinal fusion for spastic neuromuscular scoliosis: is anterior releasing necessary when intraoperative halo-femoral traction is used? Spine. 2010;35:E427–33.
28. Takeshita K, Lenke LG, Bridwell KH, Kim YJ, Sides B, Hensley M. Analysis of patients with nonambulatory neuromuscular scoliosis surgically treated to the pelvis with intraoperative halo-femoral traction. Spine. 2006;31:2381–5.
29. Watanabe K, Lenke LG, Bridwell KH, Kim YJ, Hensley M, Koester L. Efficacy of perioperative halo-gravity traction for treatment of severe scoliosis (≥100°). J Orthop Sci. 2010;15:720–30.
30. el-Shaker M, Watts HG. Acute brachial plexus neuropathy secondary to halo-gravity traction in a patient with Ehlers-Danlos syndrome. Spine. 1991;16:385–6.
31. Han X, Sun W, Qiu Y, Xu L, Sha S, Shi B, Yan H, Liu Z, Zhu Z. Clinical study halo gravity traction is associated with reduced bone mineral density of patients with severe Kyphoscoliosis. Biomed Res Int. 2016;2016:8056273.
32. Ginsburg GM, Bassett GS. Hypoglossal nerve injury caused by halo-suspension traction. A case report. Spine. 1998;23:1490–3.
33. Lewis SJ, Gray R, Holmes LM, Strantzas S, Jhaveri S, Zaarour C, Magana S. Neurophysiological changes in deformity correction of adolescent idiopathic scoliosis with intraoperative skull-femoral traction. Spine. 2011;36:1627–38.

Chapter 22
The End Game for Early-Onset Scoliosis

Benjamin Sheffer and Jeffrey R. Sawyer

Case Presentation

History and Physical Examination

A 6 + 11-year-old female presented with history of microcephaly, developmental delay, craniosynostosis requiring cranial vault expansion at age 5 years, a Chiari 1 malformation that required decompression at age 12 years, and neuromuscular scoliosis. The patient presented with a 52° right thoracolumbar curve, which was treated in a brace in an effort to delay curve progression. The brace was worn intermittently and was discontinued because of patient discomfort. Over a 3-year period, the curve progressed to 90°. At 10 years of age, the patient had dual 5.5-mm spine-based growing rods placed using pedicle screw anchors. Her spine was lengthened at 6-month intervals for the next 4 years without complications. At the conclusion of her growing rod lengthenings, her curve measured 40°, and there were no complications related to her growth-friendly treatment. At

B. Sheffer, MD • J.R. Sawyer, MD (✉)
Department of Orthopedic Surgery and Biomedical Engineering, University of Tennessee-Campbell Clinic, Memphis, TN, USA

Le Bonheur Children's Hospital, Memphis, TN, USA
e-mail: jsawyer@campbellclinic.com

R. El-Hawary, C.P. Eberson (eds.), *Early Onset Scoliosis*,
https://doi.org/10.1007/978-3-319-71580-3_22

age 14 + 3 years, she was 2 years postmenarchal with little spinal growth remaining.

The patient was alert and cooperative with the examination. She was 14 + 3 years of age, was 142 cm tall, weighed 38 kg (BMI 18.8), and was at Tanner stage 5. She had a right rib prominence on Adam's forward bending. Her previous surgical incisions were healed without implant prominence or signs of infection. Her right shoulder was elevated when compared to the left, and her trunk was shifted to the right. She had no sagittal plane imbalance and was able to ambulate without the use of assistive devices. She was neurologically intact in her upper and lower extremities.

Diagnostic Studies

Initial radiographic imaging at age 6 + 11 years showed a 52° right thoracolumbar curve with thoracic hypokyphosis and lumbar hyperkyphosis (Fig. 22.1). MRI of the spine demonstrated a Chiari malformation (Fig. 22.2), but no other neural axis abnormalities. Over the following 3 years, at age 10 + 0 years, the curve had progressed to 90°(Fig. 22.3). Spine-based distraction was utilized, and her postoperative radiographs demonstrated improvement in her curve to 65° (Fig. 22.4). Over a 4-year period, she had six lengthenings which resulted in a curve of 40° and an increase in T1-S1 height of 2.4 cm (Fig. 22.5).

Management Chosen

At age 14 + 3 years, the patient was 2 years postmenarchal and was Risser IV; therefore, lengthening was discontinued. Her T1–T12 height was 24.3 cm, and it was believed that this would be adequate for her height of 142 cm and BMI of 18.8. The patient's family consented to a definitive fusion surgery with options between in situ fusion versus deformity correction with osteotomies: if at the time of spinal fusion there was

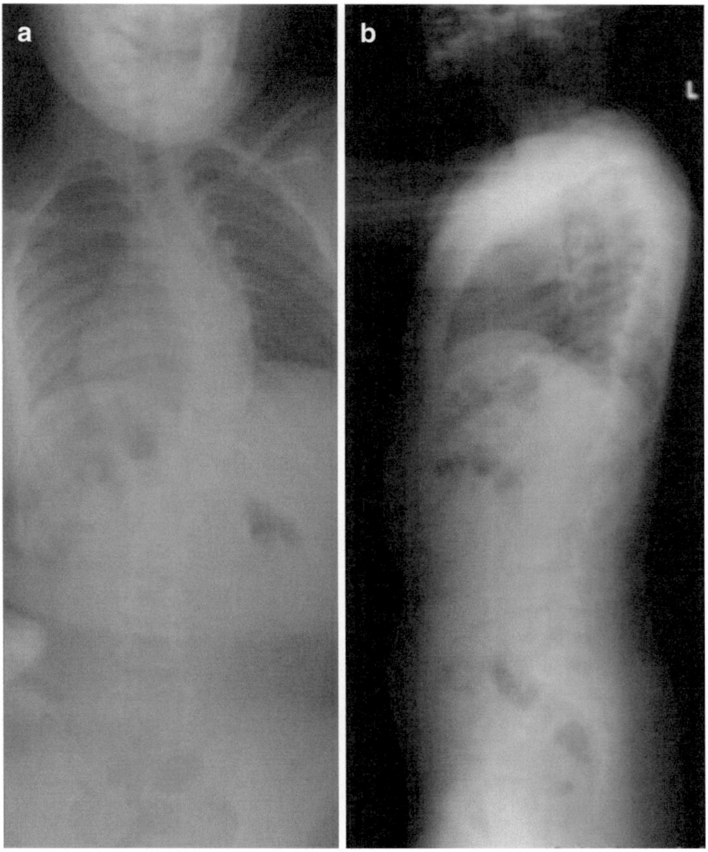

FIGURE 22.1 Anterior-posterior (**a**) and lateral (**b**) radiographs of the spine showing a right thoracolumbar curve of 52° at age 6 + 11 years

extensive autofusion, we would proceed with an in situ fusion because of the high complication rate and small correction achievable in this situation. If there were limited areas of autofusion, we would attempt to perform an osteotomy of the fusion and affected segments to gain curve correction.

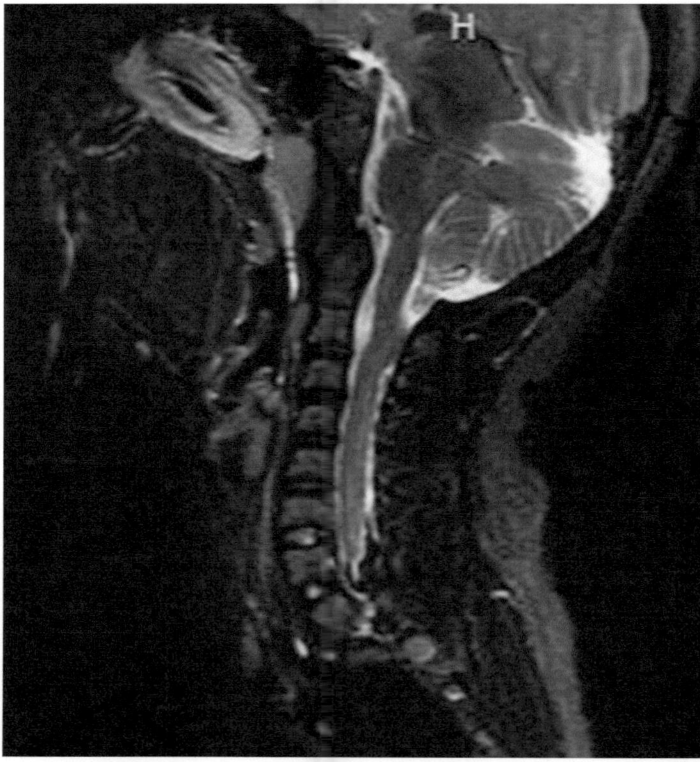

FIGURE 22.2 MRI demonstrating Chiari 1 malformation

Surgical Procedure

The patient was placed prone on a Jackson table. Preoperative antibiotics including weight based cefazolin and vancomycin were administered intravenously. A cell saver was used for the entire procedure. Preoperative motor and sensory neuromonitoring was normal and remained at baseline throughout the surgery. A midline incision connecting and including her superior and inferior scars was used to retrieve the implanted growing rods which had extensive bone growth surrounding them. A fusion mass was identified from T6 to T9 that

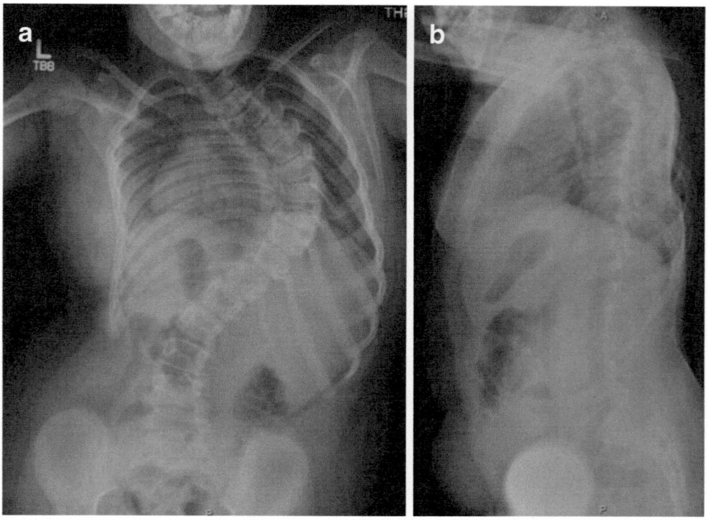

FIGURE 22.3 Anterior-posterior (**a**) and lateral (**b**) radiographs of the spine showing curve progression to 90° at age 10 + 0 years

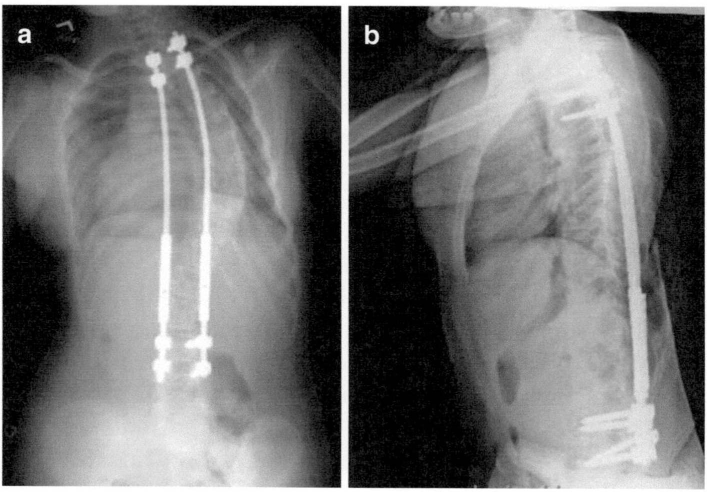

FIGURE 22.4 Anterior-posterior (**a**) and lateral (**b**) radiographs of the spine after placement of dual 5.5-mm growth rods. Thoracolumbar curve now measures 65°

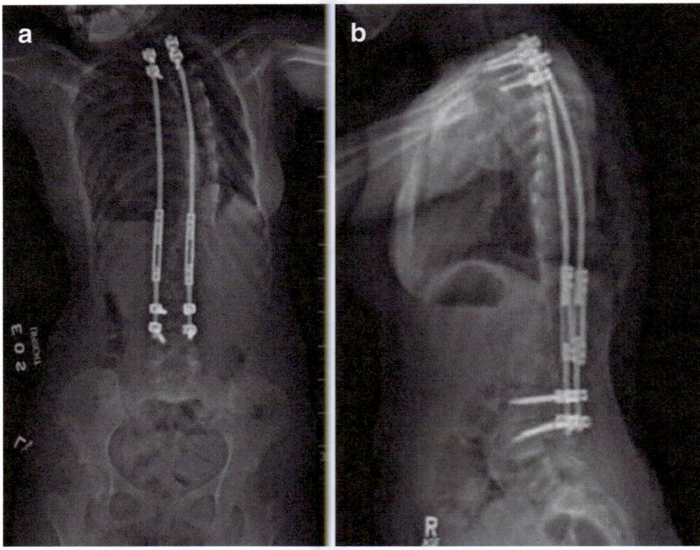

FIGURE 22.5 Anterior-posterior (**a**) and lateral (**b**) radiographs of the spine after 4 years of serial lengthenings. The thoracolumbar curve is now 40°

involved the growing rods, facets, lamina, and spinous processes. An additional fusion was identified extending two segments cephalad to the L3/4 anchors as well (Fig. 22.6). Hemostasis was obtained during this process using epinephrine-soaked sponges and Aquamantys® (Medtronic, Minneapolis, MN). The fusion masses were removed from the rods with a straight osteotome and rongeur. The growing rods were then removed; the pedicle screws were found to be well-fixed and were left in place. These were associated with very robust fusions at the anchor sites themselves (T2–3, L3–4). Facetectomies were done at all levels. By direct manipulation using apical rib pressure, it became apparent that residual deformity correction could not be achieved with the auto-fused bone in place. Uniaxial pedicle screws were placed using standard fluoroscopic-assisted technique from T4 to L2; however, during screw insertion, it was noted that there was

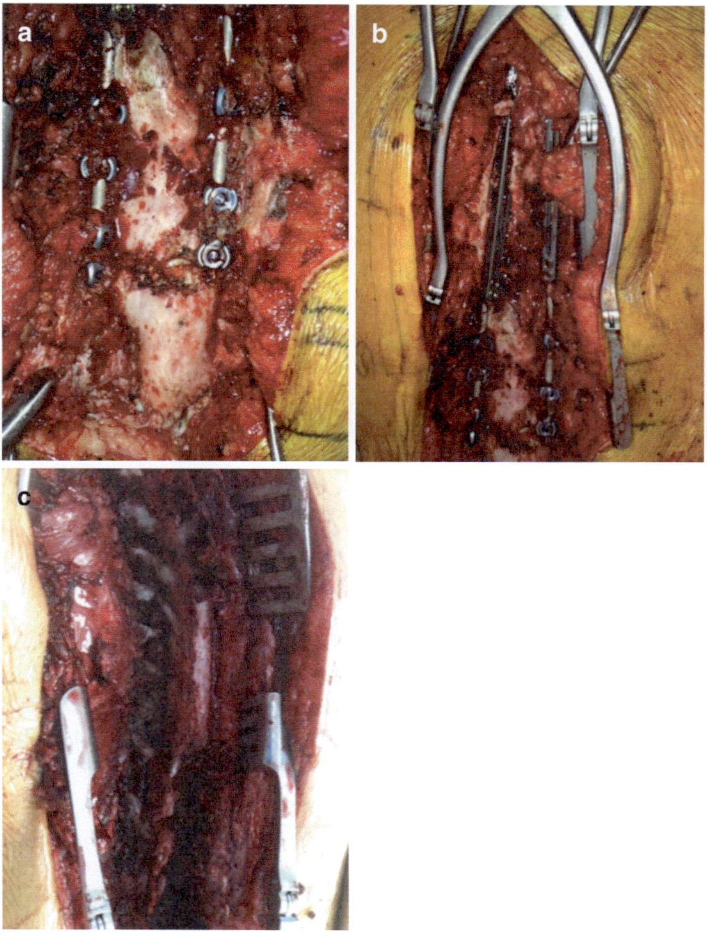

FIGURE 22.6 (**a**) Intraoperative photograph at the time of definitive fusion showing autofusion cephalad to L3/4 anchors. (**b**) Intraoperative photograph at the time of definitive fusion showing autofusion involving the growth rods. On the left side of the image, bone that had formed around the length of the growth rod was removed, exposing the implant. (**c**) Intraoperative photograph at the time of definitive fusion showing autofusion of the spinous processes of levels T6–9

some stress shielding and osteopenia of the pedicles. Extensive facetectomies, with removal of the ligament flavum, and Smith-Petersen osteotomies were performed from T6 to T9 using a high-speed burr and Kerrison rongeur through the fused facets, lamina, and spinous processes. Any additional autofusion was resected with a high-speed burr and Kerrison rongeur. These maneuvers increased spinal flexibility, and final correction was obtained by using multiple rounds of rod bending and de-rotation maneuvers. No changes in her spinal cord monitoring were noted. The spine was irrigated with warm saline containing bacitracin. Crushed cancellous allograft combined with 2 g of vancomycin powder was used for arthrodesis after decortication. The spine was closed in layers with a drain superficial to the fascia.

Clinical Course and Outcome

The patient had 850 cm^3 of blood loss during the procedure, which lasted 3 h and 51 min. One unit of packed red blood cells was transfused intraoperatively. No changes in neurologic status compared to preoperative examination were noted. She was admitted to the neurologic intensive care unit for 24 h for neurologic monitoring and was subsequently transferred to the floor and discharged home on her fourth postoperative day. Her most recent imaging, 2.5 years postoperatively, showed a stable residual curve of 19° with 1.5-cm trunk shift (Fig. 22.7). There was no evidence of proximal junctional kyphosis, distal junctional kyphosis, or sagittal imbalance either clinically or radiographically. No perioperative or postoperative complications were noted. Currently, the patient has occasional back pain approximately once monthly that is treated with nonsteroidal anti-inflammatory medications.

Clinical Pearls and Pitfalls

- In patients who have spine-based growing rods implanted and who are undergoing posterior spinal fusion, it is important to realize that the spine may have autofused segments.

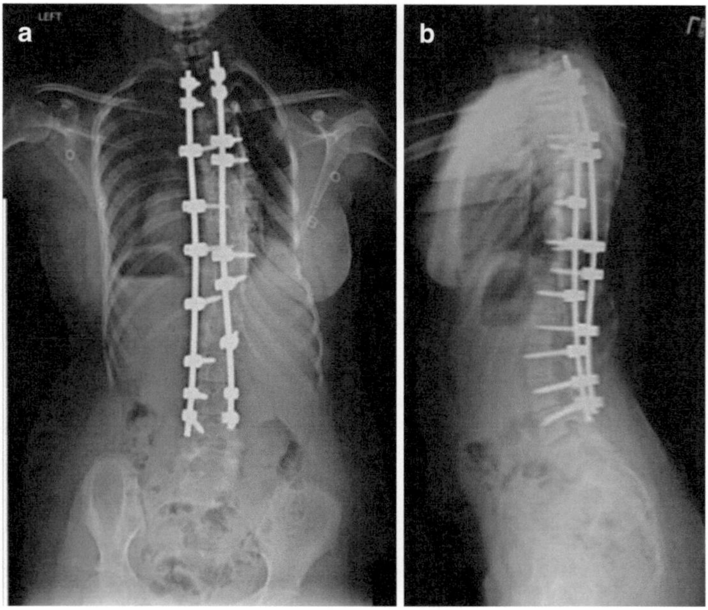

FIGURE 22.7 Anterior-posterior (**a**) and lateral (**b**) radiographs of the spine at 2.5-year follow-up showing residual curve of 19° and improvement of thoracic kyphosis and lumbar lordosis

- Preoperative advanced imaging such as CT scanning and three-dimensional modeling can help identify autofused segments before surgery and aid in preoperative planning.
- Correction of residual deformity through an autofused segment may require multiple osteotomies. This may be technically demanding if the scapula, ribs, or large segments of spine are involved (Fig. 22.8).
- The use of an anterior release in the setting of massive autofusion is controversial, and there is little information about this in the literature.
- Preoperative planning should account for increased surgical time, increased blood loss, and inability to correct the deformity.

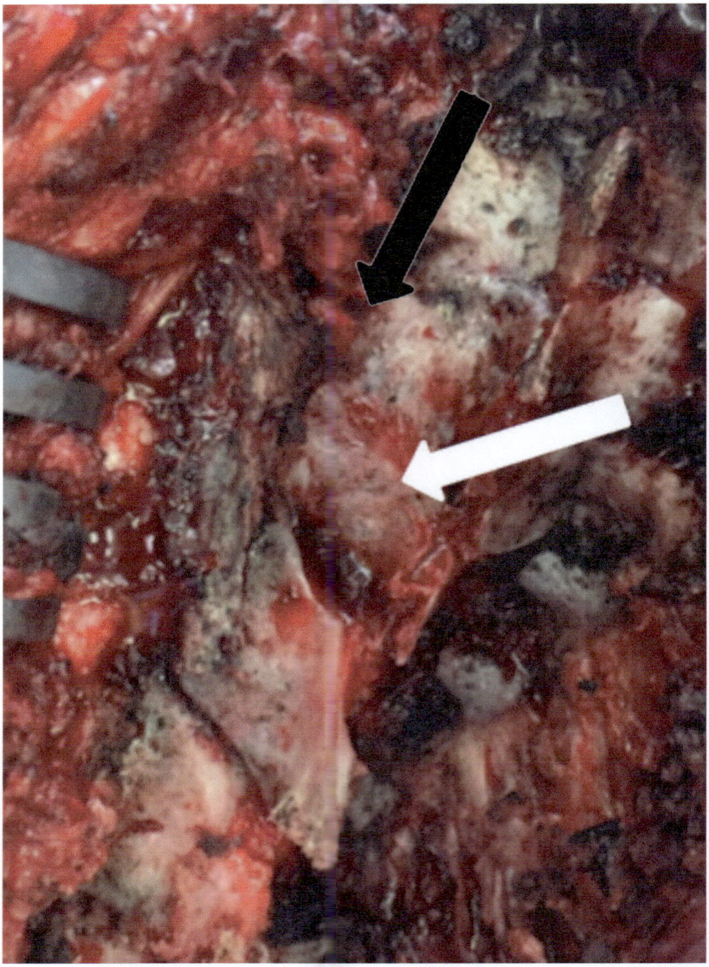

FIGURE 22.8 Intraoperative photograph of a different patient who had posterior spinal fusion after rib-based fixation. Note the fusion between the inferior pole of the left scapula (*black arrow*) and spinous process (*white arrow*)

- Certain implants, such as rib-based anchors and pelvic anchors, may have migrated from their insertion sites, and removal may be difficult, if not impossible. If asymptomatic, these can be left in place. This should be discussed with families preoperatively.
- If the residual deformity is acceptable and there is extensive autofusion, then in situ fusion or close observation without fusion should be considered.
- All patients, regardless of the treatment chosen, need to be followed long-term for deformity progression, implant failure, junctional problems, and pain.

Literature Review and Discussion

The decision to perform spinal fusion at the end of growth-friendly treatment is complicated and multifactorial. Traditionally, posterior spinal fusion has been performed at the cessation of lengthening, but, because of the rarity of early-onset scoliosis, there are few studies to guide decision-making. Recent reports of difficult and poor curve correction associated with minimal spine height/length gains and high complication rates, as well as success with long-term observation without fusion in some patients, have called this into question [1, 2]. Reoperation after "final" fusion also has been found to be frequent. In a group of 100 patients who had posterior spinal fusion after treatment with growing rods, 20 patients had 30 complications that required 57 reoperations at an average of 2 years after fusion [3]. The large cohort of patients completing their growth-friendly treatment will result in more patients, families, and surgeons who will face this complicated decision.

Posterior spinal fusion has been noted to lead to minimal curve correction and gain in spinal height. Sawyer et al. compared patients who were simply observed for more than

2 years after their final lengthening to patients who had definitive posterior spinal fusion at the end of lengthening [1]. There was no statistically significant difference in Cobb angle or kyphosis at final follow-up. Additionally, the observation group obtained 88% of the T1–T12 height of the posterior spinal fusion group. In the posterior spinal fusion group of 25 patients, 26 complications occurred in 15 patients; the observation group of 12 patients had no complications [1]. Similar findings were noted by Jain et al. in a cohort of growing rod patients [2].

Recently, it has been proposed that patients who have reached skeletal maturity and have acceptable deformity correction after growth-friendly treatment can be observed rather than undergo instrumented fusion [1, 2]. Jain et al. suggested that observation may be an acceptable treatment for patients who have satisfactory spinal alignment and trunk height, have reached skeletal maturity, and have shown minimal gain in trunk height at their last distraction [2], a conclusion similar to that noted by Sawyer et al. [1]. Longer follow-up currently underway to determine if late implant failure will occur in this subset of patients, as well as to determine factors which may be predictive of long-term success or failure of observation without fusion.

If posterior spinal fusion is planned after growth-friendly techniques, autofusion of portions of the spine and/or ribs and scapula especially with rib-based fixation must be anticipated. In addition, soft tissue scarring and/or ossification can occur around the rib- and spine-based implants which need to be taken into account. The process of autofusion in growing constructs is well documented. Cahill et al. [4] studied nine patients who were transitioned from growing constructs to definitive fusion and found an 89% rate of autofusion. This led to a Cobb angle correction of 44% during definitive fusion, and each patient averaged seven Smith-Petersen-type osteotomies. Similarly, Flynn et al. [5] noted in a multicenter study that 19% of patients undergoing definitive fusion after growth-friendly surgery had completely mobile spines, 19% had decreased flexibility with some autofusion, and 62% had completely stiff spines with extensive autofusion. Osteotomies were needed in 24% of the patients to aid in deformity correction at the time of definitive surgery. The deformity correction we were able to obtain is consistent with the findings of Cahill et al. [4]. It should be noted that the decision for spinal fusion in the patient in this chapter was made before reports of patients with successful outcomes with observation alone. Our patient may have been a good candidate for long-term observation given her low physical demand lifestyle, body habitus, and relatively good curve correction and spinal balance before posterior spinal fusion.

Many children have received growth-friendly surgery for early-onset scoliosis and are "graduating" to the next step as they reach skeletal maturity. The decision to observe or to perform a spinal fusion at the end of growth is complicated and multifactorial and should be tailored to each individual patient and surgeon. In each specific case, the benefits of a posterior spinal fusion need to be weighed against the high-risk nature of fusion in this patient population. Advanced imaging studies and three-dimensional modeling, as well as follow-up studies on patients who are observed or have fusion at the end of growth-friendly surgery, will improve decision-making at this critical time in the treatment of early-onset scoliosis.

References

1. Sawyer JR, de Mendonça RG, Flynn TS, Samdani AF, El-Hawary R, Spurway AJ, Children's Spine Study Group, et al. Complications and radiographic outcomes of posterior spinal fusion and observation in patients who have undergone distraction-based treatment for early onset scoliosis. Spine Deform. 2016;4:407–12.
2. Jain A, Sponseller PD, Flynn JM, Shah SA, Thompson GH, Emans JB, Growing Spine Study Group, et al. Avoidance of "final" surgical fusion after growing-rod treatment for early-onset scoliosis. J Bone Joint Surg Am. 2016;98:1073–8.
3. Poe-Kochert C, Shannon C, Pawelek JB, Thompson GH, Hardesty CK, Marks DS, et al. Final fusion after growing-rod treatment

for early onset scoliosis. Is it really final? J Bone Joint Surg Am. 2016;98:1913–7.

4. Cahill PJ, Marvil S, Cuddihy L, Schutt C, Idema J, Clements DH, et al. Autofusion in the immature spine treated with growing rods. Spine (Phila Pa 1976). 2010;35:E1199–203.
5. Flynn JM, Tomlinson LA, Pawelek J, Thompson GH, McCarthy R, Akbarnia BA, Growing Spine Study Group. Growing-rod graduates: lessons learned from ninety-nine patients who completed lengthening. J Bone Joint Surg Am. 2013;95:1745–50.

Index

A
Adolescent idiopathic scoliosis (AIS), 10, 299
Anterior hemivertebra excision, 153, 162
Anterior release and posterior spinal instrumentation and fusion (APSIF), 291
Anterior vertebral body tethering (AVBT)
  adequate single-lung ventilation, 127
  anterior spinal growth modulation, 129
  clinical course and outcome, 126, 127
  diagnostic studies, 118
  fusionless treatment methods, 128
  Heuter-Volkmann principle, 128
  history and physical examination, 117–118
  intraoperative fluoroscopy, 127
  irreversible growth cartilage or disc injury, 129
  management options, 118–121
  patient selection, 127
  preoperative flexibility, 127
  progressive adolescent idiopathic scoliosis, 127
  rib head localization, 127
  scoliosis porcine model, 129
  screw trajectory, 127
  segmental vessels, 127
  skeletal maturity, 130
  spine deformity, 129
  surgical procedure
    bronchial blocker, 121
    chest tube placement, 125
    with double-lumen intubation, 121
    implant, 125
    patient position, 121
    pleura, 122
    portal placement, 122, 123
    retroperitoneal dissection, 123
    standard fluoroscopy, 121
    tension, 124
    3D navigation, 121
    vertebral staple insertion, 124
    vertebral tap, 124
  vs. VBS, 131
Apical derotation, 78
Apical fusion levels, 76–77
Apical segments, 76

R. El-Hawary, C.P. Eberson (eds.), *Early Onset Scoliosis*,
https://doi.org/10.1007/978-3-319-71580-3

Autofusion, 44, 69, 309, 315, 318
AVBT, *see* Anterior vertebral body tethering (AVBT)

B

Beal's syndrome, 1

C

Cardiopulmonary function, 186
Center for Thoracic Insufficiency (CTIS), 169
C-EOS, *see* Classification of early-onset scoliosis (C-EOS)
Cerebral palsy
- contracture and stiffness, 212
- distraction procedures, 215
- dual growing rods, 218
- growing rod constructs, 217
- growing rod distraction, 214
- growing rod insertion, 213
- halo-gravity traction, 212, 213
- history and physical examination, 211
- intraoperative neural monitoring, 217
- lengthening procedures, 217
- pelvic fixation, 217
- pelvic obliquity, 215, 217
- radiographic evaluation, 212
- surgical procedure, 216
- thoracolumbar curve, 212
- treatment, 215

Chiari malformation, 308, 310
Chiari-associated scoliosis, 264
Classification of early-onset scoliosis (C-EOS), 265
- age, 9–11
- annual progression ratio, 11, 12
- clubfoot deformity, 12
- complications, 14
- etiology, 9–11
- history, 9
- interobserver and intraobserver reliability, 12
- multiple curve factors, 12
- with nemaline myopathy, 12, 13
- optimal care and prognosticate outcomes, 12
- utility and validity, 12

Clubfoot deformity, 12
Complications, 253–259, 262, 267
- axial plane deformity, 266
- casting, 263
- classification system, 263
- clinical course and outcome, 259–261
- clinical deformity, 247
- diagnostic studies, 247–249, 265
- with dual submuscular growing rods, 266
- guided growth *vs.* distraction-based techniques, 265
- idiopathic infantile scoliosis, 262
- infection, 267
- left trunk shift and thoracic prominence, 245
- lengthening, 247
- management, 249–253
- postoperative radiographs, 247
- proximal anchor failure, 264
- psychological effects, 264
- pulmonary function tests, 249
- rib anchors *vs.* spine anchors, 265
- risk of, 263
- rod fracture, 262, 266
- single concave VEPTR device, 245
- stable proximal fixation, 262
- surgical procedure
  - anterior release, 253–256
  - final fusion, 258, 259, 262, 267

growing rod distractions, 256–258
growing rod insertion with apical control, 253–256
halo-gravity traction application, 253, 262
rod revisions, 256–258
wound dehiscence, 247
Concave distraction, 188, 189, 191, 193
Congenital scoliosis
definitive fusion, 188
with fused ribs, 170
bracing, 180
casting, 180
classification system, 178
convex hemiepiphysiodesis, 180
curve progression, 170, 179, 180
derotational casting, 180
developmental anomalies, 178
developmental disturbances, 179
evaluation, 169
fusionless growing constructs, 180
hemivertebra excision, 180
hemivertebrae and block vertebra, 171
management, 169
medical history, 167
MRI evaluation, spine, 179
opening thoracostomy, 180
radiographic evaluation, 168, 169
respiratory illnesses, 168
spinal deformity, 167
surgical intervention, 180
VEPTR insertion (*see* Vertical expandable prosthetic titanium rib (VEPTR))
vertebral formation, 178
wedge resection, 180
hemiepiphysiodesis, 183–195
posteroanterior radiograph, 185
Convex growth arrest (CGA), 188, 191–193
Corrective maneuvers, 77–79
Craniosynostosis, 307

D

Definitive fusion, 39–41, 313
Deformity correction, 77
DePuy Synthes, 112
Developmental delay, 211, 307
Distraction phase, 278, 280, 281
Double windlass mechanism spring traction system, 253

E

Early-onset deformity, 236
Elongation-derotation-(lateral) flexion casting (EDF)
clinical course and outcome, 28–30
diagnostic studies, 18, 19
history and physical assessment, 17
management, 19
progressive infantile scoliosis, 32
surgical procedure
anesthesia, 20
application, 23
layer of Webril, 22
pelvic control, 21
preoperative preparation, 20
scoliosis, correction of, 23, 24
trimming, 24–28
External remote control (ERC), 92, 93

F
Facetectomies, 38, 65, 293, 312
Femoral countertraction, 296
Flexibility films, 76
Flexible thoracolumbar kyphosis, 88
Forced vital capacity (FVC), 284
Fusionless treatment methods, 128

G
Gibbus deformity, 222–225, 227
Graduation phase, 278
Gross Motor Function Classification System (GMFCS), 211
Growth-friendly treatment
  advanced imaging studies, 319
  autofusion, 309, 313, 315, 318
  Chiari malformation, 308, 310
  clinical course and outcome, 314, 315
  history, 307
  lengthenings, 308
  lumbar hyperkyphosis, 308
  management, 308–309
  physical examination, 308
  posterior spinal fusion, 316–318
  preoperative advanced imaging, 315
  residual deformity, 315, 317–319
  rib-based anchors and pelvic anchors, 317
  skeletal maturity, 319
  spine-based distraction, 308
  surgical procedure, 310–314
  thoracic hypokyphosis, 308
  three-dimensional modeling, 319

H
Halo-gravity traction (HGT)
  application, 253
  dose recommendation, 298
  efficacy, 298–299
  perioperative, 296
  technique and protocols, 297–298
Harrington rod placement technique, 98
Hemiepiphysiodesis, 153, 183–195
Hemivertebra excision
  anterior and posterior, 153
  brace treatment, 149, 152
  deformity correction, 161
  diagnosis, 151
  epidural bleeding, 159
  fixation, 155, 156
  focal kyphosis, 150
  hemivertebra cancellous bone, 159
  laminar excision, 158
  management, 152, 153
  pedicle screw position, 156, 157
  physical examination, 149
  posterior-only approach, 153
  radiographs, 164
  skin incision, 154
  stages, 157
  supine bending x-rays, 152
  transverse process, 159
Hemivertebrectomy, 188
Hemostasis, 312
Heuter-Volkmann principle, 128
Hybrid growing rod construct
  autofusion, 69
  clinical course and outcome, 67
  definitive fusion, 68
  diagnostic studies, 61
  distraction-based spinal growth constructs, 68
  EDF casting, 67
  history and physical examination, 59–61
  intraoperative positioning, 67
  magnetically lengthening rods, 67

management, 61–64
MCGR, 69
proximal rib hook anchors, 67, 69
rib hooks, 68
rib-based proximal anchors, 68
sagittal profile, 67
surgical procedure, 64–66

I

Idiopathic early-onset scoliosis
anterior vertebral body stapling
anterior procedure, 142
developmental history, 136
diagnostic studies, 137
fluoroscopy, 138
general anesthesia, 137
growth modulation treatment, 137
growth modulation with VBS, 135
intensive care unit, 139
intercostal blocks, 139
management, 137
MRI, 137
natural history, 143
neuromonitoring, 137
nighttime bracing, 143
physical examination, 136
posteroanterior and lateral radiographs, 136
preoperative measurement, 143
surgical procedure, 137–139
treatment, 143
bending radiographs, 36
bilateral rods, 43
clinical course and outcome, 41, 42
complication rates, 41
definition, 68
delaying TGR/MCGR, 41
with hybrid growing rod construct
autofusion, 69
clinical course and outcome, 67
definitive fusion, 68
diagnostic studies, 61
distraction-based spinal growth constructs, 68
EDF casting, 67
history and physical examination, 59–61
intraoperative positioning, 67
magnetically lengthening rods, 67
management, 61–64
MCGR, 69
proximal rib hook anchors, 67, 69
rib hooks, 68
rib-based proximal anchors, 68
sagittal profile, 67
surgical procedure, 64–66
lengthening, 43
management, 36
medical history, 35
nonoperative management, 41
physical examination, 36
PJK, 44
plain radiographs, 36, 37
surgical procedure
definitive fusion, 39–41
growing rod distraction, 38
intraoperative neuromonitoring, 36
postoperative PA and lateral standing radiographs, 38, 39
TGR fixation, 41
TGR instrumentation, 43
treatment options, 41, 68
two-incision technique, 43
Implantation phase, 276, 282

Infantile idiopathic scoliosis (IIS), 53–56
Instrumented spinal height gain, 114
Intraoperative skull-femoral traction (IOT), 296, 299, 300

K
Kyphoscoliosis, 231–233, 236, 241, 242
Kyphotic deformity, 153, 226

L
Low conus medullaris, 187
Lumbar hyperkyphosis, 308, 309

M
Magnetically controlled growing rods (MCGR), 43, 69, 90–94, 236
- clinical course and outcome, 94–96
- cost, 99
- deformity control, 99
- diagnostic studies, 88, 89
- with growth-friendly spinal instrumentation, 88
- Harrington rod placement technique, 98
- history, 87
- implantation, 207
- multiple treatment strategies, 98
- physical examination, 88
- surgical management, 88–89
- surgical procedure
  - Dimeglio's work, 93
  - external remote control, 92, 93
  - fusion masses and instrumentation, 90
  - gentle distraction, 90
  - lengthening, 93
  - patient position, 90
  - pre- and post-lengthening, 93, 94
  - pre- and postoperative images, 90, 91
  - rod selection, 90
  - set screws placement, 90
  - subfascial tunnels, 90
- *vs.* TGR, 99

Magnetically lengthening rods, 67
Microcephaly, 307
Modern Luque trolley
- clinical course and outcome, 108, 109
- complications, 110
- curve progression, 110
- description, 110
- flexible curves and apical translation, 109
- flexible left thoracolumbar curve, 104, 106
- history and physical examination, 103–104
- with hypotonic collapsing spinal deformities, 109
- long-term clinical follow-up, 114
- management, 104–105
- meticulous preoperative planning and execution, 110
- with new apical gliding spinal implant—trolley gliding vehicle, 114, 115
- off-label modern spinal implants, 112
- patient selection, 109
- post technique, 108
- progressive collapsing kyphoscoliotic deformity, 104, 105
- surgical procedure, 106–108
- trolley gliding vehicle, 112

Modern spinal implants, 111

Myelomeningocele
- bracing, 226
- clinical course and outcome, 224
- diagnostic studies, 222–223
- fixation points, 226
- gibbus deformity, 222, 227
- history and physical examination, 221–222
- kyphotic deformity, 226
- low-profile fixation, 227
- management, 223
- nonambulatory patients, 227
- pelvic S-hooks, 226, 227
- preoperative assessment of comorbidities, 224
- shunt malfunction, 226
- spinal deformities, 226
- surgical procedure, 223–224
- wheelchair modifications, 226

N

Nemaline myopathy
- aggressive pain control, 206
- bilateral pelvis-to-rib growing rod construct, 200–203
- cardiac and pulmonary involvement, 205
- clinical severity, 197
- collapsing parasol effect, 200
- complications, 208
- diffuse hypotonia, 198
- dysarthric, 198
- Eiffel Tower construct, 207
- fusionless model, 206
- growing rod construct, 200
- growing rod distraction, 203
- growing rod insertion, 200
- incidence, 205
- instrumentation technique, 207
- intraoperative neuromonitoring, 204
- intrathecal treatment, 206
- lengthening procedures, 203
- management, 205
- muscle relaxants, 206
- pelvic obliquity, 203, 204
- progressive thoracolumbar scoliosis, 197
- pulmonary care, 203
- pulmonary complications, 206
- radiographic evaluation, 198
- respiratory therapy program, 206
- rib engagement, 203
- sensation, 198
- static muscle architecture, 205
- supine AP traction radiographs, 199
- surgical complications, 203
- surgical management, 199, 206, 208
- surgical morbidity and mortality, 206
- thoracolumbar curve, 198
- ventilator support, tracheostomy, 197
- VEPTR instrumentation, 207
- volatile inhalational anesthetics, 206

Neurocentral synchondrosis, 4

Neuromuscular scoliosis, management, 208, 217, 218

Noninvasive lengthening procedures, 96

Normal human spinal growth
- neurocentral synchondrosis, 4
- and pulmonary function, 3
- with spinal deformity, 1, 3
- supine AP radiographs, 2
- thoracic and lumbar spine, 3–5
- VACTERL, 1

O

Off label modern spinal implants, 111

Opening wedge thoracostomy, 170, 172, 173, 177, 180, 181

P
Pediatric scoliosis, 154
Pedicle screw instrumentation, 188, 191
Pelvic obliquity, 199, 212, 215, 216
Posterior spinal instrumentation and fusion (PSIF), 291
Posterior-only hemivertebra excision, 153, 154
Prader-Willi syndrome, 87
Preoperative flexibility index, 298
Progressive adolescent idiopathic scoliosis, 127
Progressive infantile scoliosis, 32
Proximal junctional kyphosis (PJK), 44
Pulmonary function tests, 3, 249

R
Rib hooks, 68
Rib-based proximal anchors, 68

S
Sagittal spine length (SSL), 281, 282, 284
Scoliosis porcine model, 129
Scoliosis Research Society Growing Spine Committee, 274
Segmental vessel injury, 142
Self-growing rod construct, 104, 110, 112
Shilla growth guidance technique, 76–78
  clinical course and outcome, 79–81
  deformity, 83
  diagnostic studies, 74–76
  vs. distraction-based growing rod patients, 83
  history, 73
  patient criteria, 84
  physical examination, 74
  surgical procedure
    apical derotation, 78
    apical fusion levels, 76–77
    apical segments, 76
    deformity correction, 77
    growing screws, 76, 77
  treatment options, 76
SHILLA technique, 206
Shilla-guided growth system, 114
Skeletal dysplasia
  clinical course and outcome, 238
  clinical pearls and pitfalls, 238–240
  diagnostic studies, 232–233
  growth-friendly implants, 242
  history and physical examination, 231–232
  lengthening, 242
  management, 233–238
  pedicle screw fixation, 242
  surgical procedure, 236–238
SMD type I, 241
Spinal deformity, 1, 183
Spinal dysraphism, 88
Spinal traction, 296, 301
Spine growth assessment
  anthropometric data, 286
  biplanar radiographs, 286
  delay tactic, 284
  diagnostic studies, 273–274
  Dimeglio's data, 279
  distraction phase, 278, 280, 282
  expected growth rate, 279–281
  FVC, 284
  graduation phase, 278
  growth-friendly treatment, 284
  history, 271
  implantation phase, 276, 282
  law of diminishing returns, 284
  management options, 274–275
  measurements, 276

neurological examination, 272
pelvic inlet width, 283
reference data, 282
serial standing lateral radiographs, 274
serial standing PA radiographs, 273
spinal parameters, 276, 277, 279
SSL, 281, 282, 284
surgical course, 276
surgical procedure, 275
3D–TSL, 285, 286
Spine-based distraction, 200, 284, 308
Spine-based growing rods, 35, 217
Spondylometaphyseal dysplasia (SMD), 241
Spondylometaphyseal dysplasia Kozlowski type (SMDK), 231, 241
Subperiosteal exposure, 38, 154, 188

T

Thoracic hypokyphosis, 308
Thoracic insufficiency syndrome (TIS), 3, 178
Thoracolumbosacral orthosis (TLSO), 48, 59, 189
Three-dimensional true spine length (3D–TSL), 285
Traction, 296–299
advantages, 296
clinical course and outcome, 294–295
complications, 301, 304
diagnostic studies, 291
growth-friendly options, 292
HGT
efficacy, 298–299
perioperative, 296
recommended dose, 298
technique and protocols, 297–298
history and physical examination, 289–291
intraoperative skull-femoral traction, 299–300
management options, 291
skull traction options, 292
spinal traction, 296
surgical procedure, 293–294
triradiate cartilage, 293
Trolley gliding vehicle (TGV), 112
Two-stage growing rod strategy, 242

V

Vertebral body stapling (VBS)
complications, 144
detrimental effect, disc space, 145
growth modulation, 135, 137
indications, 146
posteroanterior and lateral radiographs, 139
preoperative thoracic curve, 143
radiopaque trial instrument, 138
thoracic curves, 144
Vertical expandable prosthetic titanium rib (VEPTR), 49–53, 206, 221–224, 226, 227
bone fusion, 172
clinical course and outcome, 52, 54
complication rates, 181
control of spinal deformity, 52
curvilinear incision, 171
device exchange, 175
diagnostic studies, 48, 49
distraction, 172
exchange of implants, 174
history and physical examination, 47–48
IIS, 53

Vertical expandable prosthetic titanium rib (VEPTR) (*cont.,*)
  in myelomeningocele
    bracing, 226
    clinical course and outcome, 224
    diagnostic Studies, 222–223
    fixation points, 226
    gibbus deformity, 222, 227
    history and physical examination, 221–222
    kyphotic deformity, 226
    low-profile fixation, 227
    management, 223
    nonambulatory patients, 227
    pelvic S-hooks, 226, 227
    preoperative assessment of comorbidities, 224
    shunt malfunction, 226
    spinal deformities, 226
    surgical procedure, 223–224
    wheelchair modifications, 226
  indications, 54
  lengthening procedures, 174, 175
  longitudinal incision, 174
  management, 48
  opening wedge thoracostomy, 173
  paraspinal muscles, 171
  pulmonary function, 176
  reinsertion, 177
  scoliotic deformity, 180
  skin flaps, 173
  spinal cord monitoring, 172
  surgical lengthening, concave hemithorax, 180
  surgical procedure
    exchange, 52, 53
    insertion, 49–51
    laminar hooks, 50
    lengthening, 51, 52
    postoperative images, 50
    rib cradle, 50

W

Wheelchair modifications, 294

MIX
Papier aus verantwortungsvollen Quellen
Paper from responsible sources
FSC® C105338

If you have any concerns about our products,
you can contact us on
ProductSafety@springernature.com

In case Publisher is established outside the EU,
the EU authorized representative is:
Springer Nature Customer Service Center GmbH
Europaplatz 3, 69115 Heidelberg, Germany

Printed by Libri Plureos GmbH
in Hamburg, Germany